Elemental Diets

Editor

Robin I. Russell, Ph.D.
Gastroenterology Unit
Royal Infirmary
Glasgow, Scotland

CRC Press, Inc.
Boca Raton, Florida

Library of Congress Cataloging in Publication Data

Main entry under title:

Elemental diets.

Bibliography: p.
Includes index.
1. Elemental diets. I. Russell, Robin I.
RM229.E39 615.8'54 80-25869
ISBN 0-8493-5671-7

This book represents information obtained from authentic and highly regarded sources. Reprinted material is quoted with permission, and sources are indicated. A wide variety of references are listed. Every reasonable effort has been made to give reliable data and information, but the author and the publisher cannot assume responsibility for the validity of all materials or for the consequences of their use.

Direct all inquiries to CRC Press, Inc., 2000 N.W. 24th Street, Boca Raton, Florida 33431.

International Standard Book Number 0-8493-5671-7

Library of Congress Card Number 80-25869
Printed in the United States

FOREWORD

In recent years there have been many important advances in the understanding of nutritional deficiency in association with many disease states, and many advances have been made in methods of improving nutritional insufficiency. The purpose of this book is to provide a study of one of these nutritional support methods — elemental diets. My interest, as a physician and gastroenterologist in the field of elemental diets, arose out of my interest in intestinal absorption, its physiology and pathophysiology, and in diseases associated with disturbances of absorption. Many gastrointestinal (GI) diseases may be accompanied by nutritional insufficiency, particularly those associated with malabsorption states. The function of the GI tract is basic to the principles and practice of nutrition, and is of particular importance in any form of enteral nutritional support system.

I have attempted to bring together the theory behind the use of elemental diets and to consider their clinical value as far as can be assessed at the present time. The book has been planned and laid out in four sections. The first section provides information about the normal nutritional state, digestion and absorption of nutrients, the causes and results of nutritional insufficiency, assessment and monitoring of nutritional status, and a brief resumē of methods of providing nutritional support. The second section traces the development, formulations, and properties of elemental diets with particular reference to the metabolic effects of these preparations on various aspects of GI tract function, including gastric emptying and secretion, intestinal structure and function, bile acid metabolism, pancreatic exocrine secretion, and the bacteriology of the GI tract. Section Three is devoted to detailed accounts of the clinical uses of elemental diets in a wide range of diseases such as surgical conditions, maldigestion, and malabsorption states, inflammatory bowel disease, cancer, burns and pediatrics. The problems of the administration and hazards of the use of elemental diets is also discussed in this section. Section Four summarizes the clinical uses of elemental diets and attempts to assess their place in relation to other nutritional support systems which are currently available, including other forms of enteral nutrition and i.v. nutrition.

It is my hope that this book will provide a useful balance of background theory, experimental data, and practical application in this interesting and rapidly developing field. I also hope that it will stimulate further interest in the development and clinical application of nutritional support systems in a wide range of disease states.

I have been fortunate in having a number of expert and willing contributors to this volume who have provided informative chapters on their own subject in relation to the use of elemental diets. I am grateful for their excellent contributions. I should also like to thank Benita Budd and Sandy Pearlman of the Editorial Staff of CRC Press for their assistance in planning this volume and Elisabeth King for her help during production.

Finally, I should like to thank my secretary Lynn Munro for her valuable help in the preparation of this book.

R. I. Russell

EDITOR

Robin Russell, M.D., Ph.D., F.R.C.P. (Glas.), and F.R.C.P. (Ed.) is Consultant in Charge of the Gastroenterology Unit, Royal Infirmary, Glasgow.

He qualified M.B. Ch.B. in 1960 from the University of Glasgow and obtained his M.D. degree in 1972 and Ph.D. in 1976. Formerly a member of the Scientific Staff of the Medical Research Council, Gastroenterology Research Unit in London, he took up his present post in 1970.

He is author of over 150 papers, has contributed chapters to numerous books, and edited Investigative Tests and Techniques in Gastroenterology published in 1978. He is directing an ongoing research program on various aspects of nutrition in gastrointestinal disease, experimental and clinical problems relating to absorption and malabsorption, bile acid metabolism, and the gastric mucosal barrier. He has a special interest in the development of training and teaching in gastroenterology and general internal medicine.

Dr. Russell is a member of the Association of Physicians of Great Britain, the British Society of Gastroenterology, and many other societies and organizations.

"All theory is grey, but the golden tree of actual life springs ever green."

J. W. von Goethe
Faust (1808)

CONTRIBUTORS

S. P. Borriello
Scientist
Clinical Research Center
Harrow, England

K. C. Calman, M.D., Ph.D.
Professor of Oncology
Cancer Research Campaign
Department of Clinical Oncology
Glasgow, Scotland

D. L. Christie, M.D.
Section of Pediatric Gastroenterology
Mason Clinic
Head, Gastroenterology Clinic
Children's Orthopedic Hospital and Medical Center
Clinical Associate Professor
University of Washington School of Medicine
Seattle, Washington

Michael J. Hall, M.B., M.R.C.P.
Lecturer in Medicine
University of Bristol
Bristol Royal Infirmary
Bristol, England

Michael J. Hill, Ph.D
Director
Bacterial Metabolism Research Laboratory
London, England

Michael J. Hudson
Senior Microbiologist
Bacterial Metabolism Research Laboratory
London, England

Ivan D. A. Johnston, M.Ch.
Professor of Surgery and Head of Department
University of Newcastle upon Tyne
Newcastle upon Tyne, England

Joseph A. Moylan, M.D.
Professor of Surgery
Chief, Trauma Service
Duke University Medical Center
Durham, North Carolina

Alan J. Rich
Lecturer in Surgery and
Honorary Senior Registrar
Department of Surgery
Royal Victoria Infirmary
Newcastle upon Tyne, England

Alan Shenkin, M.D., Ph.D.
Consultant in Clinical Biochemistry
Royal Infirmary
Honorary Lecturer
University of Glasgow
Glasgow, Scotland

J. M. Trotter, M.B., B.S., F.R.A.C.P.
Research Fellow
Department of Clinical Oncology
University of Glasgow
Glasgow, Scotland

TABLE OF CONTENTS

SECTION I

NUTRITION — NORMALITY AND INSUFFICIENCY

Chapter 1

THE NORMAL NUTRITIONAL STATE

A. Shenkin

TABLE OF CONTENTS

I. INTRODUCTION

It is axiomatic that "we are what we eat". In other words, the composition of the various tissues of the body is a direct result of the level of intake of nutrients in the diet. If the intake is in excess of the amount necessary to meet daily requirements, then the nutrients will either be excreted or will be deposited in some storage area. If the intake is not adequate to meet daily requirements, then a deficiency state may develop. The normal nutritional state can therefore be tentatively defined as one in which the content of each of the nutrients or their metabolites in the body is such as to maintain a normal structure and function of each of the tissues or organs.

The amount of the various nutrients in the body is the net result of the intake of each nutrient, and its rate of utilization or excretion. It is extremely difficult to indicate the normal body composition, not only because of the problem of definition of "normal" but also because of the wide variation in individuals of different age and sex. A very approximate guide would be that a 65 kg man should contain: 40 kg water (61.6%), 11 kg protein (17%), 9 kg fat (13.8%), one kg carbohydrate (1.5%), 4 kg minerals (6.1%), and small amounts of vitamins.

There have been many extensive reviews of the normal nutritional requirements in man.[1-5] In this chapter, it is proposed therefore to summarize only briefly the normal components of the diet with an indication of the functional role of each of these in the body.

II. WATER

Water is the main component in the body. Approximately 2/3 of the water is intracellular (approximately 25ℓ) and this, in turn, comprises some 70% of the total body cell mass. The 15ℓ of extracellular water is essential in maintaining blood volume and normal organ function.

Water requirements are governed, to a large extent, by the amount of losses from the body. If renal concentrating ability is good, the minimal urine volume necessary to carry the products of normal metabolism is usually about 500 mℓ, although in catabolic patients this may rise to more than 1ℓ in the absence of pyrexia, to several liters per day if sweating is profuse. The variability of such losses makes it impossible to set a rigid value for minimal water requirement. However, in the absence of excessive losses, approximately 30 mℓ/kg body weight in the adult (about 1.5 to 2.0 ℓ/day) will satisfy most individuals. Because of the fairly close relationship between intake of energy substrates and water, the water requirement can also be expressed in such individuals in terms of the energy intake — 1.0 mℓ/kcal or 0.25 mℓ/kJ should be adequate for most adults. The comparable values for children are 30 to 120 mℓ/kg body weight or 1.5 mℓ/kcal (0.4 mℓ/kJ).

III. ENERGY

Energy is required to cover resting metabolism, growth and repair of tissues, to support physical activity, and to maintain body temperature. Body size is therefore a particularly important variable in determining energy requirements. In individuals whose actual body weight is approximately equal to their ideal body weight, an estimate of resting energy requirements can be readily calculated (24 to 28 kcal/kg body weight per day.). Alternatively height can be used to provide an estimate of ideal body weight. Resting metabolic expenditure falls with age at a rate of about 2% per 10 years. On the other hand, seriously ill patients who are infected, or who have suffered a recent trauma, may well have an elevation in their resting metabolic expenditure. Moreover, depending upon their general condition, patients receiving nutritional therapy may participate in different amounts of physical activity. This corresponds to an extra consumption of about 0.4 kcal/min (1.7 kJ/min) in a sitting position and 1.4 kcal/min (5.8 kJ/min) when walking. As summarized in Table 1, the energy requirements can therefore be expected to vary between 1200 and 2000 kcal/day (5.0 to 8.4 MJ/day) or between 22 and 31 kcal/kg body weight per day (91 to 130 kJ/kg per day). In general women require less energy than men.

Energy provision is usually in the form of carbohydrate, fat and protein, and to a lesser extent from alcohol. Although protein is particularly required for repair and growth, in most individuals, the bulk of the protein intake will be metabolized to yield energy — this usually comprises some 11 to 12% of the total. The carbohydrate intake may comprise up to 80 to 90% of the remainder, but in most well-balanced diets, usually 45 to 50% of total energy is supplied by carbohydrate and 40 to 45% by fat.

IV. PROTEIN

The main function of dietary protein is to provide the amino acids necessary for synthesis of body proteins. The organic nitrogen present is also required for synthesis of certain other nitrogenous substances, e.g., nucleic acids.

Nine of the amino acids present in dietary proteins cannot be synthesized in man and they are therefore essential in the diet — these are leucine, isoleucine, valine, lysine, methionine, phenylalanine, threonine, tryptophan, and histidine. The estimated levels of requirement of the essential amino acids is shown in Table 2. The amount present in individual proteins is a major factor in the biological value of the protein and in the efficiency of its utilization. Deficiency in the level of a particular amino acid in a protein may be made good by the presence of higher levels in another protein in a mixed diet. This type of supplementary effect will not be seen in patients on artificial feeding and, hence, the amino acid content of the diet is of particular importance. However, even high quality proteins and proteins of mixed diets are probably only utilized with 65 to 70% efficiency.

Recommendations with regard to dietary protein requirements have been notoriously difficult to define. This has been due to uncertainty of the most appropriate index of protein requirement, to methodological difficulties in nitrogen balance studies, and to variations in the efficiency of protein utilization. Moreover, there are marked physiological variations, occurring as random biological variations between individuals, or associated with growth and repair, pregnancy and lactation, or stress. The interaction of energy intake with protein requirement is also very pronounced. The recommended intakes, as shown in Table 3 have attempted to allow for these factors, and are based on 70% efficiency of utilization of the dietary protein. On this basis, an average man's daily protein requirement is about 0.8 g/kg and amounts to about 7% of his energy intake.

V. FAT

Although in the well-balanced diet, 40 to 45% of the energy content is in the form of fat, only a small proportion of this is essential for health. This is due to the requirement for the essential fatty acids, linoleic and arachidonic acids (and possibly linolenic acid) which are of particular importance as precursors of prostaglandins. Most official recommendations are for about 2 to 5 g of linoleic acid per day (1 to 2% of dietary energy) but there have been some recommendations for as much as 10% of the dietary energy being supplied by essential fatty acids.[8]

Table 1
CALCULATIONS OF ENERGY REQUIREMENTS OF ADULTS

	Energy requirements of men aged						Energy requirements of women aged					
	18-35		35-75		over 75		18-55		55-75		over 75	
	kcal	MJ	kcal	MJ	kcal	MJ	kcal	MJ	kcal	MJ	kcal	MJ
Energy expenditure per 24 hr Resting metabolism	1600	6.7	1500	6.3	1350	5.6	1300	5.4	1200	5.0	1100	4.6
Sitting in or beside bed 0 to 8 hr. (8 × 60 × 0.4 = 192 kcal)	0—192	0—0.80	0—192	0—0.80	0—192	0—0.80	0—192	0—0.80	0—192	0—0.80	0—192	0—0.80
Walking 0 to 60 min (60 × 1.4 = 84 kcal)	0—84	0—0.35	0—84	0—0.35	0—84	0—0.35	0—84	0—0.35	0—84	0—0.35	0—84	0—0.35
Specific dynamic effect (6% of ingested energy)	102—120	0.43—0.50	95—113	0.40—0.47	86—104	0.36—0.44	83—99	0.35—0.41	77—94	0.32—0.39	70—88	0.29—0.37
Total energy expenditure	1,702—1,996	7.1—8.4	1595—1889	6.7—7.9	1436—1730	6.0—7.2	1383—1675	5.8—7.9	1277—1570	5.3—6.6	1170—1464	4.9—6.1
Body weight, kg	65		65		63		55		53		53	
Energy requirements per kg body weight per day	26—31	0.11—0.13	25—29	0.10—0.12	23—28	0.096—0.12	25—31	0.10—0.13	24—30	0.10—0.13	22—28	0.092—0.12
RDA (U.S.A)[2]	2300—3100	9.6—13.0	2000—2800	8.4—11.7	1650—2400	6.9—10.3	1600—2400	6.7—10.0	1400—220	5.9—9.2	1200—2000	5.0—8.4
RDA (U.K.)[3]	2510	10.5	2400	10.0	2150	9.0	2150	9.0	1900	7.9	1680	7.0

Table 2
THE REQUIREMENT OF ESSENTIAL AMINO ACIDS IN HUMAN SUBJECTS OF VARIOUS AGES[6]

Requirement	Infants mg/kg	Child 10-12 years mg/kg	Adult women mg/kg	Adult men mg/kg	Estimated for repletion[7] mg/kg
Histidine	25	—	—	—	7.4
Isoleucine	111	28	10	10	10
Leucine	153	49	13	12	39
Lysine	96	59	10	10	54
Methionine and cystine	50	27	13	12	16
Phenylalanine and tyrosine	90	27	13	14	57
Threonine	66	34	7	6	11
Tryptophan	19	3.7	3.1	2.9	4.3
Valine	95	33	11	14	20
Total essential amino acids	705	261	80	81	219

VI. MINERALS

A. Sodium

Although sodium is the major extracellular cation, and largely responsible for maintenance of extracellular fluid (ECF) volume, only about 50% of the total body sodium (4000 mmol) is, in fact, present in the extracellular fluid. Loss of sodium from the body is affected by perspiration (usually about 15 to 25 mmol/day) fecal and other intestinal fluid losses, and urinary loss. The body sodium content is maintained by ingestion of 70 to 150 mmol sodium per day, with renal regulation ensuring homeostasis in the healthy adult.

B. Potassium

Since potassium is the main intracellular cation, the total body potassium is closely related to the body cell mass. Total body potassium is about 3500 mmol, of which about 80% is intracellular in skeletal muscle. The normal dietary potassium intake is 50 to 150 mmol/day, but renal homeostasis is much less effective than for sodium.

C. Calcium

More than 99% of the total body calcium (1200 g) is present in the skeleton. A continuous supply of calcium is necessary to preserve the skeleton, as well as to maintain electrical excitability. Calcium requirements vary greatly with age and sex. The recommended dietary intake of calcium has varied with different expert panels — this ranges from 400 to 500 mg (10 to 12 mmol) per day[3] to 800 mg (20 mmol) per day.[2] The higher level appears to be more acceptable to ensure that an adequate calcium intake is achieved.

D. Phosphorus

Most of the phosphorus in the body is present in the bones as phosphate (600-900g) but there are also considerable amounts as intermediary metabolites and as nucleic acids in all cellular material. The normal recommended dietary intake is similar to that for calcium, namely about 800 mg (26 mmol) per day.

Table 3
RECOMMENDED DIETARY ALLOWANCES

Adult Values — Mean of Values for Different Age Groups

	RDA (U.S.)[a]		RDA (U.K.)[b]		Estimated safe and adequate daily levels[a]		
	Male	Female	Male	Female			
Energy	2550 kcal	1900 kcal	2450 kcal	2025 kcal	Sodium	1100—3300 mg	48—144 mmol
	10.7 MJ	7.9 MJ	10.3 MJ	8.5 MJ			
Protein (g)	56	44	60	47	Potassium	1875—5625 mg	48—144 mmol
Vitamin A (μg RE)	1000	800	750	750	Chloride	1700—5100 mg	48—144 mmol
Vitamin D (μg)	5—10		5—10		Calcium	800 mg (500 mg)[b]	20 mmol (12.5 mmol)
Vitamin E (mg, α TE)	10	8	—	—	Phosphorus	800 mg	26 mmol
Vitamin C (mg)	60	60	30	30	Magnesium	300 mg	14 mmol
Thiamin (mg)	1.4	1.0	1.0	0.8	Iron	10 mg	179 μmol
Riboflavin (mg)	1.6	1.2	1.6	1.3	Zinc	15 mg	229 μmol
B_6 (mg)	2.2	2.0	—	—	Iodine	150 mg	1.2 μmol
Niacin (mg)	18	13	18	15	Copper	2.0—3.0 mg	32—48 μmol
B_{12} (μg)	3.0	3.0	—	—	Manganese	2.5—5.0 mg	46—91 μmol
Folate (μg)	400	400	300	300	Fluoride	1.5—4.0 mg	79—210 μmol
Vitamin K (μg)	70—140		—	—	Chromium	0.05—0.2 mg	1—4 μmol
Biotin (μg)	100—200		—	—	Selenium	0.05—0.2 mg	0.6—2.5 μmol
Pantothenic Acid (mg)	4—7		—	—	Molybdenum	0.15—0.5 mg	1.6—5.2 μmol

[a] From Ref. 2.
[b] From Ref. 3.

E. Magnesium

Total body magnesium is about 25 g, the bulk of which is found in bones. It is also the second most abundant intracellular cation, after potassium, about 20% of the total being present within the cells where it is of importance as a cofactor for many enzymes. The normal daily requirements for magnesium are about 200 to 400 mg/day (8 to 17 mmol/day).

F. Iron

Total body iron in the healthy adult is about 4000 mg, of which about 70% is in hemoglobin, 20% is in iron stores, and 10% is present in other tissue proteins. The commonly accepted recommended intakes for iron are 10 mg/day for men and post-menopausal women, and 12 to 18 mg/day for women during the reproductive period. These figures are based upon an estimated absorption of 10% of orally ingested iron.

G. Zinc

Zinc has an essential role as a cofactor for many enzymes. The total body zinc is about 2000 mg (30 mmol). Based upon an estimated 20% absorption of zinc from the gut, the recommended daily intake is about 15 mg (250 μmol).

H. Copper

Copper, which is also a component of many enzyme systems, is present in the body to a total amount of 100 to 150 mg. The estimated requirement is 1 to 3 mg/day (15 to 45 μmol).

I. Chromium

Chromium is an essential nutrient, necessary for maintenance of normal glucose tolerance. The total body chromium is some 5 to 10 mg (100 to 200 μmol). The dietary requirement appears to be 50 to 200 μg (1 to 4 μmol) per day.

J. Manganese

Although manganese is known to be an essential mineral in many laboratory animals, and it is also a cofactor for many enzymes in man, no definite syndromes of manganese deficiency have been identified in man. However, adult man contains about 12 to 20 mg (200 to 400 μmol) and it is generally assumed that a regular daily provision of manganese is necessary. The suggested intake for an adult is 2.5 to 5 mg/day (50 to 100 μmol).

K. Selenium

Selenium is a cofactor for the enzyme glutathione peroxidase, which is important in maintenance of membrane function. Selenium interacts with vitamin E in maintenance of antioxidant activity, particularly in relationship to the polyunsaturated fatty acids present in cell membranes. Selenium intake is very variable and depends upon the selenium content of the soil. The recommended daily intake of selenium is 50 to 200 μg (0.6 to 2.5 μmol) per day.

L. Molybdenum

Although no deficiency syndrome is clearly associated with molybdenum deficiency in man, molybdenum is well-established as an essential part of certain enzyme systems, e.g., xanthine oxidase. The Food and Nutrition Board has recently suggested a daily intake of molybdenum as 0.15 to 0.5 mg (1.5 to 5 μmol) per day.[2]

M. Iodine

The major requirement for iodine is in the synthesis of the thyroid hormones. Total body iodine is 20 to 50 mg (160 to 400 μmol). The recommended dietary intake is 50 to 150 μg (0.4 to 1.2 μmol) per day. The best source of this in the average diet is usually fish products, but fruit, vegetables, and cereals will also provide considerable iodine.

N. Fluorine

Fluoride is necessary to increase resistance to dental caries. It does not, however, appear to be a nutrient essential to support life in man and animals. The normal daily dietary intake from sea foods and tea, in particular, is 1 to 2 mg and the Food and Nutrition Board has recommended a daily intake of 1.5 to 4 mg (80 to 210 μmol) per day.

O. Other Trace Minerals

A number of other trace elements are known to be essential in plants and animals, e.g., nickel, tin, vanadium, aluminum, and several more. However, none of these has proved essential in man. Cobalt, which is an essential trace element, is required as a constituent of vitamin B_{12}. It is unlikely that any other requirement for cobalt is necesssary, if an adequate B_{12} intake is achieved.

VII. FAT-SOLUBLE VITAMINS

A. Vitamin A

Vitamin A (retinol) is necessary for normal vision and for the maintenance of normal function of epithelial cells. In the normal diet, retinol is obtained directly from various animal products, or after conversion of carotenes which are obtained from vegetable products. The recommended daily intake for adults is 750 μg/day.

B. Vitamin D

The natural form of vitamin D is cholecalciferol (vitamin D_3). After absorption from the gut, dietary cholecalciferol is hydroxylated first in the liver and then in the kidney to form 1, 25, dihydroxy vitamin D, which is the active form of the vitamin and is necessary for regulation of calcium and phosphate metabolism. The recommended daily intake is 10 μg (400 IU) for children and 2.5 μg (100 IU) for adults.

C. Vitamin E

Vitamin E consists of a family of substances known as the tocopherols, which are found in all cell membranes and are necessary to prevent the oxidation of polyunsaturated fatty acids. Recommended intakes for vitamin E have fluctuated considerably over the years, but currently accepted values are 8 mg of α tocopherol in women and 10 mg α tocopherol in men per day.

VIII. WATER-SOLUBLE VITAMINS

A. Thiamin

Thiamin, in the form of thiamin pyrophosphate, is necessary as a coenzyme involved in carboxylation reactions. The total amount of thiamin in the body is only about 25 to 30 mg, most of which being required for active metabolism. There seems to be little capacity for storage of excess thiamin in the body. The recommended daily intake is 1.0 to 1.4 mg. Alternatively, the dietary intake can be related to the intake of energy, the FAO/WHO recommendation being 0.4 mg per 1000 kcal (96 μg/MJ).[9]

B. Riboflavin

Riboflavin is necessary as a coenzyme for many oxidation reactions. Recommended intakes range from 1.3 to 1.6 mg/day, or 0.55 mg per 1000 kcal (130 μg/MJ).[9]

C. Niacin

Niacin is necessary as a component of the coenzyme NAD, which is essential for oxidative metabolism. The dietary requirement is about 18 mg/day, or 6.6 mg per 1000 kcal (1.6 mg/MJ).

D. Pyridoxine

Pyridoxine in the form of pyridoxal phosphate is necessary for many important transamination reactions. Recommended intakes are rarely suggested, but the dietary intake of 1.5 to 2 mg/day is sufficient for the requirements of most people.

E. Ascorbic Acid

Ascorbic acid (vitamin C) is necessary for the maintenance of healthy connective tissue. Its main function appears to be in facilitating the oxidation of proline to hydroxyproline, although it may also participate in other oxidation/reduction reactions. Controversy still exists as to whether the daily requirement for vitamin C is as low as the level required to prevent scurvy, (about 10 mg/day) or as high as some of the levels proposed to be beneficial in protection against certain infectious and chronic diseases (1 to 2 g/day). The recommended dietary intake is currently 30 mg/day in the U.K., and on average 60 mg/day in the U.S.

F. Vitamin B_{12}

Vitamin B_{12} is necessary in small amounts for normal maturation of red blood cells. Only 1 to 2 μg are excreted per day in the urine and feces, whereas the normal body stores are between 2 and 5 mg, more than 50% of which is in the liver. Deficiency is therefore uncommon, except after prolonged periods of dietary deficiency or malabsorption. The recommended daily dietary intake is 3 μg.

G. Folic Acid

Folic acid is, of course, also necessary for the normal maturation of red blood cells. Folic acid is of major importance in 1-carbon metabolism, particularly with respect to methylation reactions. Folate stores in the liver are low (5 to 15 mg/kg). Recommended intakes of folate are variable and range between 200 and 400 μg/day.

IX. RECOMMENDED DIETARY ALLOWANCES (RDA)

The figures quoted in this chapter and summarized in Table 3, for RDA, have been drawn mainly from the guides issued by the National Academy of Sciences (Washington D.C.)[2] and from the Department of Health and Social Security (London).[3] However, the definitions used to clarify the meaning of the values are different for the two sets of tables. The U.S. RDA are the levels of intake of essential nutrients considered "to be adequate to meet the known nutritional needs of practically all healthy persons". Although this was the original definition also of the recommendations in the U.K. document, this has been superseded since it became clear that this type of recommendation was often not reached by the intake, and yet no signs of deficiency developed. The current U.K. edition therefore suggests the recommendation that the intake should be "the average intake of individuals in a group, and there is no intention that every person should receive the exact amount recommended". Whichever set of figures one uses, these must only be regarded as a guide, with many individuals having requirements either above or below these suggested values. This is particularly important when considering ill patients receiving some form of nutritional support, since illness is frequently associated with an alteration in the nutritional requirements. The only methods of determining what the requirement is for a particular nutrient is to test whether a certain level of intake maintains health, whether a reduction causes signs of deficiency to develop, or to perform a specific biochemical assessment.

REFERENCES

1. **Davidson, S., Passmore, R., Brock, J. F., and Truswell, A. S.,** *Human Nutrition and Dietetics,* 7th ed., Churchill Livingstone, Edinburgh, 1979.
2. Food and Nutrition Board, *Recommended Dietary Allowances,* 9th ed., National Academy of Sciences, Washington, D.C., 1980
3. Committee on Medical Aspects of Food Policy, Recommended Daily Amounts of Food Energy and Nutrients for Groups of People in the United Kingdom, Department of Health and Social Security, London, 1979.
4. Ministry of Agriculture, Fisheries and Food, Manual of Nutrition 8th ed., Her Majesty's Stationery Office, London, 1978.
5. **Goodhart, R. S. and Shils, M. E.,** *Modern Nutrition in Health and Disease,* 5th ed., Lea and Febiger, Philadelphia, 1973.
6. **Munro, H. M.,** Amino acid requirements and metabolism and their relevance to parenteral nutrition, in *Parenteral Nutrition* Wilkinson, A. E., Ed., Churchill Livingston, Edinburgh, 1972.
7. **Steffee, C. H., Wissler, R. W., Hamphreys, E. M., Benditt, E. P., Woolridge, R. W., and Cannon, P. R.,** Studies in amino acid utilization. V. The determination of minimum daily essential amino acid requirements in protein-depleted adult male albino rats, *J. Nutr.* 40, 483, 1950.
8. **Vergroesen, A. J., de Deckere, E. A. M., ten Hoor, F., Homstra, T., and Houtsmuller, U. M. T.,** in *The Essential Fatty Acids,* Nutrition Society, Toronto, Canada, 1975.
9. Food and Agriculture Organization/World Health Organization, Requirements of vitamin A, thiamine, riboflavine and niacin, *W.H.O. Tech. Rep. Ser,* 1967.

Chapter 2

DIGESTION AND ABSORPTION OF NUTRIENTS

R. I. Russell

TABLE OF CONTENTS

I. INTRODUCTION

In studying nutrition and the management of nutritional insufficiency, the mechanisms of digestion and absorption of nutrients are important. This is particularly the case when different forms of enteral nutrition are being considered. Enteral support preparations, and especially elemental diets, are based on nutritional components which are readily assimilated. A brief account of the mechanisms of digestion and absorption of individual nutrients is thus relevant to an understanding of the composition of enteral nutrition preparations such as elemental diets. Much is now known of the complex and varied processes by which individual nutrients undergo digestion and absorption in the normal subject, but information is still required on alterations of digestive and absorptive mechanisms in disease states, especially in various GI conditions. Nutritional deficiencies in GI disease may follow the impairment of one or more steps in digestion or absorption. Treatment should reflect an appreciation of the basic pathophysiological problems, and nutritional support should be tailored, if possible, to correct these abnormalities and improve the nutritional state.

The normal nutritional requirements have been considered in Chapter 1. Individual requirements vary with age, sex, activity, environment, body size, physiological state, and the presence of disease.[1] It is the purpose of this chapter to review the digestion and absorption of the principal components of food — protein, lipids, carbohydrate, minerals and trace elements, and vitamins.

II. PROTEIN

The digestion and absorption of protein is of importance in working out the composition of a synthetic diet such as an elemental diet, in view of its provision of nitrogen requirements. The normal daily ingestion of dietary protein varies between 70 and 100 g, and 35 to 120 g of endogenous protein are lost daily into the lumen of the gut. Considerable quantities of endogenous protein are also absorbed. Absorption of both dietary and endogenous sources of protein is efficient, as the daily fecal nitrogen excretion in the normal healthy adult is not more than 1 to 2 g/day.

Protein digestion starts in the stomach where denaturation of proteins occurs by gastric acid, and protein is hydrolyzed to polypeptides by pepsinogens secreted by the gastric mucosa. Only small amounts of free amino acids are released at this point and the large polypeptides enter the duodenum where further hydrolysis occurs under the influence of proteolytic enzymes produced by the pancreas and secreted into the duodenum as the inactive compounds trypsinogen, chymotrypsinogen, procarboxypeptidases, and proelastase. Trypsin is formed from trypsinogen by the action of the brush border enzyme enterokinase, and once present in small amounts, an autocatalytic activation of trypsinogen follows. The other precursor enzymes are then activated by trypsin itself. These enzymes break the internal bonds of protein and polypeptide molecules. Each enzyme preferentially splits peptide bonds within the internal structure of proteins and the sequential action of all the proteolytic enzymes produces a mixture of free amino acids, di- and tripeptides in the duodenum and upper jejunum.[2] Thus, after a protein meal the intestinal lumen contains a complex mixture of small peptides and amino acids, in which peptides predominate.

There now follows a membrane and cellular phase of peptide digestion, involving two digestive systems.[3,4] One consists of peptidases in the brush border and the other of peptidases in the cytosol of surface epithelial cells of the villi. The latter are principally involved in the mucoscal hydrolysis of dipentides in the jejunum, whereas in the ileum both brush border and cytosol peptidases are important.

Amino acids are absorbed by active group-specific transport systems, which are largely stereospecific for forms of amino acids. At least four separate carrier-mediated, sodium-dependent systems have been defined: those for neutral amino acids; basic amino acids; dicarboxylic amino acids; and a common system for proline, hydroxyproline and glycine. It is possible that amino acids can be transported by more than one carrier, and overlap probably occurs in the transport functions of individual carriers.[5]

There is now evidence that di- and tripeptides are absorbed in the small intestine independently of amino acids and it is possible that protein is principally absorbed not as free amino acids but as small peptides.[6-9] Tetrapeptides are unlikely to be absorbed in this way. It has been reported that a number of amino acids are initially absorbed faster when presented to the mucosa as peptides than as free amino acids and intestinal perfusion studies have shown faster absorption of amino acids from partial enzymic hydrolysates of casein than their equivalent amino acid mixtures.[10] However, it would appear that only certain peptide mixtures are superior to amino acid mixtures in terms of α amino nitrogen assimilation. Casein and lactalbumin hydrolysates stimulate jejuinal absorption of water and electrolytes, but fish protein hydrolysate appears to cause a net secretion of fluid and electrolytes.[11] It has been recently demonstrated using intestinal perfusion studies in normal human subjects that orally administered mixtures of peptides and free amino acids can be fully assimilated with equal efficiency. Absorption of individual amino acids from peptides was faster than that from free amino acids only in the first 2 hr after ingestion. By 3 hr, similar absorption had occurred. Secretion of fluid into the lumen of the upper small intestine was found to be less after ingestion of the peptide meal.[12] Further work is required to determine the relationships of the composition of peptide mixtures and the absorption of amino acids.

The principal advantage of direct peptide transport is the conservation of metabolic energy. It has also been shown that the ileum is important for the completion of peptide digestion and absorption,[13] but that quantitative digestion and absorption of protein is complete by the time an ingested meal has passed through the entire small intestine.

These findings may be of importance in the use of synthetic diets in which protein may be presented as a mixture of free amino acids, as a mixture of small peptides and amino acids, or as whole protein. For many purposes, diets containing protein hydrolysates may be as good as, or possibly superior to, those in which the nitrogen is derived solely from amino acids, as fuller utilization of absorptive processes may be achieved, fluid secretion may be less marked, and peptide uptake may be less adversely affected than amino acid uptake by malnutrition and GI conditions such as coeliac disease.[14] However, more data are required on the factors affecting protein absorption in health and disease, and further work is required on the optimal way of presenting protein in synthetic diets.

III. LIPIDS

Lipids are ingested as a complex mixture of triglycerides together with phospholipids, cholesterol esters, short and medium chain triglycerides, and the fat-soluble vitamins A, D, E, and K.

The first step in fat digestion is the formation of an emulsion in the stomach, which is further stabilized in the duodenum by bile acids. This is followed by hydrolysis by pancreatic lipase which breaks down the triglycerides to diglycerides, monoglycerides, sterols, and free fatty acids. In the upper small intestine, bile acid micelles and a protein known as colipase become attached to the surface of an emulsified lipid droplet. Adsorption of colipase creates a binding site for lipase, thus protecting it from the inhibitory action of bile acids. The monoglycerides and free fatty acids are then incorporated into mixed micelles with bile acids and phospholipids, rendering them water-soluble, and are subsequently transported across the unstirred water layer to the cell surface. Absorption of free fatty acid and monoglyceride occurs from this aqueous micellar solution by diffusion across the lipid-soluble cell membrane; diffusion across the unstirred layer is the rate-limiting step.[15-17] Cholesterol and fat-soluble vitamins also use the micellar route. Diffusion of long chain fatty acids across the unstirred water layer does not occur to any great extent in the absence of micelles, although short and medium chain fatty acids may undergo satisfactory diffusion across the water barrier under these conditions. Stabilization of lipid emulsions in the lumen by dietary or endogenous protein may also facilitate fat absorption.[18] After entering the cell, fatty acids and monoglycerides are reconstituted to form triglycerides. Chylomicrons are subsequently formed from a combination of triglyceride, phospholipid, and an apoprotein synthesized by intestinal microsomes. After movement to the Golgi apparatus, the lipoproteins are released into the interstitial space, then to the lymphatics.[19] Small and medium chain lipids enter the portal blood directly from the intestinal cell.[20]

Knowledge of the factors involved in fat absorption may be helpful in planning synthetic diets. Essential fatty acids are required in adequate amount, and the use of short and medium chain triglycerides may facilitate fat absorption by requiring less digestion, and may have advantages in certain situations (such as blockage of lymphatic drainage by rapidly and directly entering the portal circulation).

IV. CARBOHYDRATE

Carbohydrate is ingested mainly in the form of starch, with some disaccharides (sucrose, lactose) and monosaccharides (glucose, fructose). Large polysaccharides are hydrolyzed in the lumen by salivary and pancreatic amylases to form oligosaccharides, maltose, maltotriose, and α-limit dextrins. Further digestion occurs at the mucosal cell surface by the brush border enzymes maltase, isomaltase, sucrase, and lactase.[21] Lactose is broken down to glucose and galactose; sucrose to glucose and fructose, and malto-oligosaccharides; α-limit dextrins and trehalose to glucose. Simple sugars are absorbed efficiently and rapidly. Glucose transport is linked to sodium which may allow the cell menbranes to become more permeable to glucose.[22] The energy for the active glucose and galactose transport system is derived from the sodium pump, which moves sodium actively out of the cell by a mechanism involving the hydrolysis of ATP.[23] It is possible that sodium-independent glucose absorption may also account for some glucose absorption, using a disaccharidase-related transport mechanism. Fructose absorption occurs by facilitated diffusion. It is possible that glucose polymers are also effectively absorbed directly, although confirmation of this is required. Simple, easily absorbed carbohydrates are a useful source of energy in dietary support regimes.

V. WATER AND ELECTROLYTES

There is considerable movement of water and electrolytes in the duodenum in response to osmotic and concentration gradients, and by the time fluid reaches the upper jejunum an isotonic state has been achieved. The transfer of water across the intestinal mucosa is a passive process and depends on simple diffusion and bulk flow along osmotic pressure gradients. Water transfer accompanies net movement of solutes such as glucose and amino acids.

Sodium and potassium are absorbed in the jejunum principally by passive movement down concentration gradients associated with the movement of actively transported solutes such as glucose and amino acids.[24] Sodium is also absorbed in association with glucose by means of a common carrier protein on the brush border. Sodium is extruded out of the epithelial cells by the activity of sodium and potassium-sensitive ATPase,[25] which thereby also maintains a low intracellular sodium concentration which is required for the common carrier brush border entry mechanism.

Potassium and chloride move passively across the jejunal mucosa in relation to concentration and electrochemical gradients. Bicarbonate moves out the jejunal lumen against a concentration gradient, possible related to the production of hydrogen ions by the jejunal mucosa, which removes bicarbonate as carbon dioxide.[26] Bicarbonate in the jejunum also stimulates sodium absorption, and it is possible that an exchange system exists for sodium and hydrogen ions. Absorption of water and electrolytes in the jejunum is thus closely associated with the absorption of adequately digested (or basic synthetic) nutrients, and on bicarbonate in bile and pancreatic secretions.

In the ileum there are lower chloride and higher bicarbonate concentrations, suggesting the possibility of an ion exchange mechanism of chloride absorption for bicarbonate secretion, and a double ion exchange process involving sodium and hydrogen ions has been suggested.[27] Sodium and choloride can be absorbed actively against electrical and concentration gradients in the ileum, and are independent of the transport of other solutes as in the jejunum. In the colon active absorption of sodium and chloride occurs, the lattter probably also associated with a bicarbonate exchange as in the ileum. Potassium is secreted into the lumen of the colon. Ileal and colonic absorption of sodium and water appears to occur independently of the absorption of carbohydrate and protein digestion products, in contrast to the jejunum.

VI. MINERALS AND TRACE ELEMENTS

A. Calcium

Calcium is principally absorbed in the duodenum and jejunum by means of a two-step active transport system. A calcium-binding protein facilitates cellular uptake within the brush border of the intestinal epithelial cells. The presence of 1, 25-dihydroxycholecalciferol, the active metabolite of vitamin D, increases the protein content of the brush border, thus increasing calcium absorption.[28] Uptake then occurs across the mucosa followed by transfer to the serosa.[29] Calcium transport is enhanced by vitamin D, which also influences the diffusion of calcium into the cell, increasing mucosal to serosal transport. It is increased by the simultaneous ingestion of some sugars, especially lactose. Sodium reduces and bile acids increase calcium absorption.

B. Phosphorus

Phosphorus is absorbed by a mixture of passive and active mechanisms, occurring throughout the small intestine. Absorption of phosphate is also affected by diet and antacids which bind phosphorus within the lumen of the intestine.

C. Magnesium

Magnesium absorption occurs by means of facilitated diffusion involving a probable carrier system. More data are required on this process, but absorption appears to improve when there is increased intake of protein and lactose. It is impaired by the presence of lipids in the intestine. Magnesium absorption occurs throughout the small intestine.

D. Iron

Iron absorption occurs principally in the duodenum and to some extent in the jejunum. Dietary iron is largely protein bound and about 10% of ingested iron is available for absorption. It is partly released by gastric digestion which requires the presence of a low pH. A mucopolysaccharide gastroferrin, released by the stomach, is involved in an intraluminal transport system. Further digestion occurs in the duodenum and proximal jejunum and ionic iron is released which is chelated by cysteine, ascorbic acid, and sugars.[30] The ionic iron attaches to specific receptors in the brush border of mucosal cells and is transported into the cell by an active process. Control of iron absorption is achieved in part by the needs of the individual identified by the amount of iron accumulated in the epithelial cells at the level of serosal transfer.[31]

E. Other Trace Elements

Other essential trace elements are zinc, iodine, copper, manganese, selenium, cobalt, chromium, and molybdenum. Other trace elements such as tin, vanaduim, nickel, silicon, and fluorine are probably less essential for optimal health. Absorption of these trace elements occurs throughout the small intestine and is considered to be maximal in the proximal small intestine.[32] Absorption is partially energy dependent and binding factors in intestinal mucosa and in gastric and pancreatic secretions facilitate absorption. Other dietary constituents such as inorganic salts, phytate, and fiber may reduce absorption, but amino acid or carbohydrate complexes may enhance absorption of trace elements. In the plasma, trace elements are bound to albumin and transferrin (binding zinc, copper, chromium, and manganese) and some small amounts are bound to amino acids. Caeruloplasmin (an α_2 globulin) contains over 90% of plasma copper. Control of zinc absorption occurs at intestinal mucosal level. Copper and manganese are excreted in bile where copper is bound in complexes which reduce its reabsorption. Chromium, iodine, selenium, and molybdenum are controlled by urinary excretion as anions in the urine.

VII. VITAMINS

A. Fat-Soluble Vitamins

The fat-soluble vitamins A, D, E, and K are absorbed with lipids and are influenced by the same factors which affect lipid absorption. They require the formation of mixed micelles with bile acids to facilitate their passage across the unstirred water layer. Vitamin A is absorbed by a carrier-mediated passive mechanism in the proximal small intestine.[33] Vitamins D and E are absorbed in a similar manner to long chain fatty acids and other sterols. Vitamin K absorption occurs throughout the small intestine by passive diffusion; there is evidence that it is also absorbed in the colon where it is synthesized by bacteria.[34]

B. Water-Soluble Vitamins

Water-soluble vitamins are absorbed by active and carrier-mediated processes, mainly in the proximal small intestine. Ascorbic acid is actively transported in the ileum. Vitamin B_{12} is almost completely absorbed in the terminal ileum after combination with intrinsic factor, which is a glycoprotein secreted by the gastric parietal cells. The B_{12}-intrinsic factor complex attaches to an ileal receptor on the microvilli of the epithelial cells, this binding process requiring calcium and magnesium ions, and an alkaline pH.[35] Pancreatic proteinases are required for optimal absorption of vitamin B_{12}.[36,37]

The mechanisms involved in folic acid absorption are complex. Folic acid (pteroylglutamic acid) is not widely found in natural substances.[38] Naturally occurring folates are polyglutamates (pteroic acid conjugated with a number of glutamate residues). Hydrolytic digestion to monoglutamates by the enzyme gammaglutamyl-carboxypeptidase occurs in the upper small intestine,[39] although some hydrolysis may occur at the brush border or within the epithelial cell. Pteroylmonoglutamic acid is a weak acid, and as such may be absorbed by passive nonionic diffusion which would require its presence at least partly in the undissociated form. This would need the existence of an acid microclimate,[40] and this has been demonstrated.[41] The association of pH and pteroylmonoglutamic acid absorption has been shown.[42,43] An active process at specific receptor sites has also been postulated;[44] a saturable mechanism has been demonstrated, which does not necessarily indicate active transport. It could be a saturable passive process, possibly facilitated diffusion.[45] Metabolic conversion of monoglutamic folate to reduced methyl folate appears to occur within the intestinal cell. 5-Methyltetrahydrofolate is converted to tetrahydrofolate, which acts as an important intracellular coenzyme. Almost all folic acid absorption occurs in the jejunum.

A wide range of mechanisms are thus involved in the digestion and absorption of individual nutrients. The processes of digestion and absorption are influenced by the presence of other nutrients in various stages of digestion and by neurogenic and hormonal factors. These are complex processes with complex interrelationships. It is possible, on the basis of an understanding of normal digestion and absorption requirements of individual nutrients, to build up synthetic diets which will provide patients with adequate amounts of each of these nutrients. This is, of course, presupposing normal digestive and absorptive processes. In the presence of disease states, especially those associated with chronic GI conditions, these are likely to be abnormal. Other factors associated with normal digestion and absorption such as hormonal factors are also likely to be altered in such conditions. Further information is required on the total changes of digestive and absorptive processes and related hormonal and other factors influencing assimilation of nutrients in disease states, especially those affecting the GI tract. In any patient the specific requirements of individual nutrients must be accurately determined for adequate nutritional support to be given. In disease processes, the optimal way of presenting nutrients to the patient depends upon the pattern of damage to digestion and absorption mechanisms, and further data are required on these changes in various disease processes.

REFERENCES

1. **Berenson, M. M. and Bowers, J. H.,** Supplemental nutrition and digestive disease, *Clin. Gastroenterol.*, 8, 141, 1979.
2. **Brooks, F. P.,** Mechanisms of digestion and absorption, in, *Scientific Foundations of Gastroenterology*, Sircus, W., Ed., A. N. Smith Heinemann, London, 1980, 389.
3. **Kim, Y. S., Nicholson, J. A., and Curtis, K. J.,** Intestinal peptide hydrolysis. Peptide and amino acid absorption, *Med. Clin. North Am.*, 58, 1397, 1974.
4. **Freeman, H. J. and Kim, Y. S.,** Digestion and absorption of protein, *Annu. Rev. Med.* 29, 99, 1978.
5. **Matthews, D. M.,** Intestinal absorption of amino acids and peptides, in *The Use of Amino Acids and Oligopeptides in Dietetics*, Bassler, K. H., Fekl, W., Lang, K., Eds., *Z. Ernahrungswiss. Suppl.*, 20, 1976, 1.
6. **Adibi, S. A. and Soleimanpour, M.,** Functional characterisation of dipeptide transport system in human jejunum, *J. Clin. Invest.*, 53, 1368, 1974.
7. **Matthews, D. M.,** Absorption of peptides by mammalial intestine, in *Peptide Transport and Protein Nutrition*, Matthews, D. M., Payne, J. W., Eds., Amsterdam Associated Scientific Publishers, 1975, 61.
8. **Matthews, D. M.,** Intestinal absorption of peptides, *Physiol. Rev.*, 55, 537, 1975.
9. **Matthews, D. M. and Adibi, S. A.,** Peptide absorption, *Gastroenterology*, 71, 151, 1976.
10. **Silk, D. B. A., Clark, M. L., Marrs, T. C., Addison, J. M., Boston, D., Matthews, D. M., and Clegg, K. M.,** Jejunal absorption of amino acid mixture stimulating casein and enzyme hydrolysate of casein prepared for oral administration to normal adults, *Br. J. Nutr.*, 33, 95, 1975.

11. **Silk, D. B. A., Fairclough, P. D., Clark, M. L., Heparty, J. E., Marrs, T. C., Addison, J. M., Burston, D., Clegg, K. M., and Matthews, D. M.,** Use of a peptide rather than free amino acid nitrogen source in chemically defined "elemental" diets, *J. Parent. Ent. Nutr.*, 4, 548, 1980.
12. **Silk, D. B. A., Chung, Y. C., Berger, K. L., Conley, K., Beigler, M., Sleisenger, M. H., Spiller, G. A., and Kim, Y. S.,** Comparison of oral feeding of peptide and amino acid meals to normal human subjects. *Gut*, 20, 291, 1979.
13. **Chung, Y. C., Kim, Y. S., Shadchehr, A., Garrido, A., MacGregor, I. L., and Sleisenger, M. H.,** Protein digestion and absorption in the human small intestine, *Gastroenterology*, 76, 1415, 1979.
14. **Matthews, D. M.,** Protein absorption — then and now, *Gastroenterology*, 73, 1267, 1977.
15. **Hofmann, A. F.,** A physical-chemical approach to the intraluminal phase of fat absorption, *Gastroenterology*, 50, 56, 1966.
16. **Isselbacher, K. J.,** Biochemical aspects of lipid absorption, *Fed. Proc.*, 26, 1920, 1967.
17. **Westergaard, H. and Dietschy, J. M.,** The mechanism whereby bile acid micelles increase the rate of fatty acid and cholesterol uptake into the intestinal mucosal cell, *J. Clin. Invest.*, 58, 97, 1976.
18. **Meyer, J. H., Stevenson, E. A., and Watt, H. D.,** The potential role of protein in the absorption of fat, *Gastroenterology*, 70, 232, 1976.
19. **Sabesin, S. M. and Frase, S.,** Electron microscopic studies of the assembly, intracellular transport and secretion of chylomicrons by rat intestine, *J. Lipid Res.*, 18, 496, 1977.
20. **Schmitt, M. G., Jr., Soergel, K. H., and Wood, C. M.,** Absorption of short chain fatty acids from the human jejunun, *Gastroenterology*, 70, 211, 1976.
21. **Crane, R. K.,** Intestinal absorption of glucose, in *Biomembranes*, 4A ed., Smythe, D. H., Ed., Plenum Press, New York, 1974, 647.
22. **Olsen, W. A. and Ingelfinger, F. J.,** The role of sodium in intestinal glucose absorption in man, *J. Clin. Invest.*, 47, 1133, 1968.
23. **Gray, G. M.,** Carbohydrate digestion and absorption, *Gastroenterology*, 58, 96, 1970.
24. **Turnberg, L. A.,** Water and electrolyte metabolism, in *Scientific Foundations of Gastroenterology*, Sircus, W. and Smith, A. N., Eds., Heinemann, London, 198O, 397.
25. **Parsons, D. S.,** Salt and water absorption by the intestinal tract, *Br. Med. Bul.*, 23, 252, 1967.
26. **Turnberg, L. A., Fordtran, J. S., Carter, N. W., and Rector, F. C., Jr.,** Mechanism of bicarbonate absorption and its relationship to sodium transport in the human jejunum, *J. Clin. Invest.*, 49, 548, 1970.
27. **Turnberg, L. A., Bieberdorf, F. A., Morawski, S. G., and Fordtran, J. S.,** Interrelationships of chloride, bicarbonates, sodium and hydrogen in the human ileum, *J. Clin. Invest.*, 49, 557, 1970.
28. **Hangler, M. R. and McCain, T. A.,** Basic and clinical concepts related to vitamin D metabolism and action, *N. Engl. J. Med.*, 297, 974, 1977.
29. **Harrison, H. G. and Harrison, H. C.,** Calcium, in *Biomembranes*, 4B ed., D. H. Smythe, Ed., Plenum Press, New York, 1974, 793.
30. **Callender, S. T. and Warner, G. T.,** Iron absorption from bread, *Am. J. Clin. Nutr.*, 21, 1170, 1968.
31. **Linder M. C. and Munro, H. N.,** The mechanism of iron absorption and its regulation, *Fed. Proc.*, 36, 2017, 1977.
32. **Aggett, P. J.,** Trace elenents in medicine, *Hosp. Update*, 5, 981, 1979.
33. **Hollander, D. and Murlidhara, K. S.,** Vitamin A intestinal absorption in vivo: influence of luminal factors on transport, *Am. J. Physiol.*, 232, 471, 1977.
34. **Hollander, D., Murlidhara, K. S., and Rim, E.,** Colonic absorption of bacterially synthesised vitamin K2 in the rat, *Am. J. Physiol.*, 230, 251, 1976.
35. **Herbert, V.,** Absorption of vitamin B12 and folic acid, *Gastroenterology*, 54, 110, 1968.
36. **Toskes, P. P., Dren, J. J., and Fruiterman, J.,** Specificity of the correction of vitamin B12 malabsorption by pancreatic extract and its clinical significance, *Gastroenterology*, 65, 199, 1973.
37. **Allen, R. H. Seetharam, B., Podell, E., and Alpers, D. H.,** Effect of proteolytic enzymes on the binding of cobalamin to protein and intrinsic factor. In vitro evidence that a faiure to partially degrade a protein is responsible for cobalamin malabsorption in pancreatic insufficiency, *J. Clin. Inves.*, 61, 47, 1978.
38. **Matthews, D. M.,** Absorption of water-soluble vitamins, in *Biomembranes*, 4B ed., Smythe, D. H., Ed., Plenum Press, New York, 1974, 674.
39. **Rosenberg, I. H.,** Folate absorption and malabsorption, *N. Engl. J. Med.*, 293, 1303, 1975.
40. **Hogben, C. A. M., Tocco, J. T., Brodie, B. B., and Schanker, L. S.,** On the mechanism of intestinal absorption of drugs, *J. Pharm. Exp. Ther.*, 125, 275, 1959.
41. **Lucas, M. L. and Blair, J. A.,** The magnitude and distribution of the acid microclimate in proximal jejunum and its relation to luminal acidfication, *Proc. R. Soc. Ser. B*, 200, 27, 1978.
42. **Benn, A., Swan, C. H., Cooke, W. T., Blair, J. A., Matty, A. J., and Smith, M. E.,** Effect of intraluminal pH on the absorption of pteroylmonoglutamic acid, *Br. Med. J.*, 1, 148, 1971.

43. **MacKenzie, J. F. and Russell, R. I.,** The effect of pH on folic acid absorption in man, *Clin. Sci. Mol., Med.*, 51, 363, 1976.
44. **McIntyre, L. W., Dow, J. W., McIntyre, R. J. and Harding, N. G. L.,** Cellular acquisition of folate: a compartmental model, *J. Mol. Med.*, 1, 3, 1975.
45. **Sleisenger, M. H. and Brandborg, L. L.,** *Malabsorption,* W. B. Saunders, Philadelphia, 1977, 23.

Chapter 3

CAUSES AND RESULTS OF NUTRITIONAL INSUFFICIENCY

R. I. Russell

TABLE OF CONTENTS

I. CAUSES OF NUTRITIONAL INSUFFICIENCY

As elemental or chemically defined diets were introduced as a method of correcting nutritional deficiency by enteral means, it is relevant to consider the causes of nutritional insufficiency. Any of these causes, if associated with severe or prolonged disease, may lead to very severe nutritional deficiency, requiring correction by intravenous nutrition rather than by enteral methods. Such may also be the case in patients suffering from "alimentary failure" owing to severe and chronic gastrointestinal disease. Less severe nutritional deficiency may be amenable to treatment by oral nutritional support and in this group dietary supplements, complete oral liquid diets, or elemental diets may be of value. The metabolic consequences of severe disease initially described in association with trauma, infection, and surgery are now known to apply to a wide range of other conditions.

A. Trauma and Surgery

Metabolic changes in association with trauma were initially reported and extensively studied by Cuthbertson.[1-3] He described metabolic depression which occurs early after the traumatic episode, followed by an increased rate of metabolism with high nitrogen excretion and increased consumption of oxygen. Any traumatic episode will lead to a metabolic reaction of this kind and nutritional support may be required if the metabolic changes are severe or prolonged.[4]

Similar changes are now known to occur in association with surgery. The degree of metabolic change after surgery relates to the extent of the operation performed and the degree of nutritional deficiency which may be present prior to surgery. Preoperative nutritional support may be helpful in many patients. Metabolic alterations in association with surgery have also been well worked out.[5] Nutritional deficiency may also develop or be worsened by complications following surgery which exacerbate the catabolic response, including infections, wound rupture, the development of fistulas, prolonged paralytic ileus, and peritonitis. Nutritional deficiency is a particular problem in head and neck surgery, often associated with tumors, and nutritional support may be required in such patients.

B. Gastrointestinal and Liver Disease

A wide range of GI conditions may be associated with the development of significant nutritional deficiency. These deficiency states occur much nore widely than was formerly believed and may not be clinically apparent in many patients for some time.[6] Their occurrence depends largely on the severity and duration of the disease, and the early recognition of such problems together with their correction improves the prognosis of these patients. Many suffer from what may be referred to as "alimentary failure", but other GI conditions can also give rise to nutritional deficiency. The GI causes of nutritional deficiency can be classified in the following way:

1. Severe or chronic diarrheal states; Crohn's disease, ulcerative colitis, GI infections, tumors, of colon and rectum, GI fistulas, and chronic pancreatic insufficiency
2. Severe malabsorption states; coeliac disease, Crohn's disease, the short bowel syndrome secondary to massive small intestinal resection, and other conditions leading to malabsorption such as tropical sprue and the blind loop syndrome
3. Prolonged vomiting; this may be associated with intestinal infections, pyloric stenosis due to longstanding duodenal ulcer disease, or tumors of the upper GI tract
4. Prolonged poor oral intake; tumors, dysphagia, anorexia nervosa

5. GI surgery, GI resections may lead to nutritional deficiency, which may be exacerbated by preexisting chronic GI disease
6. Pediatric conditions of the GI tract, gut atresia and tracheo-esophageal fistulas
7. Liver disease; many patients with varying degrees of hepatic abnormality have nutritional insufficiency and there is evidence of this in patients with hepatic cirrhosis, chronic active hepatitis, primary biliary cirrhosis and other conditions; nutritional insufficiency may be exacerbated in hepatic disease if alcohol abuse is an etiological factor in the hepatic pathology

One GI disease that is particularly liable to be associated with severe nutritional deficiency is Crohn's disease. In such patients there are usually multiple causes of nutritional insufficiency, including severe malabsorption, diarrhea associated with malabsorption of fat, water, electrolytes or bile acids, chronic fistulas, and local infections. These patients may also require surgery which may necessitate resection of part of the intestine which in turn may exacerbate the malabsorption, diarrhea, and malnutrition.

C. Renal Disease

In patients with acute or chronic renal disease, there may be associated metabolic changes with increased catabolism and retention of nitrogen. Chronic nephritis, acute and chronic pyelonephritis may be associated with such nutritional abnormalities, and these may be difficult to correct.[7]

D. Tumors

Malignant disease is frequently associated with nutritional deficiency. This may be caused by anorexia, malabsorption, or protein-calorie malnutrition, and may be exacerbated by intercurrent surgery or the use of chemotherapy and radio-therapy.[8]

E. Burns

Patients with severe burns develop nutritional deficiency. Nitrogen and energy consumption are more marked in burns because of extensive skin damage, loss of body tissue and large amounts of fluid. Good nutritional support is essential in the treatment of such patients.[9]

F. Unconscious and Paraplegic Patients

Nutritional support is required in patients who are unconscious or paraplegic for whatever reason, and specific nutritional support is generally required in these patients if the abnormality persists for any length of time.

G. Other Conditions Which May Necessitate Nutritional Support

Any chronic disease state may be associated with the development of nutritional deficiency. These include chronic cardiac problems, especially those undergoing cardiac surgery, and gynecological disease, especially malignancies.

II. RESULTS OF NUTRITIONAL DEFICIENCY

The metabolic consequences of severe disease have been studied over many years and much information has now been accumulated about the pathophysiological effects of the conditions previously described. The metabolic and nutritional results are now much better understood and thus the correction of these abnormalities can be achieved more effectively.[10-14] The body has only limited reserves of immediate available energy and nitrogen sources. Carbohydrate reserves are not more than 0.15 to 9.20 kg, and are principally in the form of glycogen. Once this carbohydrate is metabolized within 8 to 12 hr, proteins and fat then proceed to be metabolized. Protein catabolism provides carbohydrate metabolic intermediates, although some amino acids are not easily converted in this way. Fat reserves are 10 to 15 kg, lasting 20 to 25 days and protein reserves 4 to 6 kg, lasting approximately 10 to 15 days. Fat is unable to provide carbohydrates and fat metabolism itself requires a steady supply of carbohydrates to prevent the development of ketoacidosis. In acute starvation states, catabolism occurs at a rate of 10 to 15 g nitrogen daily. This can be reduced to 3 to 4 g/day by giving only 100 g glucose. During such starvation states, energy supplies are derived from body fat stores which may contribute up to 50% of the calories required. During periods of reduced protein intake, the same overall rate of catabolism and anabolism occurs, but a much smaller amount of nitrogen is excreted. This adaptation explains why malnourished patients show a reduced catabolic response to stress or surgery, whereas well-nourished subjects demonstrate a greater degree of early catabolism. These metabolic changes may occur in association with any of the conditions described earlier in this chapter. The catabolic response has a number of serious pathophysiological consequences. A negative nitrogen balance develops, with resultant increased sensitivity to infections, loss of body weight, delayed wound healing, hypoproteinemia, edema, and impaired immunocompetence — humoral and cellular. A negative potassium balance may also occur. Protein breakdown releases potassium ions and fixed acids in the form of sulfates and phosphates, and acid retention may thus develop. Catabolism of 1 g nitrogen leads to a loss of 16 to 18 meq potassiun and 3 to 4 meq of acid. Nutritional deficiency is more common than previously considered, and may occur in 20 to 50% of hospital patients.[15,16]

Adequate nutritional support can reduce or even abolish these metabolic responses to severe or prolonged disease. Awareness of the causes of nutritional deficiency will lead to earlier identification and thus a more rapid and successful correction of the abnormalities. Ideally, the prevention of these metabolic changes is preferable to their correction once they have developed. Lack of awareness of the causes of protein-calorie malnutrition may delay the diagnosis and the start of adequate nutritional support. However, any patient who has lost more than 10% of his or her normal body weight must be regarded as being likely to require nutritional support. It is thus important to identify the patients at risk of developing such nutritional and metabolic problems and to correct these if possible prior to the full development of the abnormalities.

REFERENCES

1. **Cuthberson, D. P.,** The disturbance of metabolism produced by bony and non-bony injury, with notes on certain abnormal conditions of bone, *Biochem., J.*, 24, 1244, 1930.
2. **Cuthbertson, D. P.,** Certain aspects of the metabolic response to injury, *Glasgow Med. J.*, 121, 41, 1934.
3. **Cuthbertson, D. P.,** Protein requirements after injury — quality and quantity, in *Parenteral Nutrition*, Wilkinson, A. E., Ed., Churchill Livingstone, London, 1972, 4.
4. **Kinney, J. M., Duke, J. H., Long, C. L., and Gump, F. E.,** Carbohydrate and nitrogen metabolism after injury, *J. Clin. Path.*, 23, 65, 1970.
5. **Moore, F. D.,** *Metabolic Care of the Surgical Patient*, W.B. Saunders, Philadelphia, 1959.
6. **Russell, R. I.,** Intravenous nutrition and elemental diets in gastrointestinal disease, in *Scientific Foundations of Gastroenterology*, Sircus, W. and Smith, A. N., Eds., Heinemann, London, 1980, 130.
7. **Lee, H. A.,** The nutritional management of renal diseases, in *Nutrition in the Clinical Management of Disease*, ed. Dickerson, J. W. D. and Lee, H. A., Eds., Edward Arnold Limited, London, 1978, 210.

8. **Dudrick, S. J., Copeland, F. N., and MacFadyen, B. V.,** The nutritional care of the cancer patient, in *Current Concepts in Parenteral Nutrition,* ed. Soeters, P. B., Wesdorp, R. I. C., Phaf, C. W. R., and Fischer, J. E., Eds., Martinus Nijhoff Medical Division, The Hague, 1977, 187.
9. **Wilmore, D. W.,** Parenteral nutrition in burned patients, in *Current Concepts in Parenteral Nutrition,* Greep, J. M., Soeters, P. B., Wesdorp, R. I. C., Phaf, C. W. R., Fischer, J. E., Eds. Martinus Nijhoff Medical Division, The Hague, 1977, 227.
10. **Munro, H. N.,** General aspects of the regulation of protein metabolism by diet and by hormones, in *Mammalian Protein Metabolism,* Vol. 1., Allison, J. G., and Munro, H. N., Eds., Academic Press, New York, 1966, 381.
11. **Cuthbertson, D. P.,** The metabolic response to injury and its nutritional implications: retrospect and prospect, *J. Parenteral Enteral Nutr.,* 3, 108, 1979.
12. **Wretlind, A.,** Intravenous nutrition, in *Scientific Foundations of Surgery,* 2nd ed., Wells, C., Kyle, J., Dumphy, E., Eds. Heinemann, London, 1974, 626.
13. **Dudrick, S. J., McFadyen, B. D., van Buren, C. G. Ruberg, R. L., and Maynard, A. T.,** Parenteral hyperalimentation — metabolic problems and solutions, *Ann. Surg.,* 176, 259, 1972.
14. **Lee, H. A.,** Intravenous nutrition, *Br. J. Hosp. Med.,* 11, 719, 1974.
15. **Bistrian, B. R., Blackburn, G. L., Hallowell, E., and Heddle, R.,** Protein status of general surgical patients, *JAMA,* 230, 858, 1974.
16. **Bistrian, B. R., Blackburn, G. L., Vitale, J., Cochran, D., and Naylor, J.,** Prevelance of malnutrition in general medical patients, *J. Am. Med. Assoc.,* 235, 1567, 1976.

Chapter 4

ASSESSMENT AND MONITORING OF NUTRITIONAL STATUS

A. Shenkin

TABLE OF CONTENTS

I. INTRODUCTION

With the development of methods of nutritional support by oral, enteral, or i.v. routes, there has been a growing awareness of the need for quantitative assessment of nutritional status. This is a useful adjunct to clinical examination in the initial assessment of the overall nutritional state of the patient. Moreover, many of the laboratory tests performed, together with a good dietary history, give an indication of the adequacy of the recent nutritional intake. This combined assessment of actual nutritional status plus current or recent dietary intake, then permits a rational decision to be reached on the need for nutritional support.

For patients in whom a form of nutritional therapy is commenced, the initial assessment will also provide basic information with regard to the level of provision necessary for many of the nutrients. Futhermore, repeated assessments ("nutritional monitoring") will provide quantitative data which should permit an objective evaluation of the success of nutritional therapy, and hence indicate the requirement for any change in intake.

A comprehensive nutritional assessment should therefore enable a fairly accurate provision of nutrients to meet the requirements of the individual patient. Ideally, all of the components of the diet should be considered — in practice, only the major dietary components, that is protein and energy substrates (fat and carbohydrate) together with a few selected minerals and vitamins are studied.

II. ENERGY STATUS

Body weight is the single most important measurement in assessment of overall nutritional status. A "normal" body weight in comparison with published ranges[1,2] probably indicates that the total reserves of energy of the individual are satisfactory. However, normal values encompass a wide range, and an individual's ideal weight when in good health may well be higher or lower than the values quoted in tables. Moreover, the main energy store in the body is adipose tissue which normally only comprises 10 to 15% of total body weight.[3] Hence, changes in body weight do not indicate which tissue or body compartment have been affected; an alteration in fluid balance, in the amount of skeletal muscle or in the amount of depot fat, may all influence total weight. Hill and co-workers[4] have recently indicated that much of the early weight gain during nutritional support is due to water retention and is not associated with increased body fat or protein.

A more accurate method of measurement of body fat is clearly required. In healthy individuals, the best method is probably by underwater weighing which permits calculation of body density.[3] This is obviously impractical for patients, but Durnin and Womersley[5] have shown that the combined skin fold thickness at four sites (biceps, triceps, subscapular, and suprailiac), measured with skin calipers, provides an estimate of subcutaneous fat which correlates well with total body fat. Moreover, triceps skin fold thickness (TST) alone gives a reasonable estimate of body fat stores, although not as accurate as when all four measurements are used.[5] The TST is therefore of particular value when dealing with sick patients[6] and in comparison with the reference values of 12.5 mm for men and 16.5 mm for women[1] provides a convenient guide to the adequacy of fat stores. These reference values are, however, subject to marked interindividual variation and are not necessarily the ideal or target values for individual patients. The TST may therefore be especially useful when monitoring the progress of the patient — for example, in indicating the adequacy of energy intake in the severely depleted patient.[7]

The most direct method of measuring current energy requirements is to measure the rate of energy utilization. This, however, is technically difficult, requiring either direct calorimetry (rarely used in humans) or indirect calorimetry by analysis of expired air for oxygen and carbon dioxide content.[8] This currently remains a research investigation and, moreover, collection of expired O_2 and CO_2 may be technically difficult in the seriously ill.

An alternative is to estimate basal energy expenditure (BEE) using Harris-Benedict nomograms,[9] by which the BEE is computed from age, sex, height, and weight. It has been suggested that 1.75 × BEE will provide an adequate energy intake for most patients being fed i.v. and 1.5 × BEE for enterally fed patients.[9] Although this method probably correlates satisfactorily for many patients, the BEE does not allow for sepsis or severity of illness which, depending upon degree, may cause a rise of from 10% to more than 100% in the resting energy expenditure.[8,10] In the acutely ill catabolic patient, 1.75 × BEE may therefore underestimate the energy requirement in comparison to the values found from indirect calorimetry.[11] When anabolism is desired in the depleted patient, provision of energy substrates to a level of about 50% above this calculated or measured value may be required.[12]

The level of energy substrate obtained by this type of calculation, when compared with estimates derived from a careful dietary history, can give an indication of the adequacy of the current intake. A further laboratory test which may be helpful in this regard is whether the individual is accumulating ketone bodies, which are markers of mobilization and utilization of depot fat. When energy requirements are being met by dietary intake, there is no increase in metabolism of storage fat. It has been suggested that the development of ketonemia during a period of inadequate dietary intake is an adaptation by the body, leading to protein sparing and better nitrogen (N) balance.[13] However, some individuals fail to "ketoadapt" during periods of inadequate energy intake, and this may be a bad prognostic sign[14] since the body is presumably utilizing protein as an energy source.[13,15] Hence, although a rise in ketone bodies indicates inadequate energy intake the lack of such ketone response does not necessarily imply an insufficient energy supply. It is therefore mainly in those individuals known to have an inadequate intake that analysis of blood and urine for ketone bodies may be of value in indicating the extent of ketoadaptation.

III. PROTEIN STATUS

Protein nutritional status is usually considered at the same time as energy status since protein metabolism interacts very closely with energy balance.[16] The techniques used for assessment of protein status can be divided into those providing information about whole body protein, and those which investigate individual tissues or organs.

A. Protein Status of Whole Body

1. Nitrogen (N) Balance

Estimation of N balance is probably the most widely used technique for determining recent changes in total body protein. It therefore forms the basis of most methods of assessing adequacy of protein/energy intake.

Urinary N excretion can vary from less than 5 g/day in patients who are adapted to a low protein-energy intake, to 50 g/day or more in patients who are severely traumatized or septic. The level of urine N reflects the degree of catabolism of amino acids from the amino acid pool, which is derived from dietary intake of protein together with catabolism of body proteins, in particular skeletal muscle protein.

Total urine N can be fairly readily measured using a Kjeldahl method.[17] When this analysis is not available, urine urea measurement is a convenient alternative. Provided there is no urinary infection nor excess excretion of amino acids or peptides, urea-N usually comprises about 80% of total N.[18]

To compute total loss of N from the body each day, an estimate of other losses in skin, feces etc. of about 2 g/day (or more if there are large fistula or exudate losses) should be added to the urine N.

Estimates of daily N intake are very variable in their accuracy. Even with a careful dietary history, calculation of protein intake from food tables is very inaccurate. In patients receiving a defined formula oral or enteral diet, or i.v. nutrition, the daily protein or N intake can readily be calculated. The daily N balance is then derived from the difference between the N intake and N output from the body. A negative N balance is clear evidence that there is a net catabolism of body proteins.

Measurement of total N loss provides guidance as to the amount of dietary N which should be supplied to maintain balance and hence, the increased level required to achieve net anabolism. From this level, the amount of energy substrates required can be calculated, since most studies suggest that 670 to 840 kJ (150 to 200 kcal/g) dietary N will ensure optimal use of amino acid N for protein synthesis.[12,19,20] An improvement in N balance can usually be achieved either by increasing the protein (amino acid) intake, by increasing the intake of energy or by a combination of these two measures.[16]

2. Serum Ribonuclease (RNase)

Measurement of serum RNase activity has been suggested as a relatively simple method of estimating N balance, without the inconvenience of requiring urine collections, since in some clinical situations a negative N balance is associated with an elevation in serum RNase.[21-23] However, more recent studies suggest that serum RNase does not always rise when N balance is negative,[7,24] and that when there is an elevation in serum RNase there is very poor correlation with the degree of negative N balance.[25] Moreover, high levels of serum RNase may occur in many diseases, such as renal or hepatic failure.[26] There is therefore little clinical use for this measurement.

3. Plasma Amino Acids

Some fairly typical changes occur in the plasma amino acid profile in prolonged protein energy malnutrition.[27] There is a reduction in total plasma amino acids, and in particular branched-chain amino acids, whereas plasma glycine and serine levels may be increased.[27,28] The ratio of phenylalanine/tyrosine, and glycine/valine[28,29] are typically increased.

By contrast, in patients with sepsis, the total plasma amino acid level is increased,[31,32] this being mainly caused by an increased level of aromatic and sulfur amino acids. The ratio of phenylalanine/tyrosine is again elevated.[33] The possible clinical significance of these amino acid changes remains unclear. One recent observation of some interest was that in the postoperative period, patients who developed increased levels of blood ketones in response to hypocaloric feeding, had a better N balance and also had a smaller increase in the plasma levels of branched-chain amino acids than those patients who failed to show a rise in blood ketones.[13] Thus, plasma amino acid levels are not accurate indexes of nutritional status alone, but probably also serve as markers of other metabolic changes.

4. Total Body Nitrogen

Probably the most absolute method of determining body protein-status is by total body N measurement using activation analysis.[34] This technique has been used to follow the changes in body protein following surgery[4,35] but is unlikely to become a routine procedure.

5. Total Body Potassium

A further method, also unsuitable in very ill patients, is the measurement of ^{40}K from which can be calculated the total body potassium and hence, the lean body mass.[36] This technique has been used to demonstrate the increased body proteins in patients receiving elemental diets over a prolonged period.[37]

B. Protein Status of Individual Tissues

1. Skeletal Muscle

a. Midarm Muscle Circumference (MAMC)

The MAMC can be calculated from the midarm circumference (MAC) and the triceps skinfold thickness (TST) by the formula:[1] $MAMC = MAC - (\pi \times TST)$. The MAMC gives a reasonable indication of total body skeletal muscle, and the values obtained can be compared with standard tables.[1] As with the TST, the MAMC is particularly useful in monitoring the progress of the individual patient.[7]

b. Creatinine-Height Index

Conversion of creatine to creatinine in skeletal muscle is irreversible and in the absence of severe sepsis, occurs at a fairly constant rate.[38] Measurement of urinary creatinine, therefore, gives an estimate of total skeletal muscle mass.[39] This can be compared with the expected creatinine excretion for a well-nourished individual of the same height — the creatinine-height index.[40] This measurement depends upon normal renal function and upon accurate urine collections — the average value from three successive 24-hr urines greatly improves the correlation of urinary creatinine with skeletal muscle mass.[39] Sequential values over a few weeks are again of value in following changes in skeletal muscle mass.

c. Creatine

In normal individuals, creatine is excreted in urine in only small amounts (less than 1 mmol/24 hr). Creatine excretion may be influenced by many factors, including injury, sepsis, starvation, and endocrine changes.[41] In particular, high levels of excretion may occur in catabolic states, and creatinuria may correlate with potassium and N excretion, and hence, with skeletal muscle catabolism.[42] Glucose and insulin therapy can lead to an improvement in N balance[43] and also reduces the level of creatine excretion.[44] However, creatinuria is not a constant feature of net protein catabolism[25] so creatine measurements can only be used as an additional marker in assessing the metabolic state of the patient.

d. 3-Methylhistidine

N^{T}-methylhistidine (3-methylhistidine) exists largely in actin and myosin in skeletal muscle[45] and once released by catabolism of these proteins it cannot be reutilized in protein synthesis.[46] It is therefore quantitatively excreted in the urine in an amount proportional to the degree of skeletal muscle protein catabolism.[47,48] Excretion rates can be markedly increased following trauma or in sepsis.[25,49] In contrast, in prolonged starvation, as metabolic adaptation take place and urinary N excretion falls, 3-methylhistidine excretion is also much reduced[50] indicating a fall in skeletal muscle catabolism.

Taken in conjunction with N balance, knowledge of 3-methylhistidine excretion therefore permits a greater understanding of protein turnover in the different organs of the body. For example 3-methylhistidine excretion is higher in postoperative patients who do not develop a ketone body response to hypocaloric feeding,[15] confirming increased muscle catabolism in this group.[13] As Blackburn and colleagues[51] have pointed out, a net protein catabolism in skeletal muscle may not be undesirable, since it may help to maintain protein synthesis in visceral tissues such as liver, immune system, etc. Precise interpretation of 3-methylhistidine measurements must await further studies, and since its measurement is usually only available in specialized laboratories, 3-methylhistidine cannot as yet form part of a routine scheme of patient monitoring.

2. Liver

An estimate of the adequacy of provision of amino acids to the liver and the capacity of the liver to utilize them can be obtained from plasma levels of various proteins. However, the plasma level is dependent not only upon the synthetic rate of the protein, but also upon the catabolic rate and upon the distribution of the protein between intravascular and extravascular fluid.[52] The ratio of this distribution can vary markedly, especially in acutely ill patients.[53] In more stable persons, serum levels may be useful in assessing liver protein status and for monitoring therapy.[54,55]

a. Albumin

Serum albumin is the most widely used index of liver protein synthesis.[5,56] A low serum albumin is a bad prognostic sign.[56,57] Recovery from protein-calorie malnutrition can be monitored using serum albumin concentrations,[54,55] but changes in serum albumin associated with nutritional state are usually fairly slow due to its relatively long half-life.[58]

b. Transferrin

Transferrin has a shorter half-life than albumin and hence serum concentration will respond more rapidly to changes in protein nutrition.[5,60] Serum transferrin falls when protein intake is inadequate,[7,61] is low in protein malnutrition, and rises promptly on refeeding.[54,55,60] In one study, transferrin levels were normal after 15 days refeeding, whereas albumin did not reach normal levels for more than 22 days.[55]

However, the usefulness of transferrin is limited by the potentially opposite effect of iron deficiency which would tend to cause an increase in transferrin (or iron-binding capacity). A normal serum transferrin could therefore be found in a patient with both iron deficiency and protein calorie depletion.

c. Other Short Half-Life Proteins

Prealbumin, with a half-life of about 1.9 days,[62,63] and retinol binding protein, with a half-life of only a few hours,[64] have both been shown to be very sensitive to changes in protein nutritional status.[7,54,55,61] Ingenbleek and co-workers[55] have found that prealbumin was the most useful and accurate index of defining nutritional status in protein-energy malnutrition.

The levels of these proteins tend to fall during acute illness and following trauma, and in such patients there may be no correlation between the serum level and N balance.[25] The changes in plasma level at this time may therefore be a nonspecific response, possibly indicating reduced synthetic rate, which is unrelated to nutrition. However having fallen to low plasma levels, these proteins may be of value in monitoring the anabolic phase during recovery.

The low level of complement C3 has been found to be of value in monitoring recovery of chronic protein calorie malnutrition.[54] By contrast, plasma concentration may be elevated in severe illness despite markedly negative N balance.[25,44] In this situation complement C3 probably correlates better with the acute phase reaction rather than the nutritional status. With two such opposing stimuli, complement C3 is of very limited value as a nutritional index.

d. Cholinesterase

Serum level of cholinesterase is a well-established index of liver protein synthesis.[26,27,65] In common with other enzymes, however, it is subject to rapid changes in concentration associated with induction of enzyme, in response to short-term changes in diet. It may therefore be too labile to monitor the progress of individual patients.

e. Other Liver Function Tests

It is well recognized that severe malnutrition may be associated with the development of a fatty liver and abnormal liver function.[66] In patients receiving nutritional therapy, a cholestatic form of jaundice has also been reported, mainly during i.v., nutrition, but also in enteral feeding.[67] Routine checking of liver function tests therefore, is, essential in all patients receiving nutritional support.

3. Immune System

An adequate provision of dietary proteins and energy are essential for maintenance of a normal immune system.[68] Dionigi and co-workers[69] have recently reviewed the various types of host defense mechanism and indicated the effects of nutritional deficiency. Although both phagocytic activity of leukocytes[70,71] and the mass of lymphoid organs,[69] (thymus, spleen, lymph nodes) are reduced in protein-energy malnutrition, the major effect which can be routinely monitored is upon lymphocyte function.

a. Lymphocyte Count

The total lymphocyte count in peripheral blood provides an approximate estimate of the rate of development of lymphocytes, and reduced levels are suggestive of immune deficiency.[6] Seltzer and coworkers[56] have shown that a total lymphocyte count of less than 1500/mm^3 in a mixed group of patients was associated with a 4-fold increase in mortality, and when serum albumin was also reduced there was a 4-fold increase in complications and 20-fold increase in mortality. This reduction is mainly within the T groups of lymphocytes,[72,73] the percentage of B lymphocytes usually being normal or increased.[74]

b. Delayed Hypersensitivity Skin Testing

A further indication of cell-mediated immunity is the response to intradermal injections of common recall antigens, e.g., Candida, PPD, or streptokinase/streptodornase antigens.[75] In severe protein-energy malnutrition, there may be a failure to develop an erythematous response to these injections (anergy).[76,77] In hospital patients, anergy is associated with an increased susceptibility to infection and with a much higher mortality than normal reactive patients.[77] Adequate nutritional support may lead to reversal of the anergic state with a consequent improved prognosis.[76,77]

c. Immunoglobulins

Since B lymphocyte function is rarely reduced, hypogammoglobulinemia is uncommon, unless there is severe uncomplicated malnutrition.[69] However, repeated infections will often cause a rise in immunoglobulin levels, particularly of IgM and IgA.[69]

d. Complement

A defect in the complement system may also be associated with increased liability to bacterial infection.[78] Low levels of all complement components, except C4, have been observed in severe protein malnutrition.[79,80] Complement C3, however, may be elevated as part of an acute phase reaction.[25] In patients in whom complement C3 and immunoglobulins are depressed due to malnutrition, nutritional repletion usually leads to supranormal responses in these immune parameters.[68]

IV. TESTS OF PROTEIN-ENERGY STATUS — SUMMARY

Of the various tests mentioned above, only a few are of sufficient value to be consistently used for nutritional monitoring. For an assessment of overall protein-energy nutritional status at a particular time, body weight, TST and MAMC, urine creatinine, serum albumin, total lymphocyte count and skin tests to recall antigens, are likely to be most useful. Adequacy of recent intake will probably be more accurately indicated by N balance studies and serum levels of short half-life proteins, such as transferrin and prealbumin.

V. MINERAL STATUS

A large number of minerals are now known to be essential for maintenance of normal tissue function. Apart from those required in relatively large amounts (sodium, potassium, calcium, magnesium, phosphorus) there are many for which nutritional requirements are very small (e.g., iron, zinc, copper manganese, chromium).[81] For many of these, knowledge of the requirement is imprecise. Furthermore, the effects of disease upon the requirements are usually not known. There may also be problems due to malabsorption from oral or enteral nutrition. Some form of monitoring of adequacy of mineral supply is therefore essential. Uncertainties associated with transport of minerals in the blood and their uptake by the tissues, may make interpretation of such results very difficult.[52]

A. Sodium and Potassium

The methods of monitoring sodium and potassium requirements are beyond the scope of this review.[83] In essence, sodium status can be gauged from an assessment of extracellular volume, in conjunction with the plasma sodium concentration. The level of continuing requirement can be estimated from urinary plus other fluid losses (e.g., diarrhea, fistula fluid) — the urinary sodium concentration may fall to very low levels in cases of sodium depletion. An indirect estimate of potassium status is obtained from serum potassium, and therapy is usually monitored using the potassium level together with the estimate of potassium excretion in urine and body fluids.

B. Calcium

Calcium provision is rarely a problem in patients receiving nutritional support. Provided vitamin D intake is satisfactory, mobilization of calcium from the skeleton readily occurs and this only causes problems when it is very prolonged. Serum calcium levels (corrected for albumin if necessary to give a better indication of the ionized calcium level) are usually adequate for routine monitoring.

C. Magnesium and Phosphorus

Patients requiring nutritional support are often magnesium depleted due to losses from the bowel or malabsorption.[82] Moreover, both magnesium and phosphorus are liable to become depleted if there is inadequate supply, during a period of anabolism stimulated by nutritional therapy.[81] Renal control of excretion is usually very precise and a low urine level of magnesium or phosphorus is often an earlier indication of inadequate supply than is the serum level.[85,86] When the serum level falls, this is indicative of an established depletion state.

D. Iron

The best assessment of iron status is achieved from blood hemoglobin and hematocrit, together with a blood film. In more difficult cases, a marrow examination for stainable iron, or serum ferritin level may be required to assess iron stores.[87] Serum iron is rarely helpful since it is reduced nonspecifically in sepsis or trauma[88] and, moreover, is subject to very large within-day and day-to-day variation.[89] Serum transferrin also is not helpful since it is reduced in protein deficiency but increased in iron deficiency. When iron supplements are given, it is important not to exceed the binding capacity of the available transferrin since free iron may then become available for microbial growth.[90]

E. Zinc

Zinc excretion in urine is markedly increased in catabolic states.[91] Provision of large amounts of zinc at this time will probably not be helpful since it is not retained, but this should alert the clinician to the need for an increased intake when a period of anabolism ensues, with retention of zinc within growing cells.[92] If inadequate zinc is given, particularly in patients receiving i.v. nutrition, zinc deficiency can occur with hair loss and eczematous rashes.[92,93] A very low plasma zinc as well as a low urine zinc will be found in such cases.[92] A low plasma zinc level is not, however, diagnostic of zinc deficiency, since it may also fall nonspecifically in the very ill.[88] A further interesting sign of zinc deficiency is depression of cell-mediated immunity, which has been shown to be responsive to topical zinc therapy.[94]

F. Copper

Copper status is most readily checked by serum copper levels, but measurement of the copper binding protein ceruloplasmin can also be made. In cases of possible copper deficiency, a hypochromic anemia and leukopenia, unresponsive to iron therapy would support the provisional diagnosis.[95]

G. Other Trace Metals

It is unlikely that other trace metals will become deficient in individuals receiving oral or enteral intake, although deficiency of such minerals as chromium[96] and selenium[97] have been reported in patients receiving i.v. nutrition. Possible methods for investigation of such cases would be for chromium, measurement of serum chromium response to a glucose load,[98] when glucose tolerance may also be impaired;[99] for selenium, measurement of plasma or urine selenium, or measurement of red blood cell glutathione peroxidase.[100]

VI. VITAMIN STATUS

A good history is an essential part of the assessment of vitamin status. This may indicate a deficient intake before it shows as an abnormality in tissue structure or function. The laboratory investigation of vitamin status may involve a number of types of test.[101]

These include:

1. Measurement of the vitamin level in the blood
2. Measurement of the vitamin level in the urine
3. Measurement of urinary metabolites
4. Measurement in blood or urine of abnormal metabolic products resulting from vitamin deficiency
5. Measurement of changes in blood components or enzyme activity
6. Loading or isotopic tests

For routine clinical use, the tests most frequently used are the measurement of plasma or blood concentrations of the vitamin. The plasma level generally reflects recent dietary intake, whereas a better index of whole body status may be obtained from intracellular (red or white cell) levels of the vitamin, or alternatively the activity of certain red blood cell enzymes that require vitamins or their metabolites as coenzymes.[101]

A. Vitamin A (Retinol)

Serum levels of vitamin A are the only practical biochemical means of assessing the status of this vitamin.[102] The dietary intake is related to the serum level, but during periods of inadequate intake, stores of retinol, if available, are mobilized from the liver to maintain the serum vitamin A concentration.[103] This level will usually be lower than those normally found with adequate vitamin A intake.[104] Very low serum vitamin A levels therefore indicate a long-standing low intake with poor tissue reserves, whereas high serum levels suggest considerable tissue stores.[101] Interpretation of these results may be complicated when there is coexisting protein malnutrition, since retinol-binding protein levels are reduced in this condition, also leading to low serum vitamin A levels.[55,64,105,106]

B. Thiamin (Vitamin B_1)

1. Urinary excretion

The urinary level of thiamin provides a good index of recent thiamin intake[101] and will usually correlate with clinical deficiency states.[107] This does not, however, allow adequate assessment of tissue thiamin reserves.

2. Erythrocyte Transketolase

Erythrocyte transketolase activity, which represents a functional test of thiamin adequacy, has been shown to provide an early indication of thiamin insufficiency, prior to the development of clinical signs.[108,109] These methods are very suitable for routine monitoring of thiamin status.[110]

3. Blood Pyruvate

Blood pyruvate levels may be elevated in thiamin deficiency particularly during the response to a carbohydrate load.[111] This measurement may be more sensitive than the erythrocyte transketolase measurement[112] but is less convenient for routine use.

C. Riboflavin

1. Urinary Excretion

The excretion of riboflavin in the urine correlates well both with dietary intake and body reserves.[113] However, during periods of negative N balance, increased urinary levels are found.[114]

2. Erythrocyte Glutathione Reductase

The activity of erythrocyte gluthathione reductase represents a more appropriate functional test of nutritional adequacy of riboflavin.[115] The stimulation of enzyme activity due to addition of flavin adenine dinucleotide, is a measure of the degree of riboflavin deficiency. This test can be conveniently performed on patients receiving nutritional support.

D. Vitamin B_6

1. Tryptophan Load Test

In vitamin B_6 deficiency, a loading dose of tryptophan leads to increased urinary excretion of xanthurenic acid and other metabolites.[116] This test has proved very useful when such studies can be performed under controlled conditions, but many physiological factors can influence the level of metabolites excreted in the deficient subject.[101]

2. Urinary Vitamin B_6 or B_6 Metabolites

Urinary level of vitamin B_6 or 4-pyridoxic acid, the major metabolite of vitamin B_6, can provide evidence of recent intake but are of less value in assessing the possible severity of vitamin B_6 deficiency.[101]

3. Erythrocyte Transaminase Activities

Similar to the other erythrocyte enzyme tests mentioned above, erythrocyte transaminase activities provide a biochemical function test of vitamin B_6 reserves. The degree of stimulation of red cell aspartate transaminase (GOT) activity is a measure of vitamin B_6 deficiency. Transaminase analysis is widely available in clinical biochemistry laboratories and hence this test can be readily applied in monitoring vitamin B_6 status.

E. Niacin

Biochemical procedures for evaluation of niacin status are not very satisfactory. There are no suitable functional tests assessing body reserves of nicotinic acid. The best practical index available is the ratio of the urinary levels of N^1 — methylnicotinamide and N^1-methyl-2 pyridone - 5 carboxylamide,[117] but methods for such analyses are not routinely available for monitoring hospital patients.

F. Folic Acid and Vitamin B_{12}

1. Serum Folate

Low serum folic acid levels are found in folate deficiency,[118] but these are mainly of value in reflecting recent low dietary input and provide little information about tissue reserves.[119]

2. Red Cell Folate

The red cell folate level can be obtained from whole blood folate and serum folate analysis. Red cell folate is a more accurate and less variable index than serum folate as to the severity of folate deficiency.[118,119] On the other hand, red cell folate responds more slowly to changes in folate intake associated with dietary change.

3. Serum B_{12}

Investigations of folate status should usually be accompanied by an assessment of vitamin B_{12} status. This is best performed, in the first instance, by measurement of serum vitamin B_{12} level.[120]

G. Ascorbic Acid (Vitamin C)

1. Serum Ascorbic Acid

The serum level of ascorbic acid is the most commonly used and most practical method of evaluating vitamin C status. This provides information about the recent intake of vitamin C.[101,102]

2. Whole Blood Ascorbic Acid

Whole blood levels of ascorbic acid are probably a less sensitive index of vitamin C status than serum levels.[121]

3. Leukocyte Ascorbic Acid

Tissue stores of vitamin C can be fairly accurately assessed from the leukocyte ascorbic acid concentration.[101,122] This is probably the most useful test of tissue level, but is subject to considerable technical difficulty. If vitamin C intake is inadequate, serum levels fall more rapidly than leukocyte levels,[123] but a relationship continues to exist between serum and white cell concentrations.[124]

H. Vitamin D

1. Serum Alkaline Phosphatase

An adequate intake of vitamin D can be readily monitored by the serum alkaline phosphatase activity, which rises early in the development of rickets in children or osteomalacia in adults. The serum alkaline phosphatase may, however, be affected by other diseases of bone or of other tissues such as a liver, and hence other methods of vitamin D assessment may be required.

2. Plasma Vitamin D Measurement

Measurement of plasma levels of 25-hydroxy vitamin D can now be performed and these provide a satisfactory index in the majority of patients of the adequacy of vitamin D absorption and its hydroxylation by the liver.[125] This measurement, of course, does not measure the active vitamin D metabolite 1, 25 dihydroxy cholecalciferol, which is produced by further hydroxylation in the kidney.[125]

I. Vitamin E

1. Erythrocyte Hemolysis Test

The susceptibility of erythrocytes to hemolysis in hydrogen peroxide is the basis of the most widely used though indirect test of vitamin E status.[126]

2. Plasma Vitamin E

Serum or plasma levels of tocopherol have been shown to correlate well with the erythrocyte hemolysis test.[101,126,127] However, the relationship of the plasma level to α-tocopherol status of other tissues is not clear.[128]

VII. PROTOCOL FOR ASSESSMENT AND MONITORING OF NUTRITIONAL STATUS

Based upon the various clinical and laboratory tests outlined above, a protocol can be proposed for the initial assessment of patients who may require nutritional support, and for monitoring such patients if nutritional therapy is instituted. The range of tests to be performed will vary considerably depending upon the nutritional problems of the patient as well as the facilities of the local laboratories. Moreover, the frequency of performance of the various tests will also be very variable in patients with differing severity of illness. However, a tentative proposal is outlined in Table 1.

VIII. SUMMARY

A comprehensive form of nutritional assessment is necessary, both to identify patients in need of nutritional support as well as to indicate the success or otherwise of nutritional therapy. Ideally the assessment procedure should include all aspects of the diet: protein, energy substrates, minerals, and vitamins. The types of tests available have been summarized and a protocol has been tentatively proposed. It is suggested that use of such a scheme for nutritional assessment and monitoring permits rational decisions to be reached regarding the desirability, type, and amount of nutritional support required by the individual patient.

Table 1
PROTOCOL FOR ASSESSMENT AND MONITORING OF NUTRITIONAL STATUS

	Laboratory	
Clinical	**Blood**	**Urine**
Height	Na, K, Cl, CO_2,[a]	Creatinine[b]
Weight[b]	Urea and creatinine[a]	Nitrogen (urea or total)[b]
Weight % of ideal[b]	Glucose[d]	Na, K[b]
Triceps skinfold thickness[c]	Albumin, transferrin[b]	Ca, P, Mg, Zn[b]
Midarm muscle circumference[c]	Liver function tests[b]	Ward urinalysis[a]
Cell-mediated immunity by skin tests[e]	Ca, P, Mg, Zn[b]	
	Plasma vitamin A, vitamin C, folate, B_{12}[d]	
	Red cell folate[d]	
	Hemoglobin[c]	
	Total lymphocyte count[c]	
Tests to be Performed if Clinically Appropriate and if Available		
Indirect calorimetery	Other short half-life proteins	
	Immunoglobulins	Creatine
	Plasma amino acids	3-Methylhistidine
	Serum Cu, Fe, ferritin	Ketones
	Leukocyte ascorbic acid	
	Plasma vitamin E, 25-OH vitamin D	
	Erythrocyte transketolase glutathione reductase transaminase	
	Cholesterol and triglycerides	
	Ketones	

[a] Initial assessment, daily on commencing nutritional support, twice weekly when stable.
[b] Initial assessment, then twice weekly.
[c] Initial assessment, then weekly.
[d] As required.
[e] Initial assessment, then every 1 to 4 weeks.

REFERENCES

1. **Jelliffe, D. B.,** Assessment of the nutritional status of the community, W. H. O. Geneva, 1966.
2. Chicago Society of Actueries, Build and Blood Pressure Study, *Metrop. Life Ins. Co., Stat. Bull.*, 40, 1959.
3. **Davidson, S., Passmore, R., Brock, J. F., and Truswell, A. S.,** *Human Nutrition and Dietetics,* 7th ed., Churchill Livingstone, Edinburgh, 1979, chap 2.
4. **Hill, G. L., Bradley, J. A., Smith, R. C., Smith, A. H., McCarthy, I. D., Oxby, C. B., Burkinshaw, L., and Morgan, D. B.,** Changes in body weight and body protein with intravenous nutrition, *J. Parent. Ent. Nutr.*, 3, 215, 1979.
5. **Durnin, J. V. G. A. and Womersley, J.,** Body fat assessed from total body density and its estimation from skinfold thickness, *Br. J. Nutr.*, 32, 77, 1974.
6. **Blackburn, G. L. Bistrian, B. R., Maini, B. S., Schlamm, H. T., and Smith, M. F.,** Nutritional and metabolic assessment of the hospitalized patient, *J. Parent. Ent. Nutr.*, 1, 11, 1977.

7. **Shenkin, A. and Steele, L. W.,** Clinical and laboratory assessment of nutritional status, *Proc. Nutr. Soc.,* 37, 95, 1978.
8. **Kinney, J. M., Duke, J. H., Long, C. L., and Gump, F. E.,** Carbohydrate and nitrogen metabolism after injury, *J. Clin. Path.,* 23, 65, 1970.
9. **Rutten, P., Blackburn, G. L., Flatt, J. P., Hallowell, E., and Cochran, E.,** Determination of optimal hyperalimentation infusion rate, *J. Surg., Res.,* 18, 477, 1975.
10. **Gump, F. E., Martin, P., and Kinney, J. M.,** Oxygen consumption and caloric expenditure in surgical patients, *Surg. Gynecol. Obstet.,* 137, 499 1973.
11. **Gazzaniga, A. G., Polachek, J. R., Wilson, A. F., and Day, A. T.,** Indirect calorimetry as a guide to caloric replacement during total parenteral nutrition., *Am. J. Surg.,* 136, 128, 1978.
12. **Kinney, J. M.,** Energy requirements for parenteral nutrition, in *Total Parenteral Nutrition,* Fischer, J. E., Ed., Little, Brown, Boston, 1976, 135.
13. **Wedge, J. H., de Campos, R., Kerr, A., Smith, R., Farrell, R., Ilic, V., and Williamson, D. H.,** Branched chain amino acids, nitrogen excretion and injury in man, *Clin. Sci., Mol. Med.,* 50, 393, 1976.
14. **Rich, A. J. and Whitehouse, M. E.,** The relevance of preoperative nutritional assessment, *Res. Clin. Forums,* 1, 83, 1979.
15. **Williamson, D. H., Farrell, R., Kerr, A., and Smith, R.,** Muscle protein catabolism after injury in man, as measured by urinary excretion of 3-methylhistidine, *Clin. Sci. Mol. Med.,* 52, 527, 1977.
16. **Munro. H. N.,** General aspects of the regulation of protein metabolism by diet and by hormones, in *Mammalian Protein Metabolism,* Vol. 1, Munro, H. N. and Allison, J. B., Eds., Academic Press, New York, 1964, 381.
17. **Fleck, A. and Munro, H. N.,** The determination of organic nitrogen in biological materials, *Clin. Chim. Acta,*11, 2, 1965.
18. **Lee, H. A. and Hartley, T. F.,** A method of determining daily nitrogen requirements, *Postgrad. Med. J.,* 51, 441, 1975.
19. **Johnston, I. D. A.,** Metabolic foundation of intravenous nutrition, in *Advances in Parenteral Nutrition,* Johnston, I. D. A., Ed., MTP Press, Lancaster, 1978, chap 1.
20. **Woolfson, A. M. J.,** Metabolic considerations in nutritional support, *Res. Clin. Forum,* 1, 35, 1979.
21. **Albanese, A. A., Lorenze, E. J., Orto, L. A., Wein, E. H., Zavattaro, D. N., and de Carlo, R.,** Serum ribonuclease, *NY State J. Med.,* 1595, 1972.
22. **Sigulem, D. M., Brasel, J. A., Velasio, E. G., Rosso, P., and Winick, M.,** Plasma and urine ribonuclease as a measure of nutritional status in children, *Am. J. Clin. Nutr.,* 26, 793, 1973.
23. **Coombes, E. J., Shakespeare, P. G., and Batstone, G. F.,** Observations on serum and urine alkaline ribonuclease activity and urate after burn injury in man., *Clin. Chim. Acta,* 86, 279, 1978.
24. **Shenkin, A. and Bielecka, S.,** Effect of diet upon serum ribonuclease concentration in the rat, *Proc. Nutr. Soc.,* 38, 117A, 1979.
25. **Shenkin, A., Neuhauser, M., Bergstrom, J., Chao, L., Vinnars, E., Larsson, J., Liljedahl, S. O., Schildt, B., and Furst, P.,** Biochemical changes associated with severe trauma, *Am. J. Clin. Nutr.,* in press, 1980.
26. **Shenkin, A., Citrin, D. L., and Rowan, R. M.,** An assessment of the clinical usefulness of plasma ribonuclease assays, *Clin. Chim. Acta,* 72, 223, 1976.
27. **Waterlow, J. C. and Harper, A. E.,** Assessment of protein nutrition, in *Total Parenteral Nutrition – Promises and Premises,* Ghadimi, H., Ed., John Wiley & Sons, London, 1975, 1975, 231.
28. **Arroyave, G.,** Comparative sensitivity of specific amino acid ratios versus "essential to nonessential" amino acid ratio, *Am. J. Clin. Nutr.,* 23, 703, 1970.
29. **Whitehead, R. G. and Dean, R. E. A.,** Serum amino acids in kwashiorkor 1. Relationship to clinical condition., *Am., J. Clin. Nutr.,* 14, 313, 1964.
30. **Padilla, H., Sanchez, A., Powell, R. N., Umezawa, C., Swendseid, M. E., Prado., P. M., and Sigala, R.,** Plasma amino acids in children from Guadalajara with kwashiorkor, *Am. J. Clin. Nutr.,* 24, 353, 1971.
31. **Freund, H. J., Ryan, J. A., and Fischer, J. E.,** Amino acid derangements in patients with sepsis, *Ann Surg.,* 188, 423, 1978.
32. **Woolf, L. I., Groves, A. C., Moore, J. P., Duff, J. H., Finley, R. D., and Loomer, R. L.,** Arterial plasma amino acids in patients with serious post-operative infection and in patients with major fractures, *Surgery,* 79, 283, 1976.
33. **Wannemacher, R. W., Klainer, A. S. Dinterman, R. E., and Beisel, W. R.,** The significance and mechanism of an increased serum phenylalanine-tyrosine ratio during infection, *Am. J. Clin. Nutr.,* 29, 997, 1976.
34. **Oxby, C. B., Appleby, D. B., Brooks, K., Burkinshaw, L., Krupowics, D. W., McCarthy, I. D., Olroyd, B., Ellis, E., Collins, J. P., and Hill, G. L.,** A technique for measuring total body nitrogen in clinical investigations, *Int. J. App. Rad. Isotopes,* 29, 205, 1978.
35. **Collins, J. P., Oxby, C. B., and Hill, G. C.,** Intravenous amino acids and intravenous hyperalimentation as protein-sparing therapy after major surgery, *Lancet,* 1, 788, 1978.

36. **Hawkins, T. and Goode, A. W.,** The determination of total body potassium using a whole body monitor, *Phys. Med. Biol.*, 21, 293, 1976.
37. **Goode, A. W., Hawkins, T., Feggetter, J. G. W., and Johnston, I. D. A.,** Use of an elemental diet for long term nutritional support in Crohn's disease, *Lancet,* 1, 122, 1976.
38. **Waterlow, J. C., Neale, R. J., Rowe, L., and Palin, I.** Effects of diet and infection on creatine turnover in the rat, *Am. J. Clin. Nutr.*, 25, 371, 1972.
39. **Forbes, G. B. and Bruining, G. J.,** Urinary creatinine excretion and lean body mass, *Am. J. Clin. Nutr.*, 29, 1359, 1976.
40. **Bistrian, B. R., Blackburn, G. L., Sherman, M., and Scrimshaw, N. S.,** Therapeutic index of nutritional depletion in hospital patients, *Surg. Gynec. Obstet.*, 141, 512, 1975.
41. **Mack, P. B. and Montgomery, K. G.,** Study of nitrogen balance and creatine and creatinine excretion during recumbency and ambulation of five young adult human males, *Aerospace Med.*, 44, 739, 1973.
42. **Davies, J. W. L. and Fell, G. S.,** Tissue catabolism in patients with burns, *Clin. Chim. Acta,* 51, 83, 1974.
43. **Hinton, P., Allison, S. P., Littlejohn, S., and Lloyd, J.,** Insulin and glucose to reduce the catabolic response to injury in burned patients, *Lancet,* 1, 767, 1971.
44. **Shenkin, A.,** Monitoring the nutritional status of critically ill patients, *Intes. Care. Med.*, 5, 165, 1979.
45. **Haverberg, L. N., Omstedt, P. T., Munro, H. N., and Young, V. R.,** 3-methylhistidine content of mixed proteins in various rat tissues, *Biochem. Biophys. Acta.*, 405, 67, 1975.
46. **Young, V. R., Alexis, S. D., Baliga, B. S., and Munro, H. N.,** Metabolism of administered *3-methylhistidine, J. Biol. Chem.*, 247, 3592, 1972.
47. **Bilmazes, C., Uauy, R., Haverberg, L. N., Munro, H. N., and Young, V. R.,** Muscle protein breakdown rates in humans based on N-methylhistidine content of mixed proteins in skeletal muscle and urinary output of N-methylhistidine, *Metabolism,* 27, 525, 1978.
48. **Young, V. R. and Munro, H. N.,** N^{T}-methylhistidine (3-methylhistidine) and muscle turnover: an overview, *Fed. Proc.*, 37, 2291, 1978.
49. **Long, C. L., Schiller, W. R., Blackmore, W. S., Geiger, J. W., O'Dell, M., and Henderson, K.,** Muscle protein catabolism in the septic patient as measured by 3-methylhistidine excretion, *Am. J. Clin. Nutr.*, 30, 1349, 1977.
50. **Young, V. R., Haverberg, L. N., Bilmazes, C., and Munro, H. N.,** Potential use of 3-methylhistidine excretion as an index of progressive reduction in muscle protein catabolism during starvation, *Metabolism,* 22, 1429, 1973.
51. **Blackburn, G. L., Flatt, J. P., and Hensle, T. W.,** Peripheral amino acid infusions, in *Total Parenteral Nutrition,* Fischer, J.E., Ed., Little, Brown, Boston, 1976, 363.
52. **Fleck, A.,** Injury and plasma proteins, in *Metabolism and the Response to Injury,* Wilkinson, A. W. and Cuthbertson, D. P., Eds., Pitman, Kent, 1976, 229.
53. **Fleck, A.,** Protein metabolism after surgery, *Proc. Nutri. Soc.*, 39, 125, 1980.
54. **Olusi, S. O., McFarlane, H., Osunkoya, B. O., and Adesina, H.,** Specific protein assays in protein-calorie malnutrition, *Clin. Chim. Acta,* 62, 107, 1975.
55. **Ingenbleek, Y., Van den Schrieck, H.G., De Nayer, P., de Visscher, M.,** Albumin transferrin, and the thyroxine-binding prealbumin/retinol-binding protein (TBPA-RBP) complex in the assessment of malnutrition, *Clin. Chim. Acta,* 63, 61, 1975.
56. **Seltzer, M. H., Bastidas, J. A., Cooper, D. M., Engler, P., Slocum, B., and Fletcher, H. S.,** Instant nutritional assessment, *J. Parent. Ent. Nutr.* 3, 157, 1979.
57. **Whitehead, R. G., Coward, W. A., and Lunn, P. G.,** Serum albumin concentration and the onset of kwashiorkor, *Lancet,*1, 63, 1973.
58. **Beeken, W. L. , Volwiler, W., Goldsworthy, P. D. Gaeby, L. E., Reynolds, W. E., Stogsdill, R., and Stember, R. S.,** Studies of I-131-albumin catabolism and distribution in normal young males, *J. Clin. Invest.*, 41, 1312, 1962.
59. **Awai, M. and Brown, E. B.,** Studies of the metabolism of I^{131}-labelled human transferrin, *J. Lab. Clin. Med.*, 61, 363, 1963.
60. **McFarlane, H., Ogbeide, M. I., Reddy, S., Adcock, K. J., Adechina, H., Gurney, J. M., Cooke, A., Taylor, G. O., and Mordie, J. A.,** Biochemical assessment of protein-calorie malnutrition, *Lancet,* 1, 392, 1969.
61. **Shetty, P. S., Watrasiewicz, K., Jung, R. T., and James, W. P. T.,** The effects of protein and energy restriction on plasma transport proteins, *Proc. Nutr. Soc.*, 38, 56A, 1979.
62. **Socolow, E. L., Woeber, K. A., Purdy, R. H., Holloway, M. T., and Ingbar, S. H.,** Preparation of I-labelled human serum prealbumin and its metabolism in normal and sick patients, *J. Clin. Invest.*, 44, 1600, 1965.
63. **Oppenheimer, J. H., Surks, M. I., Berstein, G., and Smith, J. C.,** Metabolism of Iodine-131-labelled thyroxine binding prealbumin in man, *Science,* 149, 748, 1965.
64. **Peterson, P. A., Nilsson, S. F., Ostberg, L., Rask, L., and Vahlquist, A.,** Aspects of the metabolism of retinol binding protein and retinol, *Vitam. Horm.*, 32, 181, 1974.

65. **Schendel, H. E., Hansen, J. D. L., and Brock, J. F.,** Biochemical assessment of protein nutritional status. 1. Marginal hypoalbuminaemia. 2. Serum cholinesterase, *S. Afr. J. lab. Clin. Med.*, 8, 23, 1962.
66. **Sherlock, S.,** in *Diseases of the Liver and Biliary System,* 5th ed., Blackwell, Oxford, 1975, chap 5.
67. **Tweedle, D. E. F., Skidmore, F. D., Gleave, E. N., Knass, D. A., and Gowland, E.,** Nutritional support for patients undergoing surgery for cancer of the head and neck, *Res. Clin. Forums,* 1, 59, 1979.
68. **Law, D. K., Dudrick, S. J., and Abdou, N. L.,** The effect of dietary protein depletion on immunocompetence. The importance of nutritional repletion prior to immunologic induction, *Ann. Surg.*, 179, 168, 1974.
69. **Dionigi, R., Gnes, F., Bonera, A., and Dominioni, L.,** Nutrition and Infection, *J. Parent. Ent. Nutr.*, 3, 62, 1979.
70. **Guggenheim, K. and Buechler, E.,** Nutrition and resistance to infection, Bactericidal properties and phagocytic activity of peritoneal fluid of rats in various states of nutritional deficiency, *J. Immunol.*, 54, 349, 1946.
71. **Seelvaraj, R. J. and Bhat, K. S.,** Metabolic and bactericidal activities of leukocytes in protein calorie malnutrition, *Am. J. Clin. Nutr.*, 25, 166, 1972.
72. **Chandra, R. K.,** Rosette forming T-lymphocytes and cell-mediated immunity in malnutrition, *Br. Med. J.*, 3, 608, 1974.
73. **Ferguson, C., Lawlor, G. J., Jr., Neumann, C. N., Oh, W., and Stiehm, E. R.,** Decreased rosetteforming lymphocytes in malnutrition and intrauterine growth retardation, *J. Pediat.*, 85, 717, 1974.
74. **Bang, B. G., Mahalanabis, D., Mukherjeee, K. E., and Bang, F. B.,** T and B lymphocyte rosetting in undernourished children, *Proc. Soc. Exp. Biol. Med.*, 149, 109, 1975.
75. **Chandra, R. K.,** Interaction of infection and malnutrition, in *Intl. Congress Inmunology, Progress in Immunology,* Vol. 4, Brent, B. and Holborow, J., Eds., North-Holland, Amsterdam, 1974, 355.
76. **Bistrian, B. R., Blackburn, G. L., and Scrimshaw, N. S.,** Cellular immunity in semistarved states in hospitalized adults, *Am. J. Clin. Nutr.*, 28, 1148, 1975.
77. **Meakins, J. L., Pietsch, J. B., Bubenich, O., Kelly, R., Rode, H., Gordon, J., and MacLean, L. D.,** Delayed hypersensitivity: indicator of acquired failure of host defenses in sepsis and trauma, *Ann. Surg.*, 186, 241, 1977.
78. **Mata, L. J., Urrutia, J. J., Alberlazzi, C., Pellecer, O., and Arellano, E.,** Influence of recurrent infection on nutrition and growth of chilren in Guatemala, *Am. J. Clin. Nutr.*, 25, 1267, 1972.
79. **Suskind, R., Edelman, R., Kulapongs, P., Pariyanonda, A., and Sirinsinka S.,** Complement activity in children with protein calorie malnutrition, *Am. J. Clin. Nutr.*, 29, 1089, 1976.
80. **Chandra, R. K.,** Serum complement and immunoconglutinin in malnutrition, *Arch. Dis. Childr.*, 50, 225, 1975.
81. Recommended Dietary Allowances, Food and Nutrition Board, 8th ed., National Academy of Science, Washington, D.C., 1974.
82. **Fell, G. S. and Burns, R. R.,** Zinc and other trace elements, in *Advances in Parenteral Nutrition,* Johnston I. D. A., Ed., M.T.P., Lancaster, 1978, 241.
83. **Maxwell, M. H. and Kleeman, C. R.,** *Clinical Disorders of Fluid and Electrolyte Metabolism,* 3rd ed., McGraw-Hill, New York, 1979.
84. **Shenkin, A. and Wretlind, A.,** Parenteral nutrition, *World Rev. Nutr. Diet,* 28, 1, 1978.
85. **Main, A. N. H., Hall, M. J., Morgan, R. J., MacKenzie, J. F., Shenkin, A., Fell, G. S., and Russell, R. I.,** Magnesium status and I. V. requirements in patients with chronic inflammatory bowel disease, requiring intravenous nutrition, *Proc. Nutr. Soc.*, 39, 32A, 1980.
86. **Shenkin, A. and Fell, G. S.,** Mineral and vitamin requirements in parenteral nutrition, in *Practical Nutritional Support,* Karran, S. J. and Alberti, K. G. M. M., Eds., Pitman, Tunbridge Wells, 1979, 68.
87. **Jacobs A. and Worwood, M.,** Ferritin in serum, clinical and biochemical implications, *N. Eng. J. Med.*, 292, 951, 1975.
88. **Wannemacher, R. W., Klainer, A. S., Kigbee, G. E., and Beisel, W. R.,** in *The Biochemical Role of Trace Elements in Ageing,* Hsu, J. M., Davy, R. C., and Neithamer, R. W., Eds., Eckerd College, St. Petersburg, Florida, 1976, 175.
89. **Morrison, B., Shenkin, A., McLelland, A., Robertson, D. A., Barrowman, M., Graham, S., Wuga, G., and Cunningham, K. F. M.,** Intra-individual variation in commonly analysed serum constituents, *Clin. Chem.*, 25, 1799, 1979.
90. **Neumann, C. G., Lawlor, G. J., Steihm, E. R., Svendseid, M. E., Newton, C., Herbert, J., Ammann, A. J., and Jacob, M.,** Immunological responses in malnourished children, *Am. J. Clin. Nutr.*, 28, 89, 1975.
91. **Fell, G. S., Cuthbertson, D. P., Morrison, C., Fleck, A., Queen, K., Bessent, R. G., and Husain, S. L.,** Urinary zinc levels as an indication of muscle catabolism, *Lancet,* 1, 280, 1973.
92. **Kay, R. G., Tasman-Jones, C., Pybus, J., Whiting, R., and Black, H.,** A syndrome of acute zinc deficiency during total parenteral alimentation in man, *Ann. Surg.*, 183, 331, 1976.

93. **Bos, L. P., Volten, W. A., Smit, A. F. D., and Nube, M.**, Zinc deficiency with skin lesions as seen in acrodermatitis enteropathica, and intoxication with zinc during parenteral nutrition, *Neth. J. Med.*, 20, 263, 1977.
94. **Golden, M. H. N. and Golden, B. E.**, Zinc and immunocompetence in protein-energy malnutrition, *Lancet*, 1, 1226, 1978.
95. **Karpel, J. T. and Peden, V. H.**, Copper deficiency in long-term parenteral nutrition, *J. Ped.*, 80, 32, 1972.
96. **Jeejeebhoy, K. N., Chu, R. C., Marliss, E. B., Greenberg, G. R., and Bruce-Robertson, A.**, Chromium deficiency, glucose intolerance, and neuropathy reversed by chromium supplementation, in a patient receiving long-term parenteral nutrition, *Am. J. Clin. Nutr.*, 30, 531, 1977.
97. **Van Rij, A. M., McKenzie, J. M., Robinson, M. F., and Thomson, C. D.**, Selenium and total parenteral nutrition, *J. Parent. Ent. Nutr.*, 3, 235, 1979.
98. **Liu, V. J. K. and Morris, J. S.**, Relative chromium response as an indicator of chromium status, *Am. J. Clin. Nutr.*, 31, 972, 1978.
99. **Mertz, W. and Roginski, E. E.**, Chromium metabolism, the glucose tolerance factor, in *Newer Elements in Nutrition*, Mertz, W. and Comatzer, W. E., Eds., Marcel Dekker, New York, 1971, 141.
100. **Spooner, R. J., Campbell, R. A., Rumley, A. G., and Stromberg, P.**, Glutathione peroxidase in human selenium deficiency, *Proc. Nutr. Soc.*, 39, 37A, 1980.
101. **Sauberlich, H. E., Dowdy, R. P., and Skala, J. H.**, *Laboratory Tests for the Assessment of Nutritional Status*, CRC Press, Boca Raton, Fla. 1974.
102. **Krause, R. F.**, Laboratory aids in the diagnosis of malnutrition, in *Modern Nutrition in Health and Disease*, 4th ed., Wohl, M. G. and Goodhart, R. S., Eds., Lea and Febiger, Philadelphia, 1968, chap. 18A.
103. **Wolf, G.**, Int. Symp. Metabolic Function of Vitamin A, *Am. J. Clin. Nutr.*, 22, 897, 1969.
104. **Hodges, R. E. and Kolder, H.**, Experimental vitamin A deficiency in human volunteers, in *Summary of Proceedings of Workshop on Biochemical and Clinical Criteria for Determining Human Vitamin A Nutriture*, Bieri, J. G., Ed., Food and Nutrition Board, National Academy of Sciences, Washington, 1971, 10.
105. **Arroyave, G.**, Interrelations between protein and vitamin A — metabolism, *Am. J. Clin. Nutr.*, 22, 1119, 1969.
106. **Smith, F. R., Suskind, R., Thanangkul, O., Leitzmann, C., Goodman, D., and Olson, R. E.**, Plasma vitamin A, retinol-binding protein and prealbumin concentration in protein-calorie malnutrition, *Am. J. Clin. Nutr.*, 28, 732, 1975.
107. **Pearson, W. N.**, Blood and urinary vitamin levels as potential indices of body stores, *Am. J. Clin. Nutr.*, 20, 514, 1967.
108. **Brin, M.**, Erythrocyte transketolase in early thiamine deficiency, *Ann. N.Y. Acad. Sci.*, 98, 528, 1962.
109. **Dreyfus, P.**, Clinical application of blood transketolase determinations, *N. Engl. J. Med.*, 267, 596, 1962.
110. **Rosalki, S. B.**, Clinical biochemistry of vitamin B_6 in *The Importance of Vitamins to Human Health*, Taylor, T. G., Ed., MTP, Lancaster, 1979, 250.
111. **Thompson, R. H. S.**, The value of blood pyruvate determinations in the diagnosis of thiamine deficiency in *Thiamine Deficiency: Biochemical Lesions and Their Clinical Significance*, Wolstenholme, G. E. W., Ed., Ciba Foundation Study Group, No. 28, Churchill, London, 1967.
112. **Baines, M.**, Detection and incidence of B and C vitamin deficiency in alcohol-related disease, *Ann. Clin. Biochem.*, 15, 307, 1978.
113. **Morley, H. H., Edwards, M. A., Moller, I. I., Woodring, M. J., and Storvick, C. A.**, Riboflavin in the blood and urine of women on controlled intakes, *J. Nutr.*, 69, 191, 1959.
114. **Pollack, H. and Bookman, J. J.**, Riboflavin excretion as a function of protein metabolism in the normal, catabolic and diabetic human being, *J. Lab. Clin. Med.*, 38, 561, 1951.
115. **Tillotson, J. A. and Baker, E. M.**, An enzymatic measurement of the riboflavin status in man, *Am. J. Clin. Nutr.*, 25, 425, 1972.
116. **Sauberlich, H. E., Canham, J. E., Baker, E. M., Raica, N., Jr., and Herman, Y. F.**, Biochemical assessment of the nutritional status of vitamin B_6 in the human, *Am. J. Clin. Nutr.*, 25, 629, 1972.
117. **de Lange, D. J. and Joubert, C. P.**, Assessment of nicotinic acid status of population groups, *Ann. Rev. Med.*, 16, 359, 1965.
118. **Herbert, V.**, Folic acid, *Am. Rev. Med.*, 16, 359, 1965.
119. **Hoffbrand. A. V., Newcombe, B. F. A., and Mollin, D. L.**, Method of assay of red cell folate activity and the value of the assay as a test for folate deficiency, *J. Clin. Pathol.*, 19, 17, 1966.
120. **Baker, S. J.**, Human vitamin B_{12} deficiency, *World Rev. Nutr. Diet.*, 8, 62, 1967.
121. **Hodges, R. E., Hood, J., Canham, J. E., Sauberlich, H. E., and Baker, E. M.**, Clinical manifestations of ascorbic acid deficiency in man, *Am. J. Clin Nutr.*, 24, 432, 1971.
122. **Loh, H. S.**, The relationship between dietary ascorbic acid intake and buffy coat and plasma ascorbic acid concentrations at different ages, *Int. J. Vit. Nutr, Res.*, 42, 80, 1972.

123. **Lowry, O. H., Bessey, O. A., Brock, M. J., and Lopez, J. A.,** The interrelationship of dietary serum, white blood cell and total body ascorbic acid, *J. Biol. Chem.*, 166, 11, 1946.
124. **Andrews, J. and Brook, M.,** Leucocyte-vitamin-C content and clinical signs in the elderly, *Lancet*, 1, 1350, 1966.
125. **Deluca, H. F.,** The vitamin D system in the regulation of calcium and phosphorus metabolism, *Nutr. Rev.*, 37, 161, 1979.
126. **Binder, H. J. and Spiro, H. M.,** Tocopherol deficiency in man, *Am. J. Clin. Nutr.*, 20, 594, 1967.
127. **Horwitt, M. K., Harvey C. C., Duncan, G. D., and Wilson, W. C.,** Effects of limited tocopherol intake in man with relationship to erythrocyte hemolysis and lipid oxidations, *Am. J. Clin. Nutr.*, 8, 451, 1960.
128. **Bieri, J. G. and Poukka, R. K. H.,** Red cell content of vitamin E and fatty acids in normal subjects and patients with abnormal lipid metabolism, *Int. J. Vitam. Nutr. Res.*, 40, 344, 1970.

Chapter 5

METHODS OF PROVIDING NUTRITIONAL SUPPORT

R. I. Russell

TABLE OF CONTENTS

I. INTRODUCTION

In recent years there has been greater understanding of the need for nutritional support and in the methods of providing such support. It is the purpose of this chapter to classify the methods which are available.

Two principal methods have been developed — enteral and intravenous. In general, the enteral route should be used if the gastrointestinal tract is functioning normally. Enteral nutrition is more physiological and helps to maintain normal GI functions. The term "enteral nutrition" applies to the oral ingestion of ordinary whole food, supplemental dietary preparations, blenderized food, and special preparations such as elemental diets or complete (whole protein) liquid diets. It also applies to the administration of these preparations by nasogastric, nasoduodenal, or nasojejunal tubes, or via gastrostomies or jejunostomies.

I.v. nutrition should only be used in the presence of very severe or life-threatening nutritional insufficiency or when the GI tract is not functioning adequately — alimentary failure. In general in the past, i.v. nutrition has been used in many patients in whom adequate nutritional support could have been provided by a well-planned enteral nutrition regime, and enteral regimes should be considered as the first option in patients. Enteral nutrition regimes are generally easier to set up, are simple and flexible, cheaper and safer, and require less complex back-up services and expertise than i.v. feeding. Historically, however, i.v. nutrition was the first effective method of providing support to deficient patients, and it is only in recent years that effective enteral nutrition regimes have become available.

In planning any nutritional support regime, energy and nitrogen requirements must both be considered. In normal subjects, positive nitrogen balance can be attained with nitrogen intake of 8 to 9 g/24 hr, and a nonprotein energy to nitrogen ratio of 320:1. In the presence of disease-causing nutritional insufficiency, with low metabolic expenditure, N balance may be achieved with a nonprotein energy to nitrogen ratio of 200:1 to 250.1. In severely catabolic patients a higher nitrogen intake is necessary (up to 25 g/day) with a nonprotein energy to nitrogen ratio possibly as low as 135:1. In any individual patient, however, the optimal requirements can only be provided by determining adequate baseline nutritional data (clinical, anthropometric, biochemical, immunological) as described in Chapter 4, and continuing to monitor these these parameters during the period of treatment. In general, a nonprotein to nitrogen ratio of about 200:1 is usually adequate for most patients.

The methods of nutritional support have been classified with the aim of assessing the place of elemental diets within the range of support systems available. (Table 1).

II. ENTERAL NUTRITION

A. Dietary Supplements and Tube Feeds

Supplementary feeding with simple and palatable fluids or with normal or blenderized foods will often provide adequate nutritional support to patients in whom the alimentary tract is functioning nornally and the degree of nutritional insufficiency is not great. This method is inadequate for the management of severe or chronic problems, but in minor nutritional deficiencies and in early disease, these supplements are simple and may be very effective. They include preparations such as caloreen®, albumaid®, casilan, complan, hycal®, maxijul, aminutrin, and calonutrin.

Caloreen® — A mixture of dextrins with an average glucose chain length of 5 units. It is palatable, blends easily with most foods and readily dissolves in water. Caloreen provides 400 kcal energy per 100 g.

Table 1
CLASSIFICATION OF METHODS OF NUTRITIONAL SUPPORT

A. Enteral
1. Dietary supplements
   - Caloreen®
   - Hycal®
   - Albumaid®
   - Casilan®
   - Complan®
   - Maxijul®
   - Aminutrin®
   - Calonutrin®
2. Complete oral liquid diets
   - Isocal®
   - Clinifeed®
   - Triosorbon MCT®
   - Ensure®
   - Vital®
3. Elemental diets
   - Vivonex®
   - Vivonex® HN
   - Flexical®
   - Precision® LR
   - Precision® HN

B. Intravenous

Albumaid® — A hydrolysate of bovine serum proteins of good biological value, with a well-balanced amino acid composition. It also contains minerals, vitamins and trace elements.

Casilan — A high milk-protein food, which also contains fat as glyceryl mono-oleate, minerals, and electrolytes.

Complan — A palatable, complete food drink with a skimmed milk base. It contains casein, vegetable oil, maltodextrin, sucrose, lactose, vitamins, minerals, electrolytes, and trace elements.

Hycal® — consists of a mixture of saccharides (mainly dextrose), hexa and higher saccharides, with small amounts of electrolytes and minerals.

Maxijul — Consists of gluco-dextrins which are converted to glucose by salivary and pancreatic amylases. It provides 400 kcal/100 g, and contains small quantities of sodium and potassium.

Although these dietary supplements may be successfully taken orally by patients, they may also be administered by nasogastric tube. Combinations of complan, caloreen, and vitamins, or caloreen, albumaid, vitamins, and egg yolk, or casilan, maxijul, milk and egg are often helpful and are easily prepared and administered. The use of these feeds is relatively free from side effects although some diarrhea may occur if they are administered too quickly. Ideally they should be given in small quantities at regular intervals, or if given by nasogastric tube their intake monitored and controlled by means of a pump system.

The dietary supplements aminutrin and calonutrin (Geistlich) may be valuable in some patients requiring nutritional supplementation. Aminutrin consists of 1-amino acids in precisely defined quantities without peptides, electrolytes, carbohydrates, fats, or vitamins. It is roughage and bulk free, efficiently absorbed and thus has minimal residue. One 15 g sachet of aminutrin provides 1.8 g available nitrogen (equivalent to 11.7 g protein) and 47 kcal; only traces of minerals are present. Calonutrin is a carbohydrate supplement containing polysaccharides, disaccharides, monosaccharides, sodiun, and potassium. No fat or protein is present. One 100 g sachet of calonutrin supplies 410 kcal, and each sachet contains 4 mmol sodium, 0.3 mmol potassium and 5.4 mmol chloride. It dissolves readily in water or milk, and the monosacchardies and small chain polysaccharides are readily absorbed in the small intestine with only minimal digestive action. Aminutrin and calonutrin together provide a satisfactory dietary supplement, although a full range of basic nutrients is not present. These preparations must therefore be regarded as dietary supplements rather than complete oral liquid diets or elemental diets. Blenderized food can also be given by mouth or by nasogastric tube, and used either as a dietary supplement or as a complete feeding regime.

B. Complete (Whole Protein) Oral Liquid Diets

A range of preparations of this type has recently become available and the compositions vary widely. The aim of these preparations is to provide a complete liquid diet which can be used as a supplement to normal food or as complete nutrition by itself. They require normal digestive processes as well as normal absorptive ability in the alimentary tract. They are of value in the presence of a slight or moderately severe degree of nutritional insufficiency, provided that normal digestion and absorption are not seriously impaired. They have low residue. An assessment of their place as nutritional aids is made in Chapter 20.

Because of the wide variety of prepartions which are now available and the range of nutritional components which they contain, it is not feasible to classify these preparations in a simple way. When they are used, a full nutritional screen should be performed on the patient to assess the degree of nutritional deficiency, and a planned nutritional support program worked out so as to correct the nutritional deficiencies which are present.

Examples of commercially available complete oral liquid diets are described in this section. The principal nutritional components of the most widely used preparations are detailed in Table 2. The energy distribution from protein, fat, and carbohydrate of each preparation is shown in Table 3.

1. Clinifeed® (Roussel)

Clinifeed® consists of a range of nutritionally complete whole protein, sterilized liquid feeds. The principal preparations are Clinifeed® 400 vanilla, Clinifeed® 400 chocolate, Clinifeed® 500 vanilla, Clinifeed® LLS (low lactose, low sodium).

Clinifeed® 400 vanilla has the following ingredients — milk, corn syrup solids, whey proteins, sucrose, egg yolk, maize oil, potassium caseinate, soy oil, zinc sulfate, vitamins, glyceryl stearate, alginate, carrageen, disodium phosphate, and potassium hydroxide. Each can supplies 400 kcal. and 15 g protein. The osmolarity ranges from 306 to 370 mosmol/ℓ.

Clinifeed® 400 chocolate contains milk, corn syrup solids, cocoa powder, whey proteins, sucrose, egg yolk, maize oil, soy oil, zinc sulfate, vitamins, vanillin, glyceryl stearate, carrageen, disodium phosphate, and potassium hydroxide. Each can supplies 400 kcal and 15 g protein. The osmolarity ranges from 310 to 443 mosmol/ℓ.

Clinifeed® 500 vanilla contains milk, corn syrup, solids, sucrose whey proteins, sodium caseinate, soy oil, yeasts, potassium chloride, magnesium oxide, ferrous sulfate, zinc sulfate, vitamins, vanilla extract, vanillin, glyceryl stearate, carageen, and potassium hydroxide. Each can supplies 500 kcal and 30 g protein. The osmolarity ranges from 567 to 615 mosmol/ℓ.

Clinifeed® LLS contains corn syrup solids, chicken meat, egg yolk, isolated soy proteins, maize germ oil, sucrose, soy oil, potassium chloride, calcium carbonate, zinc sulfate,

Table 2
PRINCIPAL NUTRITIONAL COMPONENTS OF COMPLETE ORAL LIQUID DIETS

	Clinifeed® 400	**Clinifeed® 500**	**Isocal®**	**Triosorbon® MCT**	**Ensure®**
Protein	Whey protein, sodium, and potassium caseinate		Sodium caseinate, Soy protein isolate	Whey protein, casein, l-cystine	Solium and calcium caseinates: soy protein isolate
% energy contribution	15.00	24.00	13.00	16.00	14.50
Fat	Soy oil, glyceryl stearate		MCT oil Soy oil	MCT Sunflower oil	Corn oil
% energy contribution	30.00	20.00	37.00	36.00	32.50
Carbohydrate	Corn syrup solids, milk, sucrose		Corn syrup solids	Glucose, lactose, maltose, oligosaccharides	Sucrose, corn syrup solids
% energy contribution	55.00	56.00	50.00	48.00	53.50
Nonprotein energy:N ratio	142:1	79:1	170:1	130:1	147.1
Osmolarity (mosm/ℓ)	306—370	567—615	280	238—350	243

Table 3
ENERGY DISTRIBUTION IN COMPLETE ORAL LIQUID DIETS

	Energy distribution— % of total energy supply		
	Protein	Fat	Carbohydrate
Recommended distribution	10—15	20—30	55—70
Clinifeed® 400	15	30	55
Clinifeed® 500	24	20	56
Clinifeed® LLS	18	27	55
Ensure®	14	31.5	54.5
Isocal®	13	37	50
Triosorbon® MCT	16	36	48

vitamins, vegetable meat flavoring, alginate, carrageen, and potassium hydroxide. Each can supplies 500 kcal and 22.5 g protein. The osmolarity ranges from 435 to 515 mosmol/ℓ. The dose of each preparation is worked out according to the requirements of the patient and the preparation diluted according to requirements.

2. Ensure® (Abbott-Ross)

This is a general purpose, complete oral liquid diet preparation. The protein sources are sodium and calcium caseinate and soy protein isolate; the fat comes from corn oil, a low-cholesterol polyunsaturated fat which is an excellent source of essential fatty acids,. the carbohydrate source is sucrose and corn syrup solids. No lactose is present. The preparation also contains vitamin C, vitamin E, riboflavin, niacin, vitamin B_{12}, thiamin, iron, biotin, calcium, phosphorus, iodine, manganese, copper, zinc, folic acid, sodium, potassium, and chloride.

Ensure® provides 1.06 k cal/mℓ and 37.1 g protein/ℓ. The osmolarity is 243 mosmol/ℓ. It is supplied in 8 fluid oz. cans and bottles, and 32 fluid oz. cans in a variety of flavors. Ensure® powder, (vanilla flavor) is also available. As with other preparations of this type, the dose schedule should be worked out in accordance with the nutritional requirements of individual patients.

3. Isocal® (Mead-Johnson)

This is a complete liquid diet which is lactose and gluten free. The protein source is sodium caseinate and soy protein isolate, suppliing 65 g protein per 2000 kcal; fat is from medium chain triglyceride oil and soy oil, providing 85 g fat and 2000 kcal; the carbohydrate is in the form of corn syrup solids supplying 250 g carbohydrate in 2000 kcal; sodium, potassium, calcium, phosphorus, magnesium, iron, copper, zinc, manganese, chloride, iodine, vitamins A, D, E, C,, B_1, B_2, B_6 , B_{12}, K_1, nicotinic acid, pantothenic acid, choline, folic acid are also present. The osmolarity is 280 mosmol/ℓ; thus this preparation has no osmolarity problems, and is therefore not likely to lead to diarrhea. Each can contains 355 mℓ which is ready for use as a complete tube feed.

4. Triosorbon MCT® (Merck)

This preparation contains whey protein, casein and 1-cystine (19 g in 100 g sachet, providing 3.05 g nitrogen, medium chain triglycerides and a small quantity of sunflower oil containing essential fatty acid (19 g in 100 g sachet), monosaccharide (glucose), disaccharide (lactose and maltose), oligosaccharides and polysaccharides. (56 g in 100 g sachet). Sodium, potassium, calcium, magnesium, phosphorus, chloride, zinc, vitamins

A, B_1, B_2, B_6, B_{12} nicotinamide, biotin, panthothenic acid, vitamins C, D_3, K, iron and folic acid are also present. The osmolarity is 238 to 350 mosmol/ℓ depending upon dilution. The total energy contained in 100 g of the preparation is 500 kcal.

5. Precision Isotonic® (Doyle)

This is a complete oral liquid diet which contains no bulk, fiber, lactose, gluten, purine, or cholesterol, and is low in residue and sodium. The protein source is sodium caseinate and pasteurized egg white solids, and it also contains glucose oligosaccharides, sucrose, soybean oil, monoglycerides, diglycerides, calcium phosphate, potassium phosphate, citric acid, carrageen, magnesium, choline, sodium, iron, zinc, copper, manganese, vitamins A, D, E, C, K_1, B_6, B_{12} biotin, niacin, pantothenic acid and iodine.

6. Vital® (Abbott-Ross)

This preparation is fiber-free and lactose-free, and contains as its protein source hydrolyzed protein, whey, and soy protein. The fat source is sunflower oil and it also contains glucose, oligosaccharides, polysaccharides, sucrose, corn starch, calcium, phosphorus, magnesium, iron, iodine, copper, manganese, zinc, sodium, potassium, and chloride. The preparation requires digestive processes, although to a lesser extent than some of the preparations in this group. It cannot thus be regarded as an elemental diet.

C. Elemental Diets

These are semisynthetic, fiber-free liquid diets containing a full range of basic nutrients. They differ from complete oral liquid diets in that the basic nutrients — carbohydrate, protein, and fat — are presented to the GI tract in a form which does not require intact digestive capabilities. They are bulk free and have minimal residue.

The elemental diets which are available are as follows:

- Vivonex® (Eaton) — Vivonex® and Vivonex® HN
- Flexical® (Mead-Johnson)
- Precision® (or Precitene) (Doyle) — Precision® LR and Precision® HN can be regarded as elemental diets.

Two infant preparations, Nutramigen® (Mead-Johnson) and Pregestimil® (Mead-Johnson) have compositions which can be probably regarded as chemically defined diets. A full description and assessment of the composition of these preparations is to be found in Chapter 7.

III. INTRAVENOUS NUTRITION

The advent of adequate forns of i.v. nutrition in the management of patients with severe nutritional insufficiency was a major medical advance. In recent years the techniques, indications, and complications of i.v. nutrition have been assessed more precisely. Because of the risks associated with i.v. nutrition, methods of enteral nutrition were developed for patients who have reasonably good absorptive or digestive function, or less severe nutritional deficiency. The relationship of i.v. feeding to the various forms of enteral nutrition which are now available have been considered earlier in this chapter, and will be reviewed in Chapter 20.

IV. SUMMARY

The purpose of this volume is to consider in detail the place of elemental or chemically defined diets in the management of various disease processes and conditions associated with nutritional deficiency. The development, formulations, and properties of elemental diets will be considered in Section II followed by an assessment of their clinical uses in Section III. The relationship of elemental diets to other forms of enteral nutrition (dietary supplementation, complete oral liquid diets) and i.v. nutrition in clinical practice will be assessed in Section IV.

SECTION II

DEVELOPMENT, FORMULATIONS, AND PROPERTIES OF ELEMENTAL DIETS

Chapter 6

HISTORICAL BACKGROUND AND DEVELOPMENT OF ELEMENTAL DIETS

R. I. Russell

TABLE OF CONTENTS

I. DEFINITION

The term "elemental diet" or "chemically defined diet" is applied to a semisynthetic fiber-free liquid diet containing a full range of basic nutrients for the maintenance of normal physiological functions. The preparations are composed of basic nutritional components (purified l-amino acids, protein hydrolysates, or egg albumin; simple carbohydrates; essential fat; vitamins, minerals and trace elements). As they contain no polypeptides, peptones, or complex polysaccharides, they are thus presented to the gastrointestinal tract in a readily assimilable form and are absorbed without requiring full digestive processes; they contain no added bulk, and have minimal residue.[1-4] Their use allows normal growth, reproduction, and the maintenance of a satisfactory nutritional state over a period of time.

The essential features of elemental diets are their ability to provide adequate nutrition with minimal digestive requirements, and their low-residue nature. Complete oral liquid diets, on the other hand, are nutritionally complete preparations which contain complex protein, carbohydrate and fat sources which require a fully active digestive capability, although they also are of low residue.

A totally elemental diet would consist of glucose, amino acids, essential fatty acids, minerals, and vitamins in amounts proportional to normal human requirements.The term "elemental diet" is thus a misnomer as the preparations are not truly elemental. The term chemically defined which may be preferable to "elemental" was introduced during the developmental work of these preparations and used in the initial animal studies which were performed. Most of the preparations, however, contain ingredients which cannot be classified as chemically defined substances.[5] A more accurate term may be "defined formula diets", as this implies only a particular composition to a specific formula. The diets consist of well-defined chemical formulations which may be classified as foods or drugs or both. The original term "elemental diets", however, has, in spite of its inaccuracy, become widely used and is now accepted terminology for these preparations.

II. ORIGINS AND LANDMARKS OF DEVELOPMENT

The theoretical possibility of synthesizing the essential nutrients so as to provide preparations able to give complete nutritional support was considered by Emil Fischer as early as 1907[6]. The concept was further advanced by the studies of Abderhalden,[7,8] who foresaw that "science would, at one time, make such great advances that the possibility would be afforded to manufacture foodstuffs by synthetic means." Further progress was not made for some decades until the classical studies of Rose and his colleagues who demonstrated that experimental animals could grow satisfactorily, and human beings be maintained in positive nitrogen balance when mixtures of amino acids were substituted for intact protein.[9,10] The studies of Rose provided a basic understanding of protein constituents and their substitution by crystalline amino acids. Further important contributions to the physiology of nutrition were also made over this period,[11-15] and the whole subject of amino acids and nutrition was excellently reviewed by Greenstein and Winitz in 1961.[16] By the early 1950's, basic investigative work using chemically defined diets was in progress in laboratory animals and an extensive series of studies was published at this time.[17-28] The Greenstein group at NIH performed animal studies in which three generations of rats were fed chemically defined diets as their sole source of nutrition, and these diets were found to support growth, reproduction, and lactation without side effects. At about the same time, other studies using liquidized diets and formula diets were being reported.[29-31] By the early 1950's some synthetic nutrients were being manufactured and standard protein hydrolysates were available. For the first time liquid formula diets could be used which allowed consistency and control of food intake in metabolic studies.

Much basic information was now available about the use of chemically defined and formula diets in animals, and attention turned to their use in man. The amino acid requirements of initial formulas were based largely on the work of Rose[9,10,32] and Greenstein.[33,34]

The stage was now set for a series of investigations aimed at extending the use of chemically defined diets to the long-term nutritional support of normal human subjects and patients in hospital so as to study the effects on these preparations on physiological and metabolic processes. Preliminary clinical studies had shown that chemically defined diets maintained body weight in hospitalized patients.[35] These studies were performed at the California Medical Faculty on 24 normal volunteer subjects in which the diets were used to provide the sole source of nutrition for a continuous period of 22 weeks. A detailed evaluation of their nutritional efficacy was made toghether with studies on various physiological and metabolic parameters.[1,36-39] These studies have provided basic and invaluable information as to the effect of such chemically defined diets in normal human subjects and will be described in more detail in the next section.

At this time, a further impetus to the development of chemically defined diets and the investigation of their properties came from the American aerospace program. Since then, several chemically defined or elemental diets have been made available for clinical use, and much additional information has now been accumulated regarding their metabolic effects and value in a wide variety of clinical conditions.

III. INITIAL BASIC STUDIES WITH ELEMENTAL DIETS — ANIMALS AND MAN

The basic work of Rose and others allowed the development and use of amino acid mixtures of flexible composition. Studies became possible with the aim of determining normal requirements of essential components of the diet in normal subjects, together with a quantitative approach to the determination of utilization and effect of each dietary component.

A. Animal Studies

An extenisve series of aninal studies was undertaken at the NIH, and as an important landmark in the development if chemically defined diets.[18-27] Although a number of variations on the diets were utilized, they were all characterized by the provision of the essential and non essential nitrogen source solely in the form of pure 1-amino acids. They were administered as single crystal-clear aqueous solutions which were nutritionally complete. Many experiments were performed with varied proportions of 1-amino acids, which, with the addition of the necessary water-soluble and fat-soluble vitamins, mineral salts, glucose, or other simple sugars as carbohydrate source, and ethyl linoleate as a source of essential fatty acid, were nutritionally complete entities. An essential feature of these studies was that each separate component was highly purified prior to its incorporation into the diet. The exact chemical composition of each diet was thus precisely known. By varying individual aspects of the composition, either amino acid or carbohydrate, the effect of individual nutrients could be studied. The precision biochemistry which made these studies possible followed the development of enzymic resolution procedures developed by Greenstein.[33,41]

The initial studies demonstrated that the dietary solutions were stable and remained so indefinitely. The rats grew well (at a rate greater than 4 g/day) on a diet containing approxinately 20% amino acids and 80% glucose when the diet used contained nonessential amino acids modeled after casein. It was noted that no bulk was provided, intestinal contents were considerably reduced, and fecal excretion was scanty and infrequent.[18] The total urinary nitrogen and distribution of urinary nitrogen among urea, ammonia, and amino acids was determined together with the measurement of fecal nitrogen. Nitrogen balances were calculated and it was found that fecal nitrogen excretion was small and constant whatever the nature of the diet, thus indicating an adequate quantitative absorption of the nitrogenous components of the soluble diets.[19] Studies on individual amino acids added separately to the basal diet at the expense of the glucose component showed that those diets providing the best growth were those in which l-alanine, ammonium l-glutamate, l-glutamine, ammonium l-aspartate, and l-proline were used as the sole source of nonessential nitrogen.[20] Studies on the best source of carbohydrate showed that growth was greatest when sucrose-containing diets were used; d-glucose-, invert sugar-, and d-fructose-containing diets showed a decreasing order of efficacy with respect to growth and a decreased dietary intake. A progressively decreasing rate of both growth and diet intake were found when diets with progressively increasing d-glucosamine concentration were used, but the reduced growth was considered to be due to the diminished dietary intake.[21] It was also demonstrated that growth rate was greater when l-arginine was added to each diet compared with d-arginine.[22] Further studies in the same series investigated the use of chemically defined diets in mice, and differences were noted between the ideal composition of such diets in mice compared with rats. [23] This emphasizes the importance of species difference in nutritional studies. When chemically defined diets were used in tumor-bearing rats it was found that tumor growth was considerably slowed when animals were force fed diets lacking in methionine, isoleucine, or valine. Normal animals on these diets were noted to be in negative nitrogen balance.[24,25]

On the basis of those fundamental animal studies, a nutritionally adequate, chemically defined, crystal-clear liquid diet was formulated composed of 18 crystalline amino acids (excluding glycine), water-soluble and fat-soluble vitamins, ninerals, glucose, and ethyl linoleate as the source of essential fatty acid.[27] The formulation was prepared as a transparent clear, stable emulsion of fat-soluble ingredients in a 50% solution of the other ingredients in water, with the aid of a small amount of polyoxyethylene (20), Sorbitan monooleate (Tween 80). No separation of the lipid phase occurred and the diet could be stored at room temperature or in temperatures down to −20°C for an indefinite period. The dry ingredients were dissolved in distilled water to give a solution of 50 to 70% solids with a nutritive value of 2 to 3 kcal/ mℓ. The next step was to mount a series of similar studies in normal human subjects.

B. Human Studies

Preliminary clinical studies on hospitalized patients were reported in 1960. These confirmed that the diets maintained body weight, were effective in correcting protein stores lost during periods of nitrogen depeletion, and produced no abnormalities of hepatic or renal function. [35] Consistently positive nitrogen balances were achieved in these studies, and no significant clinical complications occurred.

A series of basic investigations with normal human subjects using chemically defined diets were performed between 1963 and 1964 at the California Medical Faculty in Vacaville, California and detailed evaluation of the nutritional efficacy of these diets made on a group of normal human adult males. The diets were given as sole nutriton for a continuous period of 22 weeks. The nutritional efficacy in the 15 subjects who completed the study was determined by detailed balance studies which provided information on water balance, blood chemistry, hematology and urinalysis, blood pressure, body weight and anthropometric data, GI bulk, and serum cholesterol levels. The effects on gut microflora populations were also studied together with alterations of bile pigment patterns resulting from the use of the diet.[1,37,38] The composition of the basic chemically defined diet used in the study is shown in Table 1. It provided 2.7 kcal/mℓ; the composition of the diet related to the amounts of individual nutrients present in 1800 mℓ of diet at 1.0 kcal/mℓ is shown in Table 2. Some variations in the formulations of the chemically defined diets were introduced as part of the studies. These included replacement of 25% of the glucose by an equal weight of sucrose; replacenent of the amino acids by an equal weight of glucose but keeping the two compositions isocaloric, and containing a negligible amount of nitrogen obtained from vitamins and minerals; replacement of the amino acids by 55.1 g peptone per liter of undiluted diet (isonitrogenous with the amino acids); replacement of all the glucose by an equal weight of sucrose; and variations consisting of parts of the different formulations described. The basic formulation was planned so that 1 liter of concentrated diet or 2 liters of diluted diet would provide 2700 kcal and also provide each of the essential amino acids in amounts in excess of twice the minimum levels of essential amino acids considered to be necessary for young adult males.[9,10] The chemically defined diets were provided in a concentration of 2.7 kcal/mℓ diluted with an equal volume of distilled water prior to feeding, and administered daily at four regularly scheduled 3-hr intervals. The daily amount of diet ingested by each individual was left open. Fat-soluble vitamins dissolved in 2 g of ethyl linoleate were ingested as a separate supplement in the morning. Routine weekly physical examinations were performed together with weekly blood chemistry, hematology, and urinalysis determinations. Fasting blood samples were obtained during the baseline period, once weekly during the following 22 weeks and twice weekly for the last 13 weeks, during which time the subjects were on a normal diet.

The average daily intake of chemically defined diet was about 2900 calories. All subjects remained in a satisfactory physical state with normal physiological functions and with the maintenance of normal biochemistry, hematology, and urinalysis. Adequate water balance was present during the period. After an initial weight loss in the first few weeks, the subjects' weights remained steady at satisfactory levels. It was considered that the initial weight loss may have been related to the rapid clearance of bulk from the GI tract due to the residue-free diet. Weight changes on this diet tended toward normality for an adult man. In general individuals who were overweight rapidly lost adipose tissue, and those who were underweight showed weight gains toward normal. A marked reduction in fecal excretion occurred with a reduction in average stool weight. There was an overall reduction in fecal matter of more than 80%; the stools were watery or semi-solid in consistency, and dark green or black in color.

A reduction of both systolic and diastolic blood pressure occurred in the subjects (all of whom were initially normotensive) within a few days of starting the diet. Provision of a diet in which the entire carbohydrate source was provided in the form of glucose was accompanied by a decrease in serum cholesterol levels in all individuals. These findings will be described later. Alteration of the gut microflora populations were also found and will be discussed in Chapter 9.

Other studies using chemically defined diets in nutritionally normal subjects were also being reported about this time. McKean used continuous feeding of a chemically defined diet over a period of 30 months in five children (ages 8 years 10 months to 15 years 3 months) who had mental retardation associated with phenylketonuria.[42] Satisfactory weight gains and height increases were obtained which were equivalent to, or greater than, those obtained in normal children on standard food. The same author treated a group of 24 bedridden and mentally retarded children with feeding problems for 18 months, and achieved an average weight gain of 2 kg on a mean daily elemental diet

Table 1
COMPOSITION OF CHEMICALLY-DEFINED DIET USED IN HUMAN STUDIES

(Solids content per liter of undiluted diet—2.7 kcal/mℓ)

		Per liter of undiluted diet—2.7 kcal/mℓ
	l-Lysine HCl	3.58 g
	l-Leucine	3.83 g
	l-Isoleucine	2.42 g
	l-Valine	2.67 g
	l-Phenylalanine	1.75 g
	l-Arginine HCl	2.58 g
	l-Histidine HCl H_2O	1.58 g
	l-Methionine	1.75 g
Amino acids	l-Alanine	2.58 g
	Sodium l-aspartate	6.40 g
	l-Threonine	2.42 g
	l-Proline	10.33 g
	Glycine	1.67 g
	l-Serine	5.33 g
	l-Tyrosine ethyl ester HCl	6.83 g
	l-Tryptophan	0.75 g
	l-Glutamine	9.07 g
	l-Cysteine ethyl ester HCl	0.92 g
Carbohydrates	Glucose	555.0 g
	Glucono-6-lactone	17.2 g
Fat and fat-soluble vitamins	Ethyl linoleate	2.0 g
	Vitamin A acetate	3.64 mg
	Vitamin D	0.057 mg
	α-Tocopherol acetate	57.29 mg
	Menadione	4.58 mg
Water-soluble vitamins	Thiamin HCl	1.00 mg
	Riboflavin	1.50 mg
	Pyridoxine HCl	1.67 mg
	Niacinamide	10.00 mg
	Inositol	0.83 mg
	d-Calcium pantothenate	8.33 mg
	d-Biotin	0.83 mg
	Folic acid	1.67 mg
	Ascorbic acid	62.50 mg
	Cyanocobalamin	1.67 mg
	p-Aminobenzoic acid	416.56 mg
	Choline bitartrate	231.25 mg
Minerals and trace elements	Potassium iodine	0.25 mg
	Manganous acetate $4H_2O$	18.30 mg
	Zinc benzoate	2.82 mg
	Cupric acetate H_2O	2.50 mg
	Cobaltous acetate $4H_2O$	1.67 mg
	Sodium glyccrophosphate-5½ H_2O	5.23 g
	Potassium hydroxide	3.97 g
	Magnesium oxide	0.38 g
	Sodium chloride	4.77 g
	Ferrous gluconate	0.83 g
	Calcium chloride $2H_2O$	2.44 g

Table 1 (continued)
COMPOSITION OF CHEMICALLY-DEFINED DIET USED IN HUMAN STUDIES

(Solids content per liter of undiluted diet—2.7 kcal/mℓ)

		Per liter of undiluted diet—2.7 kcal/mℓ
Minerals and trace elements	Sodium benzoate	1.00 g
	Ammonium molybdate $4H_2O$	0.42 g

Compiled from Winitz, M., Graff, J., Gallagher, N., Narkin, A., and Seedman, D. A., *Nature,* 205, 741, 1965, and Winitz, M., Seedman, D. A., and Graff, J., *Am. J. Clin. Nutr.,* 23, 525, 1970.

Table 2
COMPOSITION OF A CHEMICALLY DEFINED DIET USED IN HUMAN STUDIES

(Amounts present in 1800 mℓ of diet at 1.0 kcal/mℓ)

Essential amino acids		Electrolytes	
l-Isoleucine g	1.65	Anions	
l-Leucine g	2.61	Sodium g	2.56
l-Lysine	1.96	Potassium g	1.89
l-Methionine g	1.19	Calcium g	0.45
l-Phenylalanine g	1.19	Magnesium mg	156
l-Threonine g	1.65	Manganese mg	2.80
l-Tryptophan g	0.51	Iron mg	70.8
l-Valine g	1.82	Copper mg	0.54
l-Cysteine g	0.41	Zinc mg	0.41
Nonessential amino acids		Cobalt mg	0.27
l-Alanine g	1.76	Molybdenum mg	0.16
l-Arginine g	1.45	Cations	
l-Aspartic acid g	3.75	Chloride g	4.40
l-Glutamine g	6.19	Phosphate g	0.35
Glycine g	1.14	Acetate mg	15.7
l-Histidine g	0.80	Sulfate mg	0
l-Proline g	7.04	Iodine mg	0.13
l-Serine g	3.63	Gluconate g	13.13
l-Tyrosine g	3.43	Sorbate g	0
Vitamins		Benzoate mg	575
Vitamin A, USP units	7200	Fat	
Vitamin B_{12} ugm	1.14	Ethyl linoleate g	1.36
Vitamin C mg	42.61	Safflower oil g	0
Vitamin D_2USP units	1555	Polyoxyethylene sorbitan monooleate mg	0
Vitamin E Intl units	39		
p-Aminobenzoic acid mg	284.0	Carbohydrate	
d-Biotin mg	0.57	Glucose g	378.2
d-Calcium pantothenate mg	5.68	Sucrose g	0
Choline bitartrate mg	157.7	Fructose g	0
Choline chloride mg	0		
Folic acid mg	1.14		
Inositol mg	0.57		
Menadione mg	3.12		
Niacinamide mg	6.82		
Pyridoxine hydrochloride mg	1.14		
Riboflavin phosphate mg	1.40		
Thiamin hydrochloride mg	0.68		

Compiled from Winitz, M., Graff, J., Gallagher, N., Narkin, A., and Seedman, D. A., *Nature,* 205, 741, 1965, and Winitz, M., Seedman, D. A., Graff, J., *Am. J. Clin. Nutr.,* 23, 525, 1970.

intake of 1700 kcal.[42,43] These studies confirmed that chemically defined diets do provide adequate nutritional support for at least 6 months in human subjects.

Further basic studies have subsequently appeared which have investigated the effect of chemically defined diets on various physiological and biochemical paramenters in normal subjects. These studies have generally used commercially available elemental diets such as Vivonex® or Flexical®. In one such study in one normal subject given Vivonex® over a period of 5 days, the urinary excretion of minerals, UV absorbing compounds, phenolic acids, indoles, and phenolic amines was determined during the period of the diet and the results compared with those when a self selected diet was taken. The chemically defined diet caused a decrease in mineral excretion and also in the excretion of a number of aromatic compounds.[44] A further study in five normal volunteers using the same chemically defined diet resulted in a decrease of serum cholesterol and urea nitrogen and a rise of serum phosphate, uric acid, and creatinine. It was noted that urinary creatinine was unchanged but urinary electrolytes, urea and uric acid increased to a new stable value after 4 days on the diet.[46]

Further studies with an elemental diet of rather different composition (Flexical® formulation) have also been performed in normal human volunteers.[46] In this study, the diet was given over 12 days to normal human subjects and compared with a control diet which differed in that the protein fraction was not hydrolyzed and that no medium chain triglycerides were added to the lipid fraction. The diet was suitable for maintaining weight and nutritional parameters over the 12-day period and neither diet had significant effect on biochemical and hematological parameters. It was again noted that some weight loss occurred on the chemically defined diet during the first 4 days of treatment.

The effect of the elemental diet Vivonex® on the essential metals magnesium and zinc in normal human subjects has also been studied by measuring the daily urinary losses of these metals and knowing their exact intake in the diet. Urinary excretion of total nitrogen, urea, and creatine were also measured in the subjects. Some reduction of urea output and urinary creatine was noted and a fall in the output of sodium and chloride was observed, which reflected the reduced intake. No marked change was noted in urinary excretion of calcium and magnesium but reduced phosphate excretion was found which was probably related to the reduced intake while on the chemically defined diet. Urinary zinc output did not change.[47]

These basic studies in normal human subjects have added to our knowledge of the effects of chemically defined diets on physiology and biochemistry. They have all confirmed the adequacy of chemically defined diets in maintaining nutritional normality, but it is to be emphasized that all this data was obtained in normal human subjects with basically normal metabolism, and that most of the later studies were performed over short periods of time.

In disease states, especially those chronic conditions which may be associated with the development of nutritional deficiency, there may be increased nutritional requirements which may not be adequately met by the use of standard elemental diet. This problem will be discussed in later chapters.

These basic studies in animals and normal human subjects have provided much valuable information on chemically defined diets. On the basis of these studies, the characteristics and properties of these preparations can be identified; these are detailed and discussed in Chapter 8.

REFERENCES

1. **Winitz, M., Seedman, D. A., and Graff, J.,** Studies in metabolic nutrition employing chemically defined diets. I. Extended feeding of normal human adult males, *Am. J. Clin. Nutr.*,23, 525, 1970.
2. **Winitz, M. and Adams, R. F.,** Chemically defined diets, in *Balanced Nutrition and Therapy,* Lang, K., Fekl, W., and Berg, G., Eds., Thieme, Stuttgart, 1971, 46.
3. **Russell, R. I.,** Elemental diets — progress report, *Gut,*16, 68, 1975.
4. **Ponte, C. D., Lipman, A. G., and Moran, C. P.,** Use review of nutritionally complete liquid diets, *Am. J. Hosp. Pham.*, 35, 159, 1978.
5. **Kark, R. M.,** Liquid formula and chemically defined diets, *J. Am. Diet. Assoc.*, 64, 477, 1974.
6. **Fischer, E.,** The chemistry of proteins and its relation to biology in *Investigation on Amino Acids, Polypeptides and Proteins,* Bergmann, M., Ed., Springer, Berlin, 1923, 1.
7. **Abderhalden, E., Frank, F., and Schittenhelm, A.,** On the utilisation of completely hydrolysed protein in the human organism, *Hoppe-Seylers Z. Physiol. Chem.*, 63, 215, 1909.
8. **Abderhalden, E. and Hirsch, P.,** Feeding experiments with gelitine, ammonium salts, completely hydrolysed meat and a mixture of all known amino acids on young dogs, *Hoppe-Seylers Z. Physiol. Chem.*, 81, 323, 1912.
9. **Rose, W. C.,** Amino acid requirements of man, *Fed. Proc.*, 8, 546, 1949.
10. **Rose, W. C. and Wixom, R. L.,** The amino acid requirements of man. XVI. The role of the nitrogen intake., *J. Biol. Chem.*, 217, 997, 1955.
11. **Bassett, S. H., Woods, R. R., Shull, F. W., and Madden, S. C.,** Parenterally adninsitered amino acids as a source of protein in man, *N. Engl. J. Med.*, 230, 106, 1944.
12. **Madden, S. C., Anderson, F. W., Donovan, J. C., and Whipple, G. H.,** Plasma protein production influenced by amino acid mixtures and lack of essential amino acids. A deficiency state related to unknown factors, *J. Exp. Med.*, 82, 77, 1945.
13. **Cannon, P. R.,** Some pathologic consequences of protein and amino acid deficiencies, Charles C. Thomas, Springfield, Ill. 1948, 4.
14. **Maddy, K. H. and Elvehjem, C. A.,** Studies on growth of mice fed rations containing three amino acids, *J. Biol. Chem.*, 177, 577, 1949.
15. **Ramasarma, G. B., Henderson, L. M., and Elvehjem, C. A.,** Purified amino acids as a source of nitrogen for the growing rat, *J. Nutr.*, 38, 177, 1949.
16. **Greenstein, J. P. and Winitz, M.,** Amino acids in nutrition, in *Chemistry of the Amino Acids,* John Wiley & Sons, New York, 1961, 245.
17. **Schultze, M. O.,** Reproduction of rats fed protein-free amino acid rations, *J. Nutr.*, 60, 35, 1956.
18. **Greenstein, J. P., Birnbaum, S. M., Winitz, M., and Otley, M. C.,** Quantitative nutritional studies with water soluble, chemically defined diets. I. Growth reproduction and lactation in rats, *Arch. Biochem. Biophys.*, 72, 396, 1957.
19. **Birnbaum, S. M., Greenstein, J. P., and Winitz, M.,** Quantitative nutritional studies with water soluble, chemically defined diets. II. Nitrogen balance and metabolism, *Arch. Biochem. Biophys.*, 72, 417, 1957.
20. **Birnbaum, S. M., Winitz, M., and Greenstein, J. P.,** Quantitative nutritional studies with water soluble, chemically defined diets. III. Individual amino acids as sources of "non-essential" nitrogen, *Arch. Biochem. Biophys.*, 72, 428, 1957.
21. **Winitz, M., Birnbaum, S. M., and Greenstein, J. P.,** Quantitative nutritional studies with water soluble, chemically defined diets. IV. Influence of various carbohydrates on growth, with special reference to D-glucosamine, *Arch. Biochem. Biophys.*, 72, 437, 1957.
22. **Winitz, M., Greenstein, J. P., and Birnbaum, S. M.,** Quantitative nutritional studies with water soluble, chemcially defined diets. V. Role of isomeric arginines in growth, *Arch. Biochem. Biophys.*, 72, 448, 1957.
23. **Birnbaum, S. M., Greenstein, M. E., Winitz, M., and Greenstein, J. P.,** Quantitative nutritional studies with water soluble, chemically defined diets. VI. Growth studies on mice, *Arch. Biochem. Biophys.*, 78, 245, 1958.
24. **Sugimura, T., Birnbaum, S. M., Winitz, M., and Greenstein, J. P.,** Quantitative nutritional studies with water soluble, chemically defined diets. VII. Nitrogen balance in normal and tumour-bearing rats following forced feeding, *Arch. Biochem. Biophys.*, 81, 439, 1959.
25. **Sugimura, T., Birnbaum, S. M., Winitz, M., and Greenstein, J. P.,** Quantitative nutritional studies with water-soluble chemically defined diets. VII. The forced feeding of diet each lacking in one essential amino acid, *Arch. Biochem. Biophys.*, 81, 448, 1959.
26. **Sugimura, T., Birnbaum, S. M., Winitz, M., and Greenstein, J. P.,** Quantitative nutritional studies with water soluble, chemically defined diets IX. Further studies on d-glucosamine-containing diets, *Arch. Biochem. Biophys.*, 83, 521, 1959.

27. **Greenstein, J. P., Otley, M. C., Birnbaum, S. M., and Winitz, M.,** Quantitative nutritional studies with water soluble chemically defined diets. X. Formulation of a nutritionally complete liquid diet, *J. Nat. Cancer Inst.*, 24, 211, 1960.
28. **Winitz, M., Birnbaum, S. M., Sugimura, T., and Otley, M.C.,** Quantitative nutritional and in vivo metabolic studies with water-soluble chemically defined diets, in *Amino Acids, Proteins and Cancer Biochemistry,* Edsall, J. T., Greenstein, J. P., Eds., Mem. Symp., Academic Press, New York, 1960, 9.
29. **Robinson, C. H.,** Liquid diets, *J. Clin. Nutr.*, 1, 476, 1953.
30. **Olson, F., Michaels, G., Partridge, J. W., Bolling, L., Margens, and Kinsell, L. W.,** The use of formula diets administered via a polyethylene tube or orally for constant intake (balance) studies, *J. Clin. Nutr.*, 1, 134, 1953.
31. **Moorhouse, J. A. and Kark, R. M.,** Fructose and diabetes, *Am. J. Med.*, 23, 46, 1957.
32. **Rose, W. C.,** The amino acid requirements of adult man, *Nutr. Abstr. Rev.*, 27, 631, 1957.
33. **Greenstein, J. P.,** The resolution of racemic alpha-amino acids, *Adv. Protein Chem.*, 9, 121, 1954.
34. **Greenstein, J. P. and Winitz, M.,** Correlation of configuration, in *Chemistry of the Amino Acids,* John Wiley & Sons, New York, 1961, 86.
35. **Couch, R. B., Watkin, D. M., Smith, R. R., Rosenberg, L. E., Winitz, M., Birnbaum, S. M., Otley, M. C., and Greenstein, J. P.,** Clinical trials of water-soluble chemically defined diet, *Fed. Proc.*, 19, 13, 1960.
36. **Winitz, M., Graff, J., Gallagher, N., Narkin, A., and Seedman, D. A.,** Evaluation of chemical diets as nutrition for man in space, *Nature (London)*, 205, 741, 1965.
37. **Winitz, M., Adams, R. F., Seedman, D. A., Davis, P. N., Jayko, L. G., and Hamilton, J. A.,** Studies in metabolic nutrition employing chemically defined diets. II Effects on gut microflora population, *Am. J. Clin. Nutr.*, 23, 546, 1970.
38. **Winitz, M., Adams, R. F., Seedman, D. A., and Graff, J.,** Regulation of intestinal flora patterns with chemical diets, *Fed. Proc.*, 25, 343, 1966.
39. **Winitz, M., Graff, J., and Seedman, D. A.,** Effect of dietary carbohydrate on serum cholesterol levels, *Arch. Biochem.*, 108, 576, 1964.
40. **Greenstein, J. P.,** Resolution of DL mixtures of alpha amino acids, *Methods Enzymol.*, 3, 554, 1957.
40a. **Greenstein, J. P.,** The resolution of racemic alpha amino acids, *Adv. Protein Chem.*, 9, 121, 1954.
41. **McKean, C. M.,** Growth of phenylketonuric children on chemically defined diets, *Lancet*, 1, 148, 1970.
42. **McKean, C. M.,** Effects of totally synthetic, low phenylalanine diet on adolescent phenylketonuric patients, *Arch. Dis. Child.*, 46, 608, 1971.
43. **McKean, C. M.,** The long term effects of chemically defined diets on ambulatory phenylketonurics and bed-ridden severely retarded patients, *Balanced Nutrition and Therapy,* Lang, K., Fekl, W., Berg, G., Eds., Thieme, Stuttgart, 1971, 66.
44. **Young, D. S.,** The effects of a chemically defined diet on urinary excretion of ninerals and aromatic compounds, *Clin. Chem.*, 16, 681, 1970.
45. **Young, D. S., Epley, J. A., and Goldman, P.,** Influence of a chemically defined diet on the composition of serum and urine, *Clin. Chem.*, 17, 765, 1971.
46. **Perrault, J., Devroede, G., and Bounous, G.,** Effects of an elemental diet in healthy volunteers, *Gastroenterology,* 64, 579, 1973.
47. **Fell, G. S.,** Biochemical studies in relationship to an elemental diet, in *The Role of Elemental Nutrition,* Johnston, I.D.A., Ed., 1976, 21.

Chapter 7

FORMULATIONS OF ELEMENTAL DIETS

R. I. Russell

TABLE OF CONTENTS

I. INTRODUCTION

Following the developmental work in the 1950s on synthetic, chemically defined diets, several elemental diet preparations became commercially available. Initially, the diets were based on those used in the extensive studies of Winitz and his colleagues. The composition of these diets used in normal volunteer studies are described in the papers of Winitz, Seedman, and Graff[1] and Winitz and Adams,[2] and are described in Chapter 6. These formulas were shown to be successful in maintaining the normal nutritional state in normal volunteer subjects. No information was available at that time about their value in disease states.

It is the purpose of this chapter to describe the elemental or chemically defined diets which are at present available, to assess the differences in composition of these various diets, and to critically consider the advantages and disadvantages of the different compositions with particular references to the disease states for which they may be used.

II. FORMULATIONS

There are considerable differences in the formulations of elemental diets commercially available; variations occur in the quantity of individual nutrients, the form in which each nutrient is presented to the gastrointestinal tract, and the percentage energy distribution from the various components. Because of the differences in the formulations, after the initial decision has been made to use a chemically defined diet in any particular patient, a corresponding decision must be made with respect to the indidivual preparation to be used. Although each preparation conforms to the definition in its essential aspects of minimal digestive requirements and low residue, the formulations vary considerably and the specific benefits of any individual formulation should be considered when elemental diet therapy is being planned.

At present there are several elemental diet preparations commercially available. These include Vivonex® (Eaton), Flexical® (Mead Johsnon), Precision® (Doyle), and two formulations designed for infants, Nutramigen® (Mead Johsnon), and Pregestimil® (Mead Johsnon).

Vivonex® is based on the experimental diets of Winitz and his colleagues;[1,2] a high nitrogen preparation is also available (Vivonex HN®). The composition of Flexical® is similar to that originally used by Bounous and his colleagues[3] in their early studies. Precision® is available in the U.S. and West Germany (as Precitene®), but not in the U.K. Two of these preparations — Precision LR®, and Precision HN® can be regarded as elemental diets.

The principal nutritional components of Vivonex®, Vivonex HN®, Flexical®, Precision LR®, and Precision HN® are shown in Table 1. The composition of these various preparations has been compared in a nunber of recent publications.[4-9]

The nature of the protein content in chemically defined diets varies considerably. The amounts of amino acids present meet the recommended requirements for normal subjects, although greater amounts of essential amino acids may be required in some disease states. The essential and nonessential amino acid content of the preparations is shown in Table 2. In Vivonex® and Vivonex HN® pure synthetic amino acids are present. In Flexical®, the amino acids are derived from hydrolyzed casein although the individual amino acids tyrosine, tryptophan, and methionine are also present. In Precision® the protein source is egg albumin derived from pasteurized egg white solids. In Nutramigen® and Pregestimil®, it is hydrolyzed casein. The total amount of protein also varies in the preparations — 21 to 24 g/1000 kcal in Vivonex®, Flexical®, and Precision LR®, to 41 to 44 g/1000 kcal in Vivonex® and Precision HN®. In all the preparations, the ratio of

Table 1
PRINCIPAL NUTRITIONAL COMPONENTS OF ELEMENTAL DIETS

	Vivonex®	Vivonex HN®	Flexical®	Precision LR®	Precision HN®
Protein	Pure crystalline amino acids	Pure crystalline amino acids	Hydrolyzed casein +tyrosine, tryptophan, methionine	Egg albumin	Egg albumin
g/1000 kcal	21.10	44.79	22.40	23.70	41.70
% energy contribution	8.20	17.20	9.00	8.80	15.10
Fat	Safflower oil	Safflower oil	Soy oil, MCT, soy lecithin	Soy oil, MCT monoglycerides, diglycerides	Soy oil, MCT monoglycerides diglycerides
g/1000 kcal	1.40	0.90	34.00	0.70	0.50
% energy contribution	1.30	0.78	30.00	0.50	0.40
Carbohydrate	Glucose, glucose oligosaccharides	Glucose, glucose oligosaccharides	Sucrose oligosaccharides	Glucose oligosaccharides sucrose, and maltodextrin	
g/1000 kcal	226.30	210.30	154.00	224.70	206.70
% energy contribution	90.20	80.96	61.00	83.00	74.00
Nonprotein energy: nitrogen ratio	306:1	150:1	278:1	264:1	150:1
Osmolarlity	500—678	800—920	332—723	525	557

Table 2
ESSENTIAL AND NONESSENTIAL AMINO ACID CONTENT OF ELEMENTAL DIETS (g/1000 kcal)

	Vivonex®	Vivonex HN®	Flexical®	Precision LR®	Precision HN®
Essential (total)	7.651	16.449	11.250	10.231	18.000
l-Isoleucine	0.917	1.828	1.425	1.468	2.583
l-Leucine	1.450	2.892	2.410	1.989	3.500
l-Lysine	1.089	2.175	2.015	1.350	2.375
l-Methionine	0.939	2.017	1.060	0.876	1.542
l-Phenylalanine	1.045	3.126	1.120	1.445	2.542
l-Threonine	0.917	1.829	1.095	0.995	1.750
l-Tryptophan	0.283	0.565	0.355	0.355	0.625
l-Valine	1.011	2.017	1.770	1.753	3.083
Nonessential (total)	13.452	28.345	15.160	15.160	23.669
l-Alanine	0.978	2.280	0.845	1.705	3.000
l-Arginine	1.787	1.788	0.935	1.326	2.333
l-Aspartic acid	2.086	4.866	1.895	1.776	3.125
l-Glutamine	3.438	8.020	—	—	—
l-Glycine	1.595	4.329	0.560	0.853	1.500
l-Histidine	0.444	1.036	0.705	0.497	0.857
l-Proline	1.305	3.045	2.555	0.853	1.500
l-Serine	0.672	1.825	1.490	1.776	3.125
l-Tyrosine	1.147	1.156	0.590	0.947	1.667
l-Cystine	—	—	0.100	0.545	0.968
Glutamic acid	—	—	5.485	3.174	5.584
Total amino acids	**21.103**	**44.794**	**26.410**	**23.683**	**41.667**

essential to nonessential amino acids (35%:65%) conforms to the recommendations of Rose.[10,11] The energy contribution from protein in Vivonex®, Flexical®, and Precision LR® is 8 to 9% and from Vivonex HN® and Precision HN® 15 to 17%.

There are considerable differences in the fat content of chemically defined diets. Vivonex® preparations contain very small quantities of fat (Vivonex® 1.4 g/1000 kcal; Vivonex HN® 0.9 g/1000 kcal). The fat present in Vivonex® is purified safflower oil (80% as triglyceride of linoleic acid). Larger amounts of fat are present in Flexical® and Precision®. In Flexical®, the lipid is soy oil, medium chain triglycerides, and soy lecithin (34.0 g/1000 kcal), and in Precision® soy oil, medium chain triglycerides, monoglycerides, and diglycerides (0.5 to 0.7 g/1000 kcal). Energy contribution from fat in Vivonex® and Precision® preparations varies from 0.4% to 1.3%, but fat in Flexical provides 30% of calories. The fats used in all the formulations have adequate amounts of the essential fatty acid linoleic acid.

The principal calorie contribution in all the formulas is from carbohydrate but the nature of the carbohydrate and the percentage contribution of calories varies from formula to formula. The anounts of carbohydrate varies from 154 g/1000 kcal in Flexical® to 206 to 226 g/1000 kcal in Vivonex® and Precision.® In Vivonex® and Vivonex HN® 90.20% and 80.90%, respectively, of the calories are provided by carbohydrates but in Flexical® it is 61.00%, Precision LR® 83.00%, and Precision HN® 74.00%. The type of carbohydrate is either glucose, sucrose, or complex oligosaccharides. The presence of a large amount of glucose increases the osmolality of the preparations and may be troublesome if administered to a patient with diabetes mellitus.

The mineral, trace element and vitamin content of elemental diets is shown in Table 3. In some formulas, several vitamins such as folic acid, vitamin A, niacin, thiamin and riboflavin are present in inadequate amounts, and supplements may be required. Levels

Table 3
MINERAL, TRACE ELEMENT, AND VITAMIN CONTENT OF ELEMENTAL DIETS (per 100 kcal)

	Recommended daily intake						
	Male	Female	Vivonex®	Vivonex HN®	Flexical®	Precision LR®	Precision HN®
Sodium (mg)	1100—3300	1100—3300	860	771	350	632	933
Potassium (mg)	1875—5625	1875—5625	1170	702	1250	789	876
Chloride (mg)	1700—5100	1700—5100	1803	1858	1000	1000	1133
Calcium (mg)	800	800	445	267	600	526	333
Phosphorus (mg)	800	800	445	267	500	526	333
Iron (mg)	10	18	5.6	3.3	9.0	9.5	6.0
Magnesium (mg)	300	300	194	117	200	211	134
Zinc (mg)	15	15	6.9	4.2	10.0	7.9	5.0
Copper (mg)	2—3	2.0—3.0	1.1	0.7	1.0	1.1	0.7
Manganese (mg)	2—5	2—5	1.6	0.9	2.5	2.1	1.3
Selenium (mg)	0.05—0.20	0.05—0.02	2	1.6	28	164	294
Iodine (mg)	150	150	80	48	75	79	50
Vitamin A (IU)	5000	4000	2778	1667	2500	2632	1667
Vitamin D (IU)	400	400	222	233	200	211	133
Vitamin E (IU)	15	12	17	10	23	16	10
Vitamin K (μg)	70—140	70—140	37	22	125	—	—
Ascorbic acid (mg)	60	60	39	23	150	47	30
Folic acid (μg)	400	400	56	33	200	211	134
Vitamin B12 (μg)	3.0	3.0	2.8	1.7	7.5	3.2	2.0
Riboflavin (mg)	1.7	1.3	0.7	0.4	2.2	1.4	0.9
Thiamine (mg)	1.4	1.2	0.7	0.4	1.9	1.2	0.75
Niacin (mg)	18	13	7.4	4.4	25.0	10.5	6.7
Pyridoxine (mg)	2.0	2.0	1.1	0.7	2.5	1.6	1.0
Choline (mg)			86	51	250	53	33
Biotin (mg)	0.3	0.3	0.1	0.06	0.15	0.16	0.10
Pantothenic acid (mg)	14	14	5.6	3.3	12.15	5.3	3.3

of some trace elements and minerals are lower than recommended amounts in some elemental diets, and an adequate intake may only be attained if full dose schedules are achieved. Little is known about the requirements of minerals, trace elements, and vitamins in various disease states, and it is highly probable that increased quantities are necessary. Adequate nonitoring of mineral, trace element, and vitamin status is required in disease states before and during elemental diet therapy is started. These aspects are further discussed in this chapter.

The recommended nonprotein energy to nitrogen ratio is about 200:1. Nonprotein energy to nitrogen ratios vary from 150:1 in Vivonex HN® to 278:1 in Flexical® and 306:1 in Vivonex® standard.

The osmolarity of elemental diets depends upon the formulation, dilution, and flavoring. The range of osmolarities is shown in Table 1. Osmolarity is important in relation to diet administration. Tolerance of diet therapy depends to a large extent on osmolarity, especially the osmolar load delivered per unit of time. The osmolarity depends upon the carbohydrate and nitrogen sources — diets containing more and smaller molecules have higher osmolarities. Osmolarity is also altered by the use of flavoring agents, flavored preparations being more hypertonic than unflavored ones. The pH is also altered by the addition of flavorings, and ranges from 3.8 to 5.6.

III. CRITICAL ASSESSMENT OF ELEMENTAL DIET FORMULATIONS

A. Nutritional Efficacy

The initial experimental synthetic diets studied by Winitz and his colleagues were shown to maintain normal nutritional status in normal subjects over several months. It was demonstrated in these studies that 1.18 ft ^{3} of diet (2.7 calories/mℓ) will provide a 70 kg man with his requirements of essential and nonessential nitrogen, mineral salts, vitamins, and fat in addition to approximately 3000 calories per day and about 25% of his requirements of water for a period of one month. A diet of similar type (Vivonex)® was used successfully in phenylketonuric children with mental retardation; satisfactory weight gains and height increases with maintenance of adequate nutritional status was achieved over periods of up to 18 months.[12,13] In these studies, 1700 calories were provided daily, whereas in the studies of Winitz and his colleagues, the daily caloric intake varied from 2300 to 3400 calories. An elemental diet with a different composition — similar to that of Flexical® — was shown to maintain weight and nutritional parameters over a 12-day period in normal human volunteers.[14]

Another study has confirmed the capacity of an elemental diet to maintain normal nutritional state.[15] In this study, the nitrogen was derived from a hydrolysate of crude protein. The diets used were calculated to contain a minimal basic daily nitrogen requirement. The authors rightly emphasize that the period of adaptation required to achieve a positive nitrogen balance and other changes on an elemental diet as sole nutrition was much longer than was anticipated. This observation is important, and many of the studies reported using elemental diets, especially those studying physiological parameters, may not have administered the elemental diet for long enough to allow changes to occur.

There is now much information in the literature confirming the nutritional efficacy of the commercially available formulations of elemental diets in normal subjects, providing that the subject ingests the recommended amounts of the diet. The efficacy of elemental diets in correcting the catabolic response in various disease states depends on the severity of the nutritional deficiency which is present and the ability of the patient to ingest adequate amounts of the elemental diet. For this to be properly determined in any individual patient, a full basic nutritional assessment must be performed and monitoring continued during the course of treatment. There are few data on the degree of improvement of nutritional status in patients with nutritional deficiency which can be achieved by the use of elemental diets. They are useful in patients in whom the alimentary tract is functioning reasonably adequately and may be used for nutritional purposes as a supplement to normal food or other forms of enteral nutrition. There is no evidence to suggest that elemental diets are better than normal food in healthy individuals. It is unlikely that elemental diets alone, of whatever formulation, will be able to correct severe nutritional insufficiency. In such patients i.v. nutrition is likely to be the most effective form of therapy. Complete oral liquid diets or blenderized foods taken orally or by nasogastric tube may be as effective as elemental diets in improving the nutritional status of patients with some degree of nutritional insufficiency and are more palatable. They are also cheaper than both elemental diets and i.v. feeding. A number of studies have now been reported which indicate that effectiveness of complete liquid diets and blenderized foods in improving the nutritional state of patients, and these forms of enteral nutrition will be further discussed in Chapter 19.

B. Absorption of Elemental Diets

By definition, elemental diets are efficiently absorbed in the upper GI tract without the requirements of full digestive processes. Their formulations have thus been devised with the aim of providing nutrients which are readily assimilated. Early studies on elemental diets indicated that this was achieved satisfactorily,[1,2,14] and the maintenance or improvement of nutritional parameters implies good absorption of nutrients.

There have been few direct small intestinal absorption studies performed using elemental diets. Studies of absorption using the techniques of small intestinal perfusion are of importance in the study of nutrient absorption from elemental diets, not only in normal subjects but in disease states where intestinal absorption may be impaired. The high osmolality of many elemental diet preparations may also influence absorption. This aspect has been studied in pigs by perfusing the jejunum with Vivonex® at standard flow rates over a 75-min period.[16] Net secretion of water and electrolytes occurred in the test segment, whereas perfusion with an isotonic solution containing a higher concentration of sodium resulted in net absorption in the same segment. Glucose oligosaccharides in the elemental diet enhanced net water and electrolyte absorption compared with mannitol in the control solution. Active sugar transport stimulates sodium and water absorption, and the presence of amino acids in this formulation might also have been expected to stimulate sodium absorption; this was not demonstrated in the study, possibly due to the presence of low concentrations of sodium and amino acids in the perfusate. The importance of composition and osmolality is emphasized in these results, the latter confirming that a solution of high osmolality causes net secretion of water and electrolytes. When solutions of high osmolality are used, a concentration and rate of administration should be used which will avoid this problem and lead to better nutrient absorption.

A comparison of intestinal absorption of nutrients from isocaloric amounts of Vivonex HN®, Flexical®, Precision LR® and blenderized foods has been reported in a patient with short bowel syndrome.[17] The diets were administered by nasogastric tube at constant flow rates; net secretion occurred with Vivonex HN® and Precision LR® but not with Flexical®. Fat absorption of 61% of 87 g occurred from Flexical® and 60% from 108 g from the blenderized food preparation; Vivonex HN® and Precision LR® have very small quantities of fat. Vivonex HN® led to the highest retention of nitrogen (84% of 16.3 g), compared with 78% of 91.1 g from Flexical®. It was suggested from this study that in patients with normal pancreatico-biliary function, diets based on fat and protein hydrolysate may be the elemental diet of choice.

In more recent studies, the absorption of nutrients from Vivonex® was compared with that from a whole protein liquid meal in normal healthy subjects.[18,19] The liquid meal contained meat, egg-yolk powder, soy flour, glucose, saccharose, maltose, dextrin, maltose, corn, and wheat oil. Carbohydrate absorption increased in proportion to the quantity of carbohydrates perfused, but decreased in distal intestinal segments. Nitrogen was absorbed in the proximal intestine in proportion to the quantity perfused, but absorption decreased in the distal small intestine. Absorption of nutrients was similar for the elemental and nonelemental diet, and, for a constant amount of nutrients, was found to be independent of the osmolarity of the perfused solutions. As elemental diets have been recommended as nutrition in the short bowel syndrome, the length of intestine required for their absorption is of interest. The rate of gastric emptying is an important limiting step in intestinal absorption, and elemental and complete oral (whole protein) liquid diets are about equally assimilated in this respect. Relatively short lengths of intestine are required for adequate absorption of soluble proteins, and 60 to 75% of proteins are hydrolyzed 20 cm into the proximal jejunum. This absorption is largely dependent on slow and controlled gastric emptying. There is no adequate information on the length of intestine over which elemental diets are absorbed in normal subjects, and there are no comparative data with whole protein liquid diets or other forms of enteral nutrition.

Adequate absorption does occur from elemental diets, but further direct nutrient absorption studies are required to assess intestinal absorption from elemental diets and complete oral liquid (nonelemental) feeds, both in normal human subjects, and more particularly, in disease states when impaired intestinal absorption may be present. It is not likely that elemental diets are absorbed more easily than ordinary foods or whole protein liquid diets, except in special disease states such as pancreatic exocrine deficiency. It is possible, however, that because of delayed gastric emptying, ingested solid or whole protein meals may be absorbed more slowly than elemental diets, but not necessarily over a longer length of bowel. The effect of osmolarity and the influence of other components of the diet on the absorption of individual nutrients requires to be further studied in health and in various disease states.

C. Comparison of Elemental Diet Formulations

The energy distribution of elemental diets varies considerably (Table 4). Vivonex® and Vivonex HN® derived 80 to 90% of their energy from carbohydrate, Precision LR® and HN 74.83% and Flexical® 61%. The recoemnended level is 55 to 70%. Vivonex® and Precision® preparations derive a very low percentage of energy from fat (less than 1.5%), whereas 30% of energy in Flexical® comes from fat (recommended level 20 to 30%). Energy from protein source is 8 to 9% in Vivonex®, Flexical®, and Precision LR® (higher in HN preparations), the recommended level being 10 to 15%. From these energy distribution figures. Flexical® would appear to be the best balanced elemental diet formulation.

One study has compared the absorption and utilization of Vivonex®, Flexical®, and Precision LR®.[9] A randomized crossover design of study was used in 10 normal volunteer subjects who consumed isocaloric amounts of each diet for 10 days. Stool weight and frequency, nitrogen balance, fecal fat, ash, and moisture were determined. The stool weight on Vivonex® (43 g/day) was significantly less than on Precision LR®. (64 g/day; $p<0.01$) but not different from Flexical® (52 g/day). There was an average of one bowel movement every 2.5 days on Vivonex,® one every 1.9 days on Flexical® and one every 1.6 days on Precision LR®. The total 10-day stool weight was significantly less with Vivonex® (431 ± 1.37 g) compared with Precision LR® (639 ± 2.93 g; $p<0.01$). All subjects exhibited negative nitrogen balance during each of the experimental periods. The nitrogen intake during the Vivonex® period was significantly less than on the other

Table 4
ENERGY DISTRIBUTION IN ELEMENTAL DIETS

	Energy distribution— % of total energy supply		
	Protein	**Fat**	**Carbohydrate**
Recommended distribution	10—15	20—30	55—70
Vivonex®	8.20	1.30	90.20
Vivonex HN®	17.20	0.78	80.96
Flexical®	9.00	30.00	61.00
Precision LR®	8.80	0.50	83.00
Precision HN®	15.10	0.40	74.00

two diets ($p<0.05$), but there were no statistically significant differences in either the amount of nitrogen excreted or in the difference between intake and output. During the Vivonex® period the subjects excreted an average of 23.5 g nitrogen more than they ingested, on Flexical® they excreted 15.8 g more than they ingested, and on Precision LR® 14.5 g more than ingested. There were, however, no significant differences in stool frequency, fecal fat, ash, moisture or in nitrogen balance. The conclusion was that there were no marked differences in the parameters studied in each subject on the different elemental diets, and that the selection of these diets should be based on their particular composition, properties, and palatability. They appear to be equally effective in their nutritional support, although it should be remembered that this study was performed in normal subjects, and only over a 10-day period.

Another study comparing the responses of normal human adults maintained solely on two liquid formula diets and a commercial elemental diet (Vivonex®) has also been reported.[20] Twelve subjects received the diets as their sole source of energy using three experimental periods of 7 days, each arranged at random. The nitrogen balance was + 1.29 g and + 1.13 g on the liquid formula diets, but — 0.68 g nitrogen per day on the Vivonex®. Fecal transit time was markedly increased and fecal fat reduced on the elemental diet. It is possible that an inadequate time course was studied in these investigations as it is now realized that some time (at least 10 days) must be allowed after dietary change is made for the full effects to become apparent.

Although it would appear that all the commercially available elemental diets are nutritionally adequate in normal human subjects, they may be inadequate in the presence of marked nutritional deficiency. It is likely that there is no marked difference in the overall nutritional efficacy of individual diets, even in patients who are nutritionally depleted, provided that the recommended amounts of the diet are administered. The individual formulation to be used will depend not so much on the presence of nutritional deficiency but on other factors in relation to the causation of the disease process, or for other specific purposes especially in GI diseases. The individual formulations of the various elemental diets does, however, merit further consideration.

1. Protein

The amounts of essential amino acids expressed as g/1000 kcal or percentage of total protein in chemically defined diets meet the recommended requirements. The requirements for normal subjects, however, may be somewhat less than in chronic disease states, especially in those in which there may be protein loss either from the alimentary tract or the renal tract. The different ways in which protein is presented in elemental diets is of considerable interest and importance. Amino acids in the diets are derived from synthetic l-amino acids in Vivonex® and Vivonex HN®, hydrolyzed casein with tryptophan, tyrosine, and methionine in Flexical® and from egg albumin in Precision®. The ideal form of protein presentation in chemically defined diets, needs to be established, but there is evidence to suggest that a major part of absorption of protein occurs not as free amino acids but as di- and tripeptides.[21,22] It would appear that absorption of some amino acids may be initially faster when presented to the mucosa as di- and tripeptides rather than as free amino acids,[23,24] although normal human subjects do seem to be capable of assimilating orally administered mixtures of amino acids and peptides with equal efficiency, although at different rates initially. Secretion of fluid appears to be less after ingestion of a peptide meal. Not all peptide mixtures are superior to amino acids mixtures in respect to speed of α amino nitrogen assimilation and stimulation of sodium and water absorption.[25] Further work is required on this subject, particularly in disease states, especially those with GI pathology.

2. Fat

Vivonex® and Precision® contain only small quantities of fat. In Vivonex® it is in the form of safflower oil, but in Precision® and in Flexical® there are monoglycerides, diglycerides, and medium chain triglycerides. Mono- and diglycerides assist in holding fat particles in a finely stabilized suspension. Medium chain triglycerides are absorbed directly into the portal system, thus minimizing the requirement for mixed micelle formation and lipolysis, and also the need for subsequent reesterification of fat in the mucosal epithelial cells and transport by the lymphatic system. Although some formulas contain only small amounts of fat, there are adequate amounts of the essential fatty acid linoleic acid. The required intake of essential fatty acids to prevent deficiency is 1 to 2% of total calories.[26] However, essential fatty acid deficiency has been reported in healthy volunteers fed an elemental diet,[27] although adequate intake of the diet may not have been achieved. There are possible advantages in some disease states in the use of a chemically defined diet with a low fat content, and this will be discussed in Section III. Selection of an elemental diet on the basis of the amount and type of fat will depend upon the indication for the diet in individual patients.

3. Carbohydrate

The percentage of energy derived from carbohydrate in commercially available elemental diets differs considerably. This varies from 61% (Flexical®), to 74 to 83% (Precision®) and 80 to 90% (Vivonex®). The recommended percentage of energy derived from carbohydrate is 55 to 70, and only Flexical® is within this range. A high carbohydrate content may be troublesome in that the osmolarity of the diet is increased, possibly resulting in diarrhea or dumping. A high carbohydrate content may also be contraindicated if the diet is used in patients with chronic pancreatitis, who may have diabetes mellitus.

4. Electrolytes, Minerals, Trace Elements, and Vitamins

All elemental diet formulations contain adequate amounts of electrolytes, although it is to be noted that Vivonex® and Vivonex HN® contain considerably more sodium than Flexical®.

Although a full range of minerals, trace elements, and vitamins are present in elemental diets, some levels fall below recommended concentrations. Full dose schedules need to be achieved to avoid potential deficiencies. This may be of considerable practical importance in chronic disease states with nutritional deficiency, when deficiencies of trace elements, minerals, and vitamins are common. It is possible that deficiencies may not be corrected adequately, or even develop, during elemental diet therapy. Deficiencies depend on the underlying disease state, the degree of nutritoinal deficiency, the duration of elemental diet therapy, and whether it is used as a supplement to normal food or as a complete diet in itself. Baseline levels must be measured, and regular monitoring performed during treatment.

In one recent study the selenium content of a number of elemental diets was compared.[28] The amount of selenium depends upon the protein source. Diets containing egg albumin had the highest selenium levels (0.292 to 0.620 μ/g) but the presence of large amounts of N in the product does not guarantee a high selenium concentration. This Vivonex® was found to contain less than 0.005 μg/g dry weight. It is suggested that selenium may be lost during the manufacture of these products.

In some formulations vitamin A, niacin, riboflavin, thiamin, and folic acid are present in concentrations somewhat less than the normal amount recommended, based on normal daily intake of the diet. Vitamin K is absent from Precision LR® and Precision HN® and hypoprothrombinemia may occur during long-term therapy with this type of product.

IV. CONCLUSIONS

There are considerable differences in the formulations of elemental diets. All, however, appear to have adequate nutritional efficacy in normal subjects for short-term treatment as sole source of nutrition, or as supplements to normal food, although they may be inadequate in subjects with moderate or severe nutritional deficiency. The problem in such patients is compounded by the relative unpalability of elemental diets, and administration by nasogastric tube is used widely. More information is required on the utilization of nutrients in various disease states so that better formulations may be developed. Further data are also needed on the absorption of nutrients from various elemental diets, in normal subjects and in disease states, how absorption is altered by different osmolalities, and how the absorption of individual nutrients is altered by the composition of the diet.

There may be a relative deficiency of minerals, trace elements, and vitamins in some elemental diet formulations, which may be of considerable importance if the diets are used as the sole source of nutrition over a period of time, especially in some chronic disease states (especially GI disease) in which deficiencies of these substances may be a common feature.

When elemental diets are used in any individual patient, the formulation selected should be one which is likely to be most beneficial to the individual patient and his disease state. The regime should be carefully planned by the clinician and full cooperation of nurses, dietitians, and patient sought. A complete baseline nutritional screen is required in all subjects, together with regular nutritional monitoring throughout the period of therapy so as to plan dose schedules correctly, and avoid trace element, mineral, and vitamin deficiency.

REFERENCES

1. **Winitz, M., Seedman, D. A., and Graff, J.,** Studies in metabolic nutrition employing chemically defined diets. I. Extended feeding of normal human adult males, *Am. J. Clin. Nutr.*, 23, 525, 1970.
2. **Winitz, M. and Adams, R. F.,** Chemically-defined diets — a new approach to metabolic nutrition, in *Balanced Nutrition and Therapy*, Lang, K., Fekl, W., and Berg, G., Eds., Thieme, Stuttgart, 1971, 46.
3. **Bounous, G., Sutherland, C., McArdle, A. H., and Gurd, R. N.,** The prophylactic use of an elemental diet in experimental haemorrhagic shock and intestinal ischaemia, *Ann. Surg.*, 166, 312, 1967.

4. **Weber, H. U.**, Comparison of commercially available elemental and low residue diets, *Voeding*, 6, 330, 1974.
5. **Bury, K. D., Stephens, R. V., Cha., C., and Randall, H. T.**, Chemically defined diets, *Can. J. Surg.*, 17, 124, 1974.
6. **Young, E. A., Heulen, N., Russell, P., and Weser, E.**, Comparative nutritional analyses of chemically defined diets, *Gastroenterology*, 69, 1338, 1975.
7. **Bury, K. D.**, The use of elemental diets, in *Current Concepts in Parenteral Nutrition*, Greep, J. M., Soeters, P. B., Wesdrop, C. W. R., Fischer, J. E., Eds., Martinus Nijhoff Medical Division, The Hague, Netherlands, 1977, 243.
8. **Lipman, A. G.**, Fibre-free semi-synthetic liquid diets, *Mod. Med.*, 44, 99, 1976.
9. **McCamman, S., Beyer, P. L., and Rhodes, J. B.**, A comparison of three defined formula diets in normal volunteers, *Am. J. Clin. Nutr.*, 30, 1655, 1977.
10. **Rose,W. C.**, Amino acid requirements of man, *Fed. Proc.*, 8, 546, 1949.
11. **Rose, W. C. and Wixom, R. L.**, The amino acid requirements of man. XVI. The role of the nitrogen intake, *J. Biol. Chem.*, 217, 997, 1955.
12. **McKean, C. M.**, Growth of phenylketonuric children on chemically defined diets, *Lancet*, 1, 148, 1970.
13. **McKean, C. M.**, Effects of a totally synthetic low phenylalanine diet on adolescent phenylketonuric patients, *Arch. Dis. Child.*, 46, 608, 1971.
14. **Perrault, J., Devroede, G., and Bounous, G.**, Effects of an elemental diet on healthy volunteers, *Gastroenterology*, 64, 569, 1973.
15. **Duke, J. H., Jr., Amen, R. J., Beigler, M. A., Spiller, G. A., and Saperstein, S.**, Physiological effects of defined formula diets based on hydrolysates and intact protein, *Z. Ernahrungsiviss. Suppl.*, 20, 38, 1977.
16. **Katz, L. and Hamilton, J. R.**, Response of the young pig to intrajejunal perfusion with a hypertonic nutrient solution, *J. Pediatr.*, 87, 606, 1975.
17. **Sinko, V., and Linscheer, W. G.**, Absorption of different elemental diets in a short bowel syndrome lasting 15 years, *Dig. Dis.*, 21, 419, 1976.
18. **Vidon, P., Hecketsweiler, P., Cortot, A., and Bernier, J. J.**, Etude de l'absorption d'une solution nutritive elementaire sous perfusion jejunale continue influence du debit et de la concentration sur l'absorption des nutriments, *Gastroenterol. Clin. Biol.*, 1, 257, 1977.
19. **Hecketsweiler, P., Vidon, N., Emouts, P., and Bernier J. J.**, Absorption of elemental and complex nutritional solutions during a continuous jejunal perfusion in man, *Digestion*, 19, 213, 1979.
20. **Kies, C. and Fox, H. M.**, Orally-administered liquid formula and elemental diets as a sole source of nutrition for normal human adults, *Fed. Proc.*, 35, 261P, 1976.
21. **Matthews, D. M.**, Intestinal absorption of peptides, *Physiol. Rev.*, 55, 537, 1975.
22. **Matthews, D. M.**, Absorption of peptides by mammalian intestine, in *Peptide Transport in Protein Nutrition*, Matthews, D. M., Payne, J. W., Associated Scientific, Amsterdam, 1975, 61.
23. **Silk, D. B. A., Clark, M. L., Marrs, T. C., Addison, J. M., Boston, D., Matthews, D. M. , and Clegg, K. M.**, Jejunal absorption of an amino acid mixture assimilating casein and enzyme hydrolysate of casein prepared for oral adiministration to normal, *Br. J. Nutr.*, 33, 95, 1975.
24. **Silk, D. B. A., Chung, Y. C., Berger, K. L., Conley, K., Beigler, M., Sleisenger, M. H., Spiller, G. A., and Kim, Y. S.**, Comparison of oral feeding of peptide and amino acid meals to normal human subjects, *Gut*, 20, 291, 1979.
25. **Silk, D. B. A., Fairclough, P. D., Clark, M. L., Hegarty, J. E., Marrs, T. C., Addison, J. M., Burston, D., Clegg, K. M., and Matthews, D. M.**, Use of a peptide rather than free amino acid nitrogen source in chemically defined "elemental" diets, *J. Parent. Ent. Nutr.*, 4, 348, 1980.
26. Committee on Dietary Allowances, Food and Nutrition Board, National Research Council Recommended Dietary Allowances, Washington D.C., National Academy of Sciences, 1975, 50.
27. **Wene, J., Connor, W. E., and Denbesten, L.**, Essential fatty acid deficiency in healthy man fed fat-free diet intravenously and orally, *Clin. Res.*, 21, 890, 1973.
28. **Zabel, N. L., Harland, J., Gormican, A. T., and Ganther, H. E.**, Selenium content of commercial formula diets, *Am. J. Clin. Nutr.*, 31, 850, 1978.

Chapter 8

PROPERTIES AND METABOLIC EFFECTS

R. I. Russell

TABLE OF CONTENTS

I. INTRODUCTION

It is the purpose of this chapter to assess the basic properties of elemental diets. Because of their unusual and specific composition, and their effects on metabolic and physiological functions in the body (particularly in the gastrointestinal tract) they need to be studied. These aspects will be considered so that the full pattern of properties of elemental diets together with their physiological effects on the body can be fully explored. Thereafter, the importance of these properties and effects in relation to their clinical applications will be considered in Section III.

II. PROPERTIES OF ELEMENTAL DIETS

On the basis of extensive initial studies, the principal characteristics of elemental diets have now been defined.[1,2] These properties and other physiological effects have been reviewed in a number of recent papers.[3-13]

A. Nutritional Efficacy

The nutritional efficacy of elemental diets has been considered in Chapter 7. These diets are able to maintain normal nutritional status in normal subjects and may be helpful in improving the nutritional state of patients with a degree of nutritional deficiency. However, in patients with severe nutritional insufficiency or with alimentary failure, it is unlikely that elemental diets or any other form of enteral nutrition will be able to improve the nutritional state of the patient. In such individuals, intravenous nutrition may be necessary.

B. Minimal Digestion Requirements

It is a basic characteristic of elemental diets that they require minimal digestion and are almost totally absorbed in the upper small intestine, leaving only minimal residue in the distal small intestine and colon.[14,15] Considerations of the requirements for digestion and the absorption of elemental diets are assessed in Chapter 7. They are effective in providing dietary components in a readily assimilable form.

C. Reduced Fecal Bulk

Elemental diets contain no indigestible bulk or fibrous material and their use thus leads to a considerable reduction in GI bulk. The average stool weight is greatly reduced, the stools contain less solid matter, and frequency of elimination is decreased.

D. Reproducibility of Composition and Water Solubility

Chemically defined diets have a uniform and reproducible composition. They are water-soluble, thus allowing their administration in liquid form which may be given by nasogastric of nasoduodenal tube. Their uniform and reproducible nature also allows the establishment of stable conditions which may be suitable for metabolic studies.

E. Good Storage Capacity

Elemental diets have good storage capacity, and can be kept for up to 12 months in a dry state without appreciable deterioration when kept below 60°F. When made into solution, they need to be kept refrigerated and should be used within a few hours.

The effect of elemental diets on the following metabolic and physiological functions, particularly within the GI tract, need to be assessed in greater detail:

- Gastric secretion and emptying
- Small intestinal structure and function
- Bile acid metabolism
- Pancreatic exocrine secretion
- Lipids and blood pressure
- Immunological and hypoallergenic effects
- Bacteriology of the GI tract. The effect of chemically defined diets on the bacteriology of the GI tract is important and is considered in Chapter 9.

III. GASTRIC EMPTYING AND SECRETION

The mode of administration of elemental diets may vary. They may be given orally, or introduced directly in to the alimentary tract by tube, either intragastrically or intraduodenally. They may be given in the form of a bolus taken either orally or introduced via an intragastric or intraduodenal tube, or administered continuously.

It is thus relevant to determine the effect of the various formulations of elemental diets on both gastric emptying and gastric secretion.

A. Effect of Normal Components of Food on Gastric Emptying and Gastric Secretion

1. Gastric Emptying

Factors involved in influencing gastric emptying have been the subject of studies by Hunt and his colleagues.[16,17] They found that gastric emptying was influenced by the presence of sugars, long chain fatty acids, hydrogen ions, and some specific amino acids in the gastric lumen or the duodenum. It has been postulated that they may activate receptors which respond to osmotic pressure, hydrogen ion concentration, amino acids and the chain length of lipids, thus allowing only a specific amount of calories to enter the small intestine in a certain time.

The effects of carbohydrates on gastric emptying was studied by Elias et al.[18] who demonstrated a slowing of gastric emptying in test meals containing monsaccharides and disaccharides. Slowing of gastric emptying by amino acids has also been demonstrated,[19] and a relationship between the chain length of fatty acids and the slowing of gastric emptying was further investigated by the same authors.[20]

The effect of five amino acids on gastric emptying has been studied in normal volunteer subjects.[21] The amino acids were given in the form of test meals containing varying concentrations of the amino acids. They were introduced directly into the stomach by means of an intragastric tube. It was found that all the amino acids studied in concentrations of 0.2 *M* delayed emptying significantly. The delay in gastric emptying was related to the molar concentration of the amino acid in the test meal rather than to the molecular weight of the amino acid or to the amount of gastric acid secreted. These results are of significance in relation to elemental diets containing individual amino acids

It was noted in this study that glucose on a molar basis caused roughly the same delay in gastric emptying as the amino acid test meals. It has also been demonstrated that glycine and glucose have similar effects on gastric emptying when compared on an osmolar basis.[22]

2. Gastric Secretion

Food of course, is the normal physiological stimulus for acid secretion, and ingestion of a meal rich in protein produces high acid secretion. Protein digestion products stimulate oxyntic cell secretion. Little specific information is available on the effect of individual amino acids on gastric acid secretion, but in one study it was found that glycine and 1-alanine caused a greater increase in gastric acid response than the other amino acids studied, although this tended to decrease with increasing concentration. These two amino acids are potent liberators of the hormone gastrin.[23] Intraduodenal fat (and i.v. fat) has been shown to be a potent inhibitor of i.v. amino acid stimulated gastric acid secretion,[24] and inhibition of acid secretion by i.v. fat occurs without changes in serum cholecystokinin or gastrin. This study suggests that circulating as well as alimentary lipid may be an important regulator of acid secretion in man, the results having implications for both elemental and i.v. nutrition. This is also of considerable relevance to the composition and clinical uses of elemental diets. However, further information is required regarding the effect of individual components of food on gastric acid secretion in the normal human subject.

B. The Effect of Elemental Diets on Gastric Emptying and Secretion

1. Gastric Emptying

The effect of the elemental diets Vivonex® and Flexical® on gastric emptying in normal human volunteers was investigated in one study.[25] Two volumes of four test meals were used, the meals being introduced by bolus into the stomach by means of a nasogastric tube. The test meals consisted of Vivonex®, Flexical®, blenderized food, and water. Each meal was given in two volumes — 300 mℓ and 600 mℓ. Gastric emptying was determined by the method of George,[26] and gastric acid secretion was also studied. This method of measuring gastric emptying involves a double-sampling test meal technique, is practical, avoids cumulative error, but allows serial measurements to be made as the stomach empties. It is best used with fluid test meals. The blenderized whole food diet was also fluid and hypertonic, and had a fat, protein, and carbohydrate composition similar to that of the elmental diets. The main difference, however, was that the elemental diets contained pure 1-amino acids (Vivonex®) and hydrolyzed casein with 1-amino acids (Flexical®) as their nitrogen source whereas the blenderized meal contained whole egg protein. The results indicated that both the elemental diets delayed gastric emptying compared with the control diet, but there were no significant differences in the degree of gastric emptying induced by the two elemental diets. The calculated final emptying times were 30 to 60 min longer than the documented emptying times for normal diets. It was noted that there was no further delay in gastric emptying when fat was present in the test meal. Slowing of gastric emptying by fat is well documented but depends on the presence of long-chain fatty acids. In Flexical®, fat is present principally as medium chain triglycerides and the fat content of Vivonex® is very low indeed. The difference in fat composition between Flexical® and Vivonex® did not result in any difference in gastric emptying time between the two elemental diets. It is possible that the presence of the amino acids in the elemental diet was the principal factor in slowing gastric emptying. This study thus demonstrates that gastric bolus feeding of the elemental diets Flexical® and Vivonex® significantly slows gastric emptying. This suggests that the diets should be ingested by continuous feeding so as to avoid the effect on gastric emptying, and would also favor the direct intraduodenal installation of elemental diets in clinical use.

2. Gastric Secretion

The effect of elemental diets on gastric secretion has been studied both in animals and in man. Using Pavlov pouches in dogs, Rivilis and his colleagues studied the effect of the elemental diet Flexical® on gastric acid secretion, the results being compared with animals given standard control dog feed.[27,28] The day before the diet experiment, the dogs were fed only with the elemental diet, and test meals of the diet were administered on the next three consecutive days in liquid form. Two 15-min collections of gastric juice were made before control and elemental diet tests, and collections subsequently made every 15 min for 3 hr after each feed. The total 3-hr volume output was reduced from a control value (mean ± SEM) of 47.46 mℓ ± 3.23 to 10.07 ± 1.11 ($p<0.002$) and the total 3-hr hydrogen ion output reduced from the control values of 6.17 meq ± 0.50 to 0.71 meq ± 0.15 ($p< 0.001$). The individual volume and hydrogen ion output of comparable 15-min collections were also significantly different. This study thus indicated that the elemental diet Flexical® markedly decreases gastric acid secretion in dogs with Pavlov pouches.

The comparative effect of Vivonex® and Flexical® on gastric acid secretion in man was also studied by Bury and Jambunathan,[25] the results again being compared with test meals containing blenderized food and water. Compared with the blenderized food diet, both elemental diets Vivonex® and Flexical® (300 mℓ and 600 mℓ) significantly reduced the total gastric acid output over the period of the study. No significant difference was noted in the effect of gastric acid output between Vivonex® and Flexical®. The gastric acid measurements in this study (by pH electrode) may not be accurate, as they may be affected by binding of secreted hydrogen ion by the monomeric amino acids.

Although the predigested nature of the elemental diets may be a factor, a reduction in the cephalic phase of secretion may be the principal cause, possibly associated with the relative unpalatability of elemental diets.

C. Conclusions

The elemental diets Vivonex® and Flexical® have both been shown to slow gastric emptying significantly, but to about the same extent. It is probable that the amino acid content of the elemental diet is important in this, rather than the fat content which differs markedly between these two prepartions.

These elemental diets have also been shown to cause a marked decrease of gastric acid secretion, both in animals and in man. The decrease in acid secretion was similar with each elemental diet. To avoid slowing of gastric emptying with possible subsequent adverse effects, direct intraduodenal instillation of elemental diets may be desirable when used clinically in man.

IV. INTESTINAL STRUCTURE AND FUNCTION

The components of elemental diets are absorbed largely in the upper small intestine, without the full requirements of the normal digestive processes. Their absorption is considered in detail in Chapter 7. They have also been postulated as being of value in providing luminal nutrition to the small intestine, and may thus be helpful in the management of the short bowel syndrome when intestinal adaptation is required. The nature of the luminal nutrition provided may be of importance in maintaining normal structure and function of the small intestine. This, however, is only one of many interrelating factors involved in maintaining normal small intestinal structure and function. It is thus important to assess the effect of the various formulations of chemically defined diets on intestinal structure and function.

A. Factors Involved in the Maintenance of Normal Intestinal Structure and Function

Major alterations of diet have been shown to have a profound effect on the small intestine. Thus, fasting decreases epithelial cell size and renewal of the small intestine[29-33] resulting in decrease of small intestinal mass, mitotic index, and villus height.[29,31,34,35] Disaccharidase activity in the small intestinal mucosa is also sensitive to the nature of oral intake.[36-39] Most of the studies reported relate to studies in rats, and marked alterations in the numbers of small intestinal epithelial cells and their renewal have been reported in protein-depleted or starved rats.[33,34] Hyperplasia also leads to alterations in the small intestine.[40] Lack of dietary intake and the probable effect of consequent reduction of normal digestive secretions may lead to atrophy of the small intestine.[41] As fasting and protein deprivation both result in structural and functional damage to the small intestine, it was unclear for some time if the lack of oral intake or the presence of a negative nitrogen balance was responsible for the damage to the small intestine. This problem was resolved to some extent by a study reported by Levine et al.[42] who demonstrated that depriving rats of oral intake while maintaining positive nitrogen balance by i.v. feeding leads to significant decreases in intestinal mass, protein, DNA, and disaccharidase activities; hypoplasia occurred in addition to atrophy. Confirmation that luminal nutrition is necessary to maintain the structural and functional integrity of the normal small bowel was reported in a study aimed primarily at investigating the effect of oral and i.v. nutrition on intestinal adaptation after small intestinal resection.[43]

Further evidence of the importance of luminal nutrition comes from studies in rats in which bypass of small intestinal segments or isolation as separate Thiry-Vella loops leads to atrophy of the intestinal mucosa, and a reduction of intestinal absorptive function.[44-46] There has been little work in man on this particular aspect, and data are needed particularly in view of conflicting reports appearing in the literature — some reporting lack of mucosal atrophy in human small intestine, after jejunoileal bypass surgery for obesity.[47,48] The theory that intraluminal nutrition is important in maintaining small intestinal structure and function demands the presence of food in the small intestine without necessarily implying that the nutrients must be absorbed to exert their effect.[44,49,50] Support for the trophic effect of luminal nutrients is also provided by the absence of morphological or functional adaptation of the small intestine after jejunectomy in rats and dogs receiving i.v. nutrition.[43,51] It has also been suggested that a mechanism based on the functional workload of the epithelium may be a factor rather than the sole presence of intraluminal nutrition, and some evidence favoring this theory has been reported in rats.[52] Further work is required, particularly in man.

Intraluminal nutrition is not the sole factor in the maintenance of adequate small intestinal structure. GI secretions, notably biliary and pancreatic, appear to be important in maintaining normal gut structure and function. Oral intake of food stimulates the flow of bile and pancreatic juice and thus the absence of exogenous nutrients may modify normal small intestinal structure and function by preventing adequate stimulation of these secretions. There is evidence from a number of studies that adaptive hyperplasia following jejunectomy is stimulated, at least in part, by biliary and pancreatic secretions.[46,53-57] Chronic stimulation of pancreatic of biliary secretion by secretin and cholecystokinin has been shown to prevent intestinal hypoplasia in dogs maintained in adequate nutritional state by i.v. feeding.[58]

Neurovascular and hormonal stimuli also have a part to play in the maintenance of intestinal structure and function.[59-62] There has been considerable interest recently in the effect of hormonal stimuli and it is probable that these are of importance in relation to the maintenance of normal small intestinal structure and function, and also in adaptation after intestinal surgery. The subject has recently been extensively reviewed.[63,64] Enteric hormones may be either stimulatory or inhibitory and a balance of these hormones is required for maintenance of normal intestinal structure and function. A variety of hormones is likely to be involved, including gastrin, prolactin, corticosteroids, pituitary hormones, thyroxine, testosterone, enteroglucagon, and others; antitrophic effects have been reported with secretin and vasoactive intestinal polypeptide (VIP). It is also possible that the bacterial content of the intestine has an influence on the maintenance of normal small intestinal structure and function. Differences between germ-free and conventional animals suggest that the bacterial flora of the gut is important in this respect.[65,66]

It is clear therefore that normal small intestinal structure and function is maintained by an interlinking of many factors, one of the most important is the presence of intraluminal nutrients, but also modified by biliary and pancreatic secretions, neurovascular, hormonal, and possibly bacteriological factors.

Many of the same factors also influence the structure of the colon. It has recently been demonstrated in rats that colonic growth is stimulated by the presence of luminal contents, nonabsorbable bulk, and circulating gastrin.[67] As the colon is beyond the influence of "luminal nutrition", other mechanisms must be responsible, but there is a link with a luminal factor. Other interrelated influence similar to those in the small intestine are likely to be involved.

Little information has been available on the specific effect of individual nutrients or combinations of nutrients on intestinal structure and function. The advent of chemically defined diets has stimulated interest in this aspect and indeed the whole subject of the factors involved in luminal nutrition.

B. Effects of Elemental Diets on Intestinal Structure and Function

There have been few published reports to date of studies investigating the effects of various elemental diets on the structure and function of the small intestine. This aspect is of relevance in view of the potential value of elemental diets as intraluminal nutrition in the promotion of intestinal adaptation after surgery.

1. Effects on Intestinal Structure

Much of the information available provides conflicting results which may be related to the widely differing compositions of the diets used and the duration of adminstration. The relationship between structure and function is also unclear. It has been reported that structural changes in the mucosal mitochondria may occur during amino acid absorption,[68] thus suggesting that active absorptive function may alter the mucosal structure per se. The effects of the elemental diets Vivonex® and Flexical® on small intestinal morphology have been studied in normal rats, and jejunal histology examined after 1 or 3 months.[69,70] The body weights of rats receiving the diets were significantly greater than control rats receiving normal rat chow. Crypt height to villus height ratio was significantly lower in rats fed both Vivonex® and Flexical® compared with rats receiving the control diet, the villi being long and thin, but with no marked change in cellular infiltration. (Table 1.) Although rats on Flexical® showed less marked morphological changes than those receiving Vivonex®, the differences were not statistically significant. Cell kinetic studies were not performed in this study, but the appearances did suggest improved survival of the mature enterocyte population: it is noteworthy that changes in the crypt height to villus height ratio similar to those in rats fed an elemental diet were reported in germ-free rats, and 3H thymidine labeling showed increase in villus transit time in germ-free animals.[71] There thus may be reduced cell turnover in rats fed an

Table 1
EFFECT OF VIVONEX® AND FLEXICAL® ON BODY WEIGHTS, LENGTH, AND MORPHOLOGY OF RAT JEJUNUM AND ILEUM (MEAN ± SEM)

		Control group (n = 12)	Vivonex® group (n = 12)	Flexical® group (n = 12)
Initial body weight (g)		162 ± 5	161 ± 6	161 ± 6
Final body weight (g)		370 ± 10	412 ± 10[a]	388 ± 11
Length of small intestine (cm)		128 ± 2	122 ± 2	123 ± 2
Villus height (μm)	Jejunum	394 ± 23	506 ± 21[b]	495 ± 19[b]
	ileum	383 ± 20	531 ± 26[b]	505 ± 17[b]
Crypt height (μm)	Jejunum	117 ± 3	109 ± 5	107 ± 5
	ileum	137 ± 5	117 ± 7[a]	119 ± 5[a]
Crypt height	Jejunum	0.31 ± 0.02	0.22 ± 0.01[b]	0.22 ± 0.11[b]
Jejunal height	ileum	0.36 ± 0.02	0.23 ± 0.02[b]	0.24 ± 0.01[b]

[a] $p<0.05$
[b] $p<0.02$
Significance of difference from control value.

elemental diet, which may be due to alteration of bacterial flora. Hypoplasia with reduced villus height in bypassed loops of dog jejunum was prevented in one study by saline perfusion, and perfusion of Vivonex® was found to increase villus height.[72]

A study comparing Vivonex®, Vivonex HN®, and Flexical® on the mucosal mass of the small bowel in the rat has also been reported.[73] In this study animals were fed isocaloric amounts of the elemental diet (61 kcal/day) by continuous intragastric infusion. All the animals given the defined formula diets gained significant amounts of weight compared with rats given ordinary rat chow. After 2 weeks, the mucosal weight and the DNA were significantly decreased in most bowel segments of rats fed all the elemental diets. No data were reported on the morphology of the intestime in this study, and it was to be noted that the animals only received the elemental diet for a period of 2 weeks before the small intestine was examined. Another short-term study (8 days) has shown reduced crypt height to villus height ratio after Vivonex® although small bowel mass was also reduced. [74] It has been shown that no marked change in morphology of the small intestine occurs in early weeks of treatment with the elemental diet,[70] and these differing results may be related to duration of therapy. There may also be a species difference in that no alteration of small intestinal morphology was reported in mice given Vivonex®.[75]

In a long-term study of a hydrolyzed casein-based elemental diet on the morphology and structure of the small intestine of adult mice, it was found that the absorptive cells of the jejunal villi exhibited a proliferation of the smooth endoplasmic reticulum in the supranuclear region in animals given the elemental diet. After 6 or 12 months of the diet this was no longer observable.[76] It was considered that this proliferation of the smooth endoplasmic reticulum in the absorptive villus cells may be related to the high content of sucrose in the elemental diet used in the study, as similar changes had been found after prolonged use of a fructose diet.[77,78]

Another study investigated the effect of Vivonex® on the intestinal mucosa of rats following jejuno-ileal bypass operations;[79] the results indicated that the elemental diet is capable of stimulating compensatory adaptive changes, but not to any greater extent than a normal diet. Ileal changes have also been reported in rats fed an elemental diet.[70] The crypt height to villus height ratio is reduced in the ileum as well as the jejunum, these being more marked with Vivonex® than with Flexical®. Colonic changes may also occur—a loss of colonic weight and a decline of DNA synethesis has been reported in animals fed an elemental diet.[67]

The differences in the studies reported to date on the effect of elemental diets on the morphology and ultrastructure of the small intestine can probably be explained by the differing types of diets, differing durations of the studies, and possibly species differences. There is evidence, however, that elemental diets of different compositions when given to animals over some weeks and months, do have an effect on the small intestine, reducing crypt height to villus height ratios, producing long thin villi, and possibly reducing cell turnover. Alterations also occur in the colon. Further information is clearly required on the effect of different elemental diets on intestinal morphology, especially in man.

2. *Effects on Intestinal Function*

Changes in small intestinal morphology need not imply changes in function. There is, however, little information on the effect of various elemental diets on absorptive function. Various parameters have been suggested as providing information on the function of the small intestine. These include measurement of enzymes, such as disaccharidases, alkaline phosphatase, and peptidases, specific measurement of intestinal absorption using a perfusion technique, and motility measurements.

a. Enzyme Studies

The measurement of various brush border and cellular enzymes in the small intestine may give an indirect measurement of function of the intestine.[37,42,59] An elemental diet of Flexical® type caused a decrease in the activities of two mucosal dipeptidases,[80] but a more recent study has shown that the response of intestinal peptidase hydrolase activities to elemental diets depends on the nitrogen source and on the particular hydrolase studied.[81] The lack of correlation between peptidase activity (which is markedly influenced by dietary composition) and absorption rates reduces the value of these estimations as an index of intestinal absorptive activity.[82]

The effects of the elemental diets Vivonex® and Flexical® on the activity of alkaline phosphatase, lactase, sucrase, and maltase over 3 months in nornal rat jejunum have also been studied.[69,70] No differences were noted in enzyme activity between control animals and those fed Vivonex® and Flexical® after 3 months for any of the disaccharidases studied, but a statistically significant increase in total alkaline phosphatase activity was noted after 3 nonths of feeding with both chemically defined diets (Table 2). The significance of this observation needs to be determined, but it is noteworthy that increase of disaccharidase and alkaline phosphatase activities have been reported in germ-free rats. [83,84] A more direct indicator of intestinal absorptive capacity is required.

b. Perfusion Studies of Intestinal Absorption

An intestinal perfusion system has been used to study the effect of elemental diet on rat jejunal and ileal function.[85] In this particular study, using a standard gas-lift recirculation method,[86] animals were divided into groups who received either a control diet, Vivonex® or Flexical®. Water absorption was determined with a segmental perfusion system using 14 C polyethylene glycol as a water-soluble marker. After 1-month of treatment with the elemental diets, no significant differences in water and glucose absorption were observed in the Vivonex®-treated group, but significantly less absorption was found in the Flexical® treated rats, compared with control animals both in jejunum and ileum. Jejunal water absorption from 30 to 60 minutes was 77 ± 13 (SEM) $\mu l \cdot cm^{-1}$ in Flexical®-fed rats, which was significantly less than in Vivonex®-fed animals (137 ± 12 $\mu l \cdot cm^{-1}$; $p<0.05$) and in rats fed a normal diet (138 ± 15 $\mu l \cdot cm^{-1}$;

Table 2
EFFECT OF ELEMENTAL DIETS ON ENZYME ACTIVITY IN RAT JEJUNUM (MEAN ± SEM)

	Control group (n = 12)	Vivonex® group (n = 12)	Flexical® group (n = 10)
Protein (mg/cm)	6.57 ± 0.22	6.89 ± 0.28	—
Alkaline phosphatase (munits/cm)	671 ± 27	809 ± 50[a]	744 ± 52
lactase (munits/cm)	116 ± 4	115 ± 13	98 ± 23
sucrase (munits/cm)	589 ± 34	530 ± 39	484 ± 45
maltase (munits/cm)	2.32 ± 0.13	2.35 ± 0.11	2.27 ± 0.16

[a] $p<0.0$ 5— Significance of difference from control value.

$p<0.05$). A similar reduction of water absorption in the ileum was also found in animals fed Flexical® compared to those given Vivonex® and a normal diet. Over this period, the morphology of the jejuman and ileum showed a significant reduction in crypt height to villus height ratio. These morphological changes therefore were not accompanied by a marked change in intestinal absorption at three months.[87] Thus, the morphological changes after Vivonex® did not appear to be accompanied by a significant alteration in intestinal absorptive function. Similar results were reported for the effects of Vivonex® perfusion after Thiry-Vella bypass of the jejunum in the dog.[72] Another study, using a whole bowel perfusion technique in rats fed Vivonex® or Vivonex HN®, reported an increase of glucose and water absorption after 1 week of treatment.[80]

The differences observed in the reported data are probably related to differences in technique, composition of the elemental diet, and duration of dietary therapy. Nutritional demand may be a more important determinant of absorptive function per unit length of intestine than surface area, as indicated by villus height. This would explain the lack of change of absorptive function in the rat jejunum. Further studies are required to investigate the specific effects of particular elemental diets of different compositions on animal and human intestinal morphology and with specific information regarding intestinal function, before any definite conclusions can be drawn.

c. Motility Measurements

The effect of an elemental diet (Flexical®) on electrical activity of the small intestine in dogs has been reported, with the aim of providing information on the effects of the elemental diet on intestinal motility.[88] The electrical activity of the smooth muscle of the small intestine can be monitored to determine the patterns of motility of the bowel. The results from the three dogs studied indicated that the myoelectric activity of the small intestine was significantly greater than in the fasting state. Elemental diets thus do not appear to offer the same degree of bowel rest as indicated by myoelectric activity than can be attained by complete i.v. nutrition.

C. Conclusions

There are data from animal studies that elemental diets, over a period of time, do alter the morphology of the jejunum, ileum, and colon. The balance of evidence favors a reduced crypt height to villus height ratio with the production of long villi and a probable reduction of cell turnover. There is evidence of intestinal adaptation after intestinal resection or bypass, as effective as with normal diet, suggesting a basis for the use of elemental diets in the management of the short bowel syndrome in man. Although some changes in intestinal function also occur, from enzyme measurements and perfusion studies, these do not correlate well with the morphological changes.

The intestinal changes associated with the use of elemental diets seem unrelated to the composition of the elemental diet. Variability in the results of different studies appears to be related to the duration of diet therapy, differences in technique, and species difference. More information is required on the effect of different elemental diets on intestinal structure and function, especially in man. Data are also required on the effect of these diets on factors related to the maintenance of normal intestinal structure and function, notably hormonal and neurovascular factors and the bacteriology of the GI tract.

V. BILE ACID METABOLISM

It is probable that elemental diets have effects on bile acid metabolism. This aspect needs to be studied in view of the potential clinical uses of elemental diets and their effects on the GI tract.

Bile acids are syntesized in the liver and enter the alimentary tract through the biliary duct system after storage in the gallbladder. In the GI tract they are involved in promoting emulsification of lipids, activating lipase, forming mixed micelles with monoglycerides, and free fatty acids, and are also involved in the intracellular reesterification of fatty acids.

The release of bile into the duodenum following gall bladder contraction is related to digestion of food and the nature of the diet itself. The products of digestion influence the extent of gall bladder contraction and thereby the entry of bile acids into the duodenum. It is probable also that the nature of the diet influences bile acid metabolism, ranging from the hepatic synthesis of bile acids to the maintenance of the enterohepatic circulation of bile acids. This has important implications with respect to the effect of chemically defined diets on bile acid metabolism, and the available evidence on this subject is reviewed in this chapter.

A. Factors Involved in the Maintenance of Normal Bile Acid Metabolism

Bile acids are synthesized in the liver from cholesterol, the two primary bile acids being cholic acid and chenodeoxycholic acid. Deoxycholic acid and lithocholic acid are secondary bile acids which are formed in the lumen of the intestine after 7α dehydroxylation by anaerobic intestinal bacteria.[89] Free bile acids do not normally occur in bile, and bile acids are secreted as taurine or glycine conjugates.

The formation of cholic and chenodeoxycholic acid from cholesterol involves a number of changes to the sterol molecule. The first step is the introduction of 7α hydroxyl group into the cholesterol molecule, catalyzed by the enzyme cholesterol 7α hydroxylase (a microsomal mixed-function oxidase requiring cytochrome P450, Na DPH, and oxygen.) This enzyme is the rate-limiting step in bile acid synthesis. Cholesterol synthesis is under the control of a rate-limiting enzyme, HMG CoA reductase. Interruption of the enterohepatic circulation of bile acids causes a rise in bile acid synthesis and cholesterol 7α hydroxylase activity, and the activity of HMG CoA reductase also increases.[90] Bile acid synthesis is under negative feedback control which varies inversely with hepatic bile acid flux.[89,91]

Bile acids undergo an enterohepatic circulation and are thereby effectively conserved. Conjugated bile acids are absorbed in a large part by an active transport mechanism in the terminal ileum, returning to the liver in the portal circulation.[92,93] Small amounts of bile acids, especially unconjugated bile acids and the glycine conjugates of dihydroxy bile acids, are absorbed by passive nonionic diffusion throughout the small intestine.[94] In the liver free bile acids are conjugated with glycine or taurine and secreted into the bile canaliculi by a specific active transport process which has considerable excess capacity.

Bacterial alterations of bile acids occurs under normal circumstances mainly in the colon and distal part of the ileum. The principal modifications are deconjugation and 7α dehydroxylation.[95] The deconjugating enzyme is widely distributed among anaerobic intestinal bacteria such as *Bateroides, Veillonella,* bifido bacteria, and some strains of clostridia.[96,97] The efficiency of intestinal absorption of bile acids thus depends upon the nature of the individual bile acids and the extent of bacterial deconjugation and dehydroxylation; it is also influenced by the rate of intestinal transit,[98] the amount and nature of unabsorbed dietary residue which may bind bile acids,[99] and ileal sphincter function.

The dynamics of the enterohepatic circulation have been extensively studied in recent years. The pool size of bile acids is normally constant and fecal loss is balanced by the synthesis of new bile acids in the liver. In man there is a total bile acid pool of 3 to 5g which circulates six to ten times per day with the daily loss in the feces of 200 to 600 mg. Studies in the Rhesus monkey with controlled interruption of the enterohepatic circulation have shown that 20% interruption can be adjusted for by a ten-fold increase in the hepatic synthesis of bile acids, but greater interruption results in a marked duction in bile acid secretion.[100] Resection or severe damage to the terminal ileum, as in Crohn's disease, results in bile acid malabsorption with a markedly increased turnover. This is compensated for, to some extent, by an increase in hepatic synthesis of bile acids. With large resections, the liver cannot keep pace with increased fecal loss and steatorrhea may occur. Prior to this stage, however, severe watery diarrhea (cholerheic diarrhea) occurs, which has been shown to be due to the effect of dihydroxy bile acids on the colon resulting in water and electrolyte secretion.[101] A number of interrelated factor may affect the metabolism of bile acids. One such factor is the quantity and nature of the diet.

B. Effects of Dietary Alterations on Bile Acid Metabolism

Diets with a high glucose or sucrose content cause a fall in biliary bile salt concentrations and a rise in cholesterol concentration;[102] such diets have been reported to cause cholesterol-rich gall stones in hamsters. The effects are reduced or abolished by substituting uncooked starch for glucose or sucrose.

Fat-free and fiber-free diets also appear to reduce biliary bile salt concentration in animal leading to a rise of cholesterol concentration, resulting in an increased predilection to the development of cholesterol gall stones. Fiber content may be of particular importance as it has been reported that germ-free rats pass carmine markers very slowly on a fiber-free, chemically defined diet, but at a normal rate of a fiber-containing pelleted diet.[103] In this study the half-line of cholic acid was found to be considerably prolonged on the fiber-containing diet in germ-free rats. This suggests that fiber is more important than bacterial flora in determining the fate of bile acids. These authors also reported a reduced fecal bile acid excretion in the rats on the chemically defined diet, in both conventional and germ-free rats.

It has been shown in rats[104] and in rabbits[105] that semisynthetic, low residue diets containing a high proportion of sugar or processed starch result in lower bile acid turnover than is found in animals on oridinary food. It has also been reported in man that a low residue diet results in reduced fecal bile acid excretion compared with individuals on a normal high roughage diet.[106] By adding roughage to the diet a considerable increase in bile acid turnover was demonstrated in rats initially fed on a refined diet.[104,107] Increased fecal bile acid excretion has also been reported in young women on a hypocholesterolemic regime,[108] and the addition of an artificial bulk-forming agent to the diet of young men on normal diet markedly increased fecal bile acid excretion;[109] this has also been reported in rats.[110] It would thus appear that a constant intake of refined, fiber-depleted diets may result in reduced bile acid synthesis and reduced bile acid turnover, and results in reduced fecal bile acid excretion.

C. Effect of Elemental Diets on Bile Acid Metabolism

It would be expected that there would be alterations in bile acid metabolism in animals and man when chemically defined diets are administered as the sole neans of nutritional support. Stephens and Randall[111] reported a patient with pancreatic insufficiency and a biliary fistula in whom the fistula drainage decreased markedly during a 21-day period of treatment with Vivonex®, and the fluid changed from a dark viscous black-green biliary composition to a thin yellowish-green paler material. The same elemental diet, Vivonex®, on being given to three healthy male medical students, resulted in a reduction of fecal steroids and fecal flora in a study reported by Crowther et al.[112] However, in 18 healthy volunteers who were administered an elemental diet of Flexical®-type there was found to be no alteration in the hepatic secretion of bile acids.[113]

Portman and his colleagues[114,115] found that rats eating a semisynthetic, nonelemental diet which was nutritionally complete and allowed normal growth, had a smaller bile acid pool size and lower fecal excretion of bile acids than rats on normal diet. The half-life of labelled cholic acid was prolonged, indicating that the bile acids were being absorbed more efficiently than normal or circulating less frequently. The small pool size and turnover rate implied decreased synthesis of bile acids. Decreased bile acid excretion and prolonged cholate half life was reported in rats on a starch-based semisynthetic diet[104] and similar findings have been reported in rabbits.[105]

A 12% reduction of bile acids in duodenal content was reported after administration of an elemental diet over 3 hr to normal human subjects, compared with an isocaloric, isonitrogenous standard.[116] The effect of elemental diets of different composition on bile acid metabolism in rats has also been studied recently.[117] Three groups of rats were fed Vivonex®, Flexical® or a standard rat diet respectively for three months. Fecal bile acid excretion (median with range) was reduced from 1094 (855-1115) μmol/kg body weight/week in control animals to 541 (407-695) in those given Flexical® ($p < 0.002$) and 207 (126-280) in those given Vivonex® ($p < 0.002$). Cholic acid half-life increased from 2.8 (2.5-3.7) days in control rats to 4.2 (3.3-7.5) days in rats fed Flexical® and 10.5 (8.8-11.6) days in rats fed Vivonex® ($p < 0.03$). A significant increase of liver cholesterol was also noted in the Vivonex®-fed rats. Reduced fecal bile acid excretion during elemental diet feeding does not thus result from a reduced bile acid pool, but reduced turnover of a normal sized pool. Elevation of liver cholesterol reflects reduction of bile acid synthesis. The results of these studies suggest that the low fiber nature of Vivonex® may be more important than its low fat content in reducing fecal bile acid excretion in rats since a similar, although less marked, reduction was found with Flexical® which contains much more fat than Vivonex®. Liver histology in this study showed marked fatty change in five of six rats given Vivonex®, and slight fatty change in five of six rats given Flexical®. It has also been reported that feeding Vivonex® premixed with methylcellulose restores fecal weight to control values.[118] The differences in the fecal excretion of bile acids and cholic acid turnover between rats fed conventional food and elemental diets (especially Vivonex®), are similar to the difference observed between conventional and germ-free rats fed the same diet.[103,119] It is suggested that the bile acids excreted on feeding elemental diets represent a smaller proportion of a normal sized pool rather than reflecting a reduced pool size.

It has been reported that deoxycholic acid is absent from the bile in most patients taking a liquid formula diet although in very few on a solid diet.[120] On transition from solid to liquid diets, the deoxycholic acid content of the bile appears to fall. As deoxycholate is principally produced in the colon under normal conditions, this suggests that there may be reduced entry of bile acids into the colon when a liquid formula diet is given.

The effect of the elemental diet Vivonex® on fecal bile acid excretion has been studied in man. Six patients with cholerhic diarrhea following ileal resection, normal control subjects, and four patients with noncholerheic diarrhea were studied.[121] The total fecal bile acid excretion in the patients with bile acid induced diarrhea was significantly reduced from 6.37 ± 1.64 mmol/24 hr (mean ± SEM) to 2.70 ± 1.12 mmol/24 hr during Vivonex® therapy (see Chapter 12). Similar reductions in man of bile acid output in ileal fistula drainage have been reported in patients treated solely with Vivonex.[122,123]

The factors involved in these changes in bile acid metabolism induced by chemically defined diets need to be further investigated. The diets are low in fiber and high in refined carbohydrate, and it is possible that one factor is a direct effect of rapidly available carbohydrate on hepatic bile acid synthesis. A reduction of bile acid secretion was noted in monkeys by diets with a low fat content[124] and diets with restricted fat and protein content have been shown to reduce the frequency of enterohepatic cycling of bile acids in man.[125] Increase reabsorption of bile acids might result from a reduction of stool residue, prolonged transit time and increased stool alkalinity during ingestion of the elemental diet, or be related to alteration of gut flora.[112,126] The principal factors, however, may, be the low fiber content and the high proportion of readily available carbohydrate.

D. Conclusions

Chemically defined diets alter bile acid metabolism in animals and man. Fecal bile acid excretion is reduced with both Vivonex ® and Flexical®. This suggests that the low fat content is not its most important property in this respect. It is probable that the low fiber content of elemental diets may be an important factor. The high, readily available carbohydrate content may also be important. A reduction of bile acid turnover appears to occur without any change in pool size and reduced bile acid synthesis may occur with elemental diets, although earlier work with semisynthetic, nonelemental diets suggests a reduction of pool size. Further data are needed on the cause of the alterations of bile acid metabolism induced by dietary changes, and especially by the use of elemental diets. The effect of specific dietary composition on hepatic bile acid synthesis and secretion, transit time, stool residue, and alkalinity, GI bacterial activity, and bile acid absorption requires further study. More information is also required on the possible effects of elemental diets in altering biliary lipids. The reduction of fecal bile acid excretion by elemental diets has specific clinical applications in the management of cholerheic diarrhea, and this will be further discussed in Chapter 12.

VI. PANCREATIC EXOCRINE SECRETION

The provision of nutrients in a readily assimilable form with minimal digestive requirements suggests that chemically defined diets may be of value in patients with limited or impaired digestive abilities. The possibility thus arises that these diets may be of value in the management of patients with pancreatic dysfunction. This has led, in turn, to interest in the effect of elemental diets on exocrine pancreatic secretion.

A. Effects of Components of Food on Pancreatic Exocrine Secretion

The secretion of pancreatic enzymes and contraction of gallbladder after the ingestion of food is stimulated by the hormones or cholecystokinin and secretion which are released from the mucosa of the upper small intestine by acid chyme in the duodenum and proximal jejunum. Vagal stimulation and antral gastrin release also play a part.[127,128] It was shown that secretion of pancreatic enzymes can be stimulated in this hormonal system in the dog by certain amino acids, peptone, and fatty acid soaps when infused intraduodenally.[129] Similar investigations have shown increases in intraduodenal concentrations of lipase, amylase, and proteolytic enzymes after the intraduodenal instillation of triglycerides and peptone; dextrose gave a reduced response.[130] Important information was provided about the effect of individual nutrients on the production of pancreatic enzymes in a study by Go et al.[131] Using an intraduodenal perfusion system in healthy volunteer subjects, they studied the effect of isotonic saline, amino acids, micellar fatty acid, and dextrose on exocrine pancreatic secretion. It was found that pancreatic enzyme production was significantly higher in response to a mixture of essential and nonessential amino acids than that produced by micellar fatty acid, and was equivalent to an i.v. injection of cholecystokinin. A sustained secretion of pancreatic enzymes following perfusion with the amino acid mixture was noted during the second hour. Perfusion with essential amino acids produced enzyme outputs equivalent to those induced by the amino acid mixture, but perfusion with non essential amino acids had no effect on pancreatic enzyme production. The essential amino acids were also tested individually but only phenylalanine, methionine, and valine increased pancreatic enzyme secretion significantly. However, pancreatic enzyme output was less in response to these three essential amino acids than to mixtures containing all of them. Trypsin output in response to dextrose fell rapidly after 40 min and in the second hour was no different from that induced by isotonic saline itself. It is to be noted that the amino acids which were most effective in this study were alpha amino monocarboxylic essential acids with an unchanged side chain. These are probably absorbed by the same transport mechanism as cholecystokinin, and are indeed present in the polypeptide chain of cholecystokinin.[132,133]

It would appear from that study that exocrine pancreatic secretion is stimulated by the presence of intraduodenal amino acids. Similar results were reported in man by Ertan et al.[134] using the technique of jejunal amino acid perfusion, and later in animals by Veyer and Grossman.[135]

B. The Effect of Elemental Diets on Pancreatic Exocrine Secretion

A number of workers have studied the effect of the elemental diets Vivonex® and Flexical® on pancreatic exocrine secretion, both in animals and in man. A variety of methods have been used, both in the administration of the diet and in the methods used to assess their effect.

1. Animal Studies

A summary of the results of animal studies is shown in Table 3. The first investigation of elemental diets on pancreatic function was reported in dogs by Bounous et al.[136] They used a homemade chemically defined diet which subsequently formed the basis of the formula of Flexical®. Reduced pancreatic enzyme secretion was found when the dogs were fed the elemental diet solution.

A further study using dogs given an elemental diet containing protein in the form of essential and non essential amino acids (17.12%), fat (medium chain triglycerides 14.22%), and carbohydrate (sucrose and glucose, 57.10%), vitamins and minerals, was reported by Brown et al.[137] These workers reported a decrease in pancreatic trypsinogen in dogs given the elemental diet for 3 days, the levels being less than one third of the values found on a normal diet. Ultrastructural studies showed that pancreatic acinar cell granules were principally in the prezymogen form whereas dogs on a normal diet showed few granules of this type.

Dogs fed Flexical® for 3 days showed a marked reduction of pancratic trypsinogen levels (by over 50%) in the pancreas than animals fed the elemental diet.[138] Although no difference in zymogen granules was found between the two groups on light microscopy,

Table 3
EFFECT OF ELEMENTAL DIETS ON PANCREATIC ENZYME SECRETION IN ANIMALS

Animals	Elemental diet	Route of administration	Effect	Ref.
Dogs	Flexical®	Oral	Inhibits enzyme secretion	136
Dogs		Oral	Inhibits pancreatic trypsinogen	137
Dogs	Flexical®	Oral	Inhibits pancreatic trypsinogen and reduced secretion	138
Dogs	Vivonex®	Intrajejunal Intragastric	Inhibits secretion Stimulates secretion	140
Dogs	Vivonex®	Intraduodenal	Stimulates volume and protein output	142
Dogs	Vivonex®	Oral	Stimulates pancreatic stimulation	144
Dogs	Vivonex®	Oral and intraduodenal	Stimulates protein response — reduced water and bicarbonate production	145
Dogs	Vivonex®	Oral	Stimulates pancreatic stimulation	147
Dogs	Vivonex®	Oral	Inhibits enzyme response	148
Dogs	Flexical® Vivonex®	Oral	Both stimulate enzyme response, least stimulation occurring with Vivonex	150
Rats	Flexical® Vivonex®	Oral	Both inhibit amylase activity in pancreas and reduce serum amylase levels	73

electronmicroscopy showed that in the Flexical®-fed animals, a greater number of storage granules was in the prezymogen form. This study thus appeared to demonstrate a depression of the formation of storage enzymes in the pancreas and a reduction of pancreatic secretion when animals were given Flexical® for a 3-day period.

Levenson et al.[139] found that chemically defined diets appeared to cause minimal stimulation of pancreatic exocrine function in rats, although indirect methods of measurement were used in this study.

Using the elemental diet Vivonex® in dogs, Ragins et al.[140] found that perfusion of the diet at neutral pH through a Thiry-Vella loop resulted in no significant pancreatic secretion, although secretion was stimulated when the diet was instilled into the stomach. They also found that a mixture of essential and nonessential amino acids and a mixture of phenylalanine, leucine, and tryptophan (strong stimulators of pancreatic secretion in the dog), when perfused through the Thiry-Vella loop at neutral pH, and in the concentrations present in Vivonex®, caused minimal pancreatic secretion. When the same amino acid mixtures acidified to pH 3.5 were perfused, strong pancreatic stimulation occurred. These data emphasize the importance of bypassing the stomach and minimizing acid secretion thus allowing minimal pancreatic stimulation. The importance of acid is also emphasized in a report by Konturek et al.[141] who found that the amount of cholecystokinin released by intraluminal perfusion of the intestine with amino acid is reduced correspondingly to the distance the solution is perfused distally to the pylorus.

A further study in dogs compared the effect of the same elemental diet (Vivonex®) on exocrine pancreatic secretion by infusing the diet into the dog duodenum, and comparing the effect with that achieved by infusing a nearly equimolar dose of an 1-form neutral amino acid (1-Phenylalanine), 0.16 *N* hydrochloric acid saline control, and cholecystokinin, infused at 2 units per kg/hr.[142] Intraduodenal infusion of Vivonex® produced significant increases in pancreatic volume and protein output compared to the control solution and similar to those produced by the amino acid solution. This carefully performed study suggests that the elemental diet does stimulate pancreatic function, and that these stimulatory properties are primarily due to its amino acid content. Another study in dogs reported that a chemically defined diet of Flexical® type induced a brisk pancreatic secretory response, but the fluid was watery and enzyme concentration lower than with a normal diet.[143]

Dogs fed Vivonex® for 6 months showed no changes on light or electronmicroscopy in the pancreas compared to control animals on normal chow diets.[144] This study suggests that the elemental diet does not rest the pancreas to any significant extent.

When Vivonex® was administered orally and intraduodenally to dogs intraduodenal administration caused reduced water and bicarbonate production from the pancreas compared with oral administration, but this did not prevent a normal protein response.[145] It was considered that the different results obtained after oral and duodenal administration in relation to volume and bicarbonate outputs were probably due to the addition of secreted acid to the intragastric contents. This is consistent with Grossman's observation that postcibal volume and bicarbonate output in dogs vary with the flow of gastric juice into the duodenum. Enzyme or protein output is independent of duodenal acidification or bicarbonate secretion from the pancreas. Meyer and Kelly[146] reported that peptic digests of bovine serum albumin were potent stimuli of pancreatic enzyme secretion when perfused into the duodenum of dogs with chronic pancreatic fistulas. Mixtures of oligopeptides and amino acids caused as much pancreatic secretion as the peptic digests. I.v. nutrition in these animals caused only minor exocrine pancreatic secretion compared to the elemental diet.

The ability of the elemental diet Vivonex® to act as a prophylactic and therapeutic agent in bile-induced pancreatitis was studied in dogs by Kerstein and Tonkens.[147] There were no histological or ultrastructural differences in modification of zymogen granules by pretreatment with Vivonex®, nor was there any significant difference in the severity of pancreatitis among animals previously treated with Vivonex® and those not given the elemental diet. Mortality figures showed that Vivonex® did not prevent pancreatitis in dogs. Some reduction in the enzyme response in dogs on Vivonex® measured by cannulation of the pancreatic duct through a duodenocutaneous fistula compared to controls was observed in one study.[148]

The two elemental diets Vivonex® and Flexical® were compared by Lewis and Freeman[149,150] in four dogs with pancreatic pouches in which pancreatic exocrine secretion was studied. A control diet using isocaloric meat-based blenderized food was used. Each of the three diets was infused three times on different days to each of the four animals and the volume, total protein, and total bicarbonate concentrations measured together with amylase and lipase estimations. The results suggested that Vivonex® stimulated the least pancreatic exocrine response of the three diets tested.

2. Human Studies

There have been fewer adequate studies of the effect of elemental diets on exocrine pancreatic secretion in man than in animals, but the results which are available are summarized in Table 4. The first study of the effect of an elemental diet on exocrine pancreatic secretion in normal human volunteers was reported by Perrault et al.[113] The elemental diet Flexical® and a control diet were given to two groups of volunteers for 12 days. The principal difference between the control and chemically defined diet was nonhydrolysis of the protein fraction and the absence of medium chain triglycerides in the lipid fraction of the control diet. The output of pancreatic enzymes was measured on the 12th day by means of duodenal intubation and infusion of cholecystokinin. The 20-min duodenal aspirates were analyzed for lipase, amylase, and trypsin activities. There was no difference in the pancreatic secretion of these enzymes in the subjects on the control diet compared with those on the elemental diet.

A further study in normal human subjects measured the pancreatic secretion of lipase and chymotrypsin in response to continuous jejunal perfusion of the elemental diet

Table 4
EFFECT OF ELEMENTAL DIETS ON EXOCRINE PANCREATIC SECRETION IN NORMAL HUMAN SUBJECTS

Elemental diet	Route of administration	Effect	Ref.
Flexical®	Oral	Stimulates enzyme secretion to same level as control diet	113
Vivonex®	Intraduodenal	Stimulates enzyme secretion	151
Vivonex®	Oral	Stimulates enzyme secretion	152

Vivonex® and an equicaloric infusion of crushed food homogenate.[151] The solutions were infused at the duodeno-jejunal junction; the results showed that the crushed food homogenate caused greater pancreatic enzyme secretion than the elemental diet but that this could be directly related to is greater nitrogen content. Pancreatic enzyme secretion was shown to increase with the calorific and nitrogenous loads infused but was not affected by volume or osmolality of the infused solutions.

Another study compared the trypsin concentrations in duodenal juice following the ingestion of a standard Lundh test meal with that obtained after oral ingestion of the elemental diet Vivonex® in the same normal human subjects.[152] The mean tryptic activity over the 2-hr collection period was less in the Vivonex® group compared with the Lundh test group in four of the five subjects studied, but the difference was not statistically significant. During the first hour, the mean tryptic activity following Vivonex® was less in three subjects than that following the Lundh meal, but again the differences were not statistically significant (Table 5). However, the mean tryptic activity during the second hour was significantly less following Vivonex® than the Lundh meal in all five subjects studied. The results of this study agree with those of previous human studies that elemental diets in normal human subjects do stimulate exocrine pancreatic secretion. This is probably related to the presence of amino acids in the upper small intestine which are important stimulators of pancreatic secretion. In the last study described, the reduced tryptic activity in the second hour of the test may indicate that intragastric administration of amino acids alone or as components of an elemental diet may result in less marked stimulation of pancreatic secretion. Perhaps more likely, however, is the lower nitrogen content of the Vivonex® compared with the Lundh test meal. It may also have been related to the observation that intrajejunal glucose inhibits pancreatic secretion in man, and the high glucose content of Vivonex® may thus be a factor in the reduced tryptic activity found in the second hour of that study.

A further recent study showed that the elemental diet Vivonex®, given over a 3-hr period by duodenal perfusion to normal volunteer subjects, led to a statistically significant reduction of 26% in trypsin concentration $p<0/001$) and in 12% in duodenal bile acid content ($p<0.001$) compared with an isocaloric, isonitrogenous standard breakfast.[116]

3. Conclusions

There has been a large number of studies which have looked at the effect of various elemental diets on the stimulation of exocrine pancreatic secretion, both in animals and in man. Many of the early animal studies suggested a reduction or absence of exocrine pancreatic stimulation with chemically defined diets. Some later animal work, however, has shown that pancreatic stimulation does occur. In human studies, there has been shown to be pancreatic stimulation with Vivonex® and Flexical®, and significant stimulation of trypsin and lipase has been demonstrated.

Clearly, differing results would be expected in such a widely varying series of studies; different formulations and concentrations of elemental diets have been used; different

Table 5
MEAN TRYPTIC ACTIVITY AFTER LUNDH MEAL AND VIVONEX

	Mean tryptic activity (± SEM) (ueq H^+/min/mℓ)		
	Lundh meal	Vivonex®	
First hr	15.4 ± 3.1	14.5 ± 5.6	N.S.
Second hr	23.6 ± 3.1	7.4 ± 1.9	$p<0.025$

rates of infusion have been utilized; the results may vary as to whether or not the diet was given orally, intragastrically, or by direct intraduodenal or intrajejunal infusion; and finally different ways of measuring exocrine pancreatic secretion have been employed in many of these studies. However, the consensus of the results, especially in studies in normal human volunteers, suggests that the principal elemental diets Vivonex® and Flexical® do stimulate exocrine pancreatic secretion, although it is possible that stimulation may not be as much as with normal food. Amino acids are stimulators of pancreatic secretion when infused into the upper small intestine but intragastric administration of amino acids causes less marked pancreatic stimulation. Intrajejunal glucose inhibits pancreatic secretion. However, there is no clear indication that less pancreatic stimulation occurs when elemental diets are administered directly into the duodenum compared with the oral route. Any reduction of pancreatic enzyme activity after elemental diets (compared to control diets) may be related to the lower nitrogen content of the elemental diet, although further work is required on this aspect.

It also seems unlikely that elemental diets will be of value in the management of acute pancreatitis by resting the pancreas, although they may be of value in providing easily absorbed nutrients and thereby improving nutritional insufficiency in patients with chronic pancreatic insufficiency. This will be further discussed in Chapter 12.

VII. LIPIDS AND BLOOD PRESSURE

In one of the early studies reported, the effect of dietary carbohydrate on serum cholesterol levels were studied.[1] The chemically defined diet used in this study contained less than 0.5% ethyl linoleate as the sole source of dietary fat but had a high carbohydrate content. It resulted in a marked reduction of serum cholesterol levels in normal adult males after 4, 7, 8, and 19 weeks on the diet. Diets with glucose as their principal carbohydrate source caused a significant reduction in serum cholesterol levels; an increase in serum cholesterol was found with partial substitution of the glucose by sucrose. The reduction of serum cholesterol level with sucrose however, was statistically significant compared with normal levels.

Further studies on dietary alteration of serum lipid levels was reported by McDonald.[153,154] He found that an increase of dietary glycerol raised the serum triglycerides of men 1 to 2.5 hr after the ingestion of cholesterol. Supplementation of glycerol to the free diet caused a rise of fasting serum glyceride concentration in men but not in women.[153] In investigating the effect of amino acid and carbohydrate on fasting serum lipid levels over 5 days, the same author studied a complete amino acid mixture as the nitrogen source (Vivonex®) and used different carbohydrate sources in the form of sucrose, glucose, lactose, or a partial hydrolysate of starch; only small quantities of fat were present in the diet.[154] A marked fall in serum cholesterol was seen with all the carbohydrates used and was considered to be due to a cholesterol-free intake. The fall in cholesterol on the sucrose diet was no less than occurred with the other diets, but a rapid rise in fasting serum triglyceride level was observed on the sucrose diet which had not been found in normal subjects when the protein used was either a casein hydrolysate or normal solid protein intake (as obtained from meat and fish).

Winitz and colleagues[1,2] also resported changes in serum lipid levels and blood pressure secondary to dietary alterations, using chemically defined diets. During the first 4 weeks on the diet, the entire carbohydrate source was provided in the form of glucose. This diet led to a marked decrease in serum cholesterol levels in all subjects, the average serum level for the group being reduced from a baseline of 227 mg% to 161 mg% at the end of the fourth week. The largest fall occurred during the first week. At the end of the fourth week, 25% weight of the glucose was replaced by an isocaloric amount of sucrose and over the following 3 weeks a progressive increase in serum cholesterol levels to an average value of 208 mg% for the group was noted. Reinstitution of the glucose-based diet at the end of the seventh week was accompanied by a marked drop in serum cholesterol levels within a week. This study demonstrates that the nature of the dietary carbohydrate can exert a marked effect on serum cholesterol levels.

A further study by Young et al[155] in five normal subjects confirmed that a diet with a high glucose content (Vivonex®) leads to a reduction of serum cholesterol levels.

Similar observations were made by Perrault et al.[113] using a diet of Flexical® type, and by Persson[156] who studied the effect of Vivonex® on lipid metabolisn in Ethiopian children with kwashiorkor. In the latter study, prior to treatment, a slight increase of triglyceride levels was noted in serum but when treatment was started a fall of free fatty acids and cholesterol levels occurred.

Data have also been reported on the effect of various chemically defined diets on blood pressure levels in normotensive subjects.[1,2] Daily systolic and diastolic blood pressure readings were obtained from each subject during the last week of each phase of the study. Statistically significant differences were found with the use of the diet with a high glucose content, the blood pressure being significantly lower when the elemental diet was used. This mainly affected the systolic blood pressure, although a small decrease in diastolic levels was also observed. About 10 days of continuous elemental diet therapy was required before significant decreases in both systolic and diastolic blood pressure levels were achieved.

A. Conclusions

It can be seen from these studies that a chemcially defined diet with a high carbohydrate content tends to reduce the serum cholesterol and plasma lipid levels, and that a reduction in blood pressure may also be achieved. These findings emphasize the importance of diet and dietary manipulation. These observations may be of little practical value in relation to the management of hyperlipoproteinemia and blood pressure abnormalities; convincing data on the reduction of these parameters in patients with abnormal levels are not yet available. The principal interest in the findings, however, is the confirmation that diet does appear to be important in the control of blood lipid and blood pressure levels, and that dietary manipulation may lead to improvement in these parameters within a relatively short period of time. Further work is required in this field.

VIII. IMMUNOLOGICAL AND HYPOALLERGENIC EFFECTS

The experimental chemically defined diet used by Winitz and colleagues[1] was considered to be hypoallergenic. There was little experimental clinical evidence supporting this statement at that time, and little investigative work has been performed on the effect of the various chemically defined diets on immunological mechanisms, either in animals or in man. The presence of basic food elements such as amino acids without the presence of complicated protein is the theoretical basis of the considered hypoallerginicity of elemental diets.

Elemental diets have been used in the investigation of food allergies and other immunological conditions, and the suggestion has been made that they may be of some value in the management of diseases which are considered to have an immunological basis, such as food hypersensitivity, coeliac disease, and the nephrotic syndrome.

The immunogenicity of the elemental diet Vivonex® has been studied in rabbits by immunization with milk, egg, and Vivonex®, and the animals evaluated for the production of precipitin and passive cutaneous anaphylactic antibodies.[157] Some 25 mg of the milk and egg albumin and Vivonex® were injected sequentially in multiple s.c. sites every 4 days over a 3-week period. After the series was completed the rabbits were bled and the sera tested using the Ouchterlony technique to detect precipitin antibodies to the food antigens.[158] Passive cutaneous anaphylaxis was studied using Hartley guinea pigs passively sensitized by intradermal injections with 0.1 mℓ of the rabbit sera used in the precipitin tests and by nonspecific rabbit control sera. Four hours later the injection areas were challenged by the i.v. injection of 0.5 mℓ of egg or Vivonex® and 0.15 mℓ 1% Evans blue dye. Reaction sites were evaluated by the size of dye extravasation 15 to 20 min after injection of the antigen. Milk and egg albumin produced many precipitin antibodies in the rabbit but no precipitins were produced by Vivonex®. In addition, Vivonex® did not precipitate with the antibodies formed to the milk and egg albumin. The passive cutaneous anaphylaxis evaluation showed that all skin test sites were negative. From this study, it would appear that Vivonex® is not immunogenic in these animals by either the precipitin reaction or passive cutaneous anaphylactic response. The hypoallergincity of this elemental diet as suggested by early workers was thus supported.

The effect of the removal of food antigens by the use of an elemental diet while maintaining a normal amount of microbial antigens has been studied in animals, but no adequate human work has yet been published on this subject. The immune status of mice fed Vivonex® from shortly after birth has been compared with those fed a standard diet and has been reported.[159] By comparison with mice reared on a normal diet, animals reared on the elemental diet were less aggressive, lighter, the spleen and thymus were smaller, and peripheral white blood counts were lower. Serum antibody responses to a protein antigen were impaired but cell mediated immunity was normal. Multifactorial aspects of imnunity were studied by infection with the helminth parasite *Nippostrongylus brasiliensis.* Infection with the parasite in mice fed the elemental diet led to wasting and a delay in parasite expulsion, indicating impaired antiparasite immunity.

A further study of the immunological status of mice reared on an elemental diet has shown greater villous atrophy and crypt hypertrophy in animals fed Vivonex® who were infected with either *Giardia muris* or *Nippostrongylus brasiliensis.*[75] Although it would appear that the elemental diet alters the host-parasite relationship to the detriment of the host, it is possible that improved nutrition of the parasites themselves due to the elemental diet was a factor, rather than any marked alteration of the immune status of the animals due to the presence of the elemental diet; more information is required on this aspect.

A. Conclusions

Elemental diets do seem to be hypoallergenic, thus raising the possibility of their use in the diagnosis and management of allergic conditions such as food allergy or in diseases associated with immunological disturbance.

Further data are still required on their possible alteration of immune mechanisms. The effect of elemental diets on immune mechanisms in man needs to be studied, together with their possible value in diseases in man associated with immunological abnormality. This latter aspect will be further discussed in Chapter 17.

REFERENCES

1. **Winitz, M., Seedman, D., and Graff, J.,** Studies in metabolic nutrition employing chemically defined diets. I. Extended feeding of normal human adult males, *Am. J. Clin. Nutri.,* 23, 525, 1970.
2. **Winitz, M. and Adams, R.F.,** Chemically defined diets: a new approach to metabolic nutrition, in *Balance Nutrition and Therapy,* Lang, K., Fekl, W., and Berg, G., Eds., Thieme, Stuttgart, 1971, 46.
3. **Glotzer, D. J.,** Space diets: comment, *Gastroenterology,* 61, 405, 1971.
4. **Beigler, M. A.,** The elemental diet: a new concept in nutritional support of the debilitated patient, *Surg. Dig.,* 6, 18, 1971.
5. **Randall, H. T.,** Diet and nutrition in the care of the surgical patient, in *Modern Nutrition in Health and Disease,* Goodheart, R. S., and Shils, M. E., Eds., Lea and Febiger, Philadelphia, 1973, 961.
6. **Bury, K. D., Stephens, R. V., Cha, C., and Randall, H. T.,** Chemically defined diets, *Can. J. Surg.,* 17, 124, 1974.
7. **Russell, R. I.,** Elemental diets *Gut.,* 16, 68, 1975.
8. **Voitk, A. J.,** The place of elemental diet in clinical nutrition, *Br. J. Clin. Prac.,* 29, 55, 1975.
9. **Editorial,** Elemental diets, *Lancet,* 2, 68, 1975.
10. **Freeman, J. B., Egan, M. C., and Millis, B. J.,** The elemental diet, *Surg. Gynaecol. Obstet.,* 142, 925, 1976.
11. **Kaminski, M. V.,** Enteral hyperalimentation, *Surg. Gynaecol. Obstet.,* 143, 12, 1976.
12. **Russell, R. I. and Hall, M. J.,** The practical value of elemental diets, *Practitioner,* 222, 631, 1979.
13. **Russell, R. I.,** Intravenous nutrition and elemental diets in gastrointestinal disease, in *Scientific Foundations of Gastroenterology,* Sircus, W. and Smith, A. N., Eds., Heinemann, London, 1980, 130.
14. **Winitz, M., Birnbaum, S. N., Sugimura, T., and Otley, M. C.,** Quantitative nutritional and in vivo metabolic studies with water-soluble chemically defined diets, in *Amino Acids, Proteins and Cancer Biochemistry,* (Greenstein Mem. Symp. Edsell, J. G. and Jessie, P., Eds., Academic Press, New York, 1960, 9.
15. **Morgan, A., Filler, R. M., and Moore, F. D.,** Surgical nutrition *Med. Clin. North Am.,* 54, 1367, 1970.
16. **Hunt, J. N.,** The duodenal regulation of gastric emptying, *Gastroenterology,* 45, 149, 1963.
17. **Hunt, J. N. and Knox, M. T.,** Control of gastric emptying, *Am. J. Dig. Dis.,* 13, 372, 1968.
18. **Elias, G., Gibson, G. J., and Greenwood, L. F.,** The slowing of gastric empyting of monosaccharides and disaccharides in test meals, *J. Physiol. (London),* 194, 317, 1968.
19. **Hunt, J. N. and Knox M. T.,** The slowing of gastric emptying by amino acids, *J. Physiol. (London),* 201, 161, 1969.
20. **Hunt, J. N. and Knox, M. T.,** A relationship between the chain length of fatty acids and the slowing of gastric emptying, *J. Physiol. (London),* 194, 327, 1968.
21. **Cooke, A. R. and Moulang, J.,** Control of gastric emptying by amino acids, *Gastroenterology,* 62, 528, 1972.
22. **Hunt, J. N. and Knox, M. T.,** The control of gastric emptying, *Gastrointestinal Motility,* Demling, L., and Ottenjam, R., Eds., Academic Press, New York, 1971, 46.
23. **Elwin, C. E. and Uvnas, B.,** Distribution and local release of gastrin, in *'Gastrin,'* Grossman, M. I., Ed., University of California Press, Los Angeles, 1966, 69.
24. **Varner, A. A., Isenberg, J. I., Elashoff, J. D, Lamers, C. B., and Shulkes, A. A.,** Intravenous fat inhibits amino acid (AA) stimulated gastric acid secretion (GAS) in man, *Abstr. Gastroenterology,* 76, 1264, 1979.
25. **Bury, K. D. and Jambunathan, G.,** Effects of elemental diets on gastric emptying and gastric secretion in man, *Am. J. Surg.,* 127, 59, 1974.
26. **George, J. D.,** New clinical method for measuring the rate of gastric emptying: the double sampling test meal, *Gut,* 9, 237, 1968.
27. **Rivilis, J., McArdle, H., Wlodek, G. K., and Gurd, F. N.,** The effect of an elemental diet on gastric secretion, *Ann. R. Coll. Phys. Surg. Can.,* 5, 57, 1972.
28. **Rivilis, J., McArdle, H., Wlodek, G., and Gurd, F. N.,** Effects of an elemental diet on gastric secretion, *Ann. Surg.,* 179, 226, 1974.

29. **McManus, J. P. A. and Isselbacher, K. J.,** Effect of fasting versus feeding on the rat small intestine, *Gastroenterology,* 59, 214, 1970.
30. **Steiner, M., Bourges, H. R., Freedman, L. A., and Gray, S. J.,** Effect of starvation on the tissue composition of the small intestine of the rat, *Am. J., Physiol.,* 215, 75, 1968.
31. **Altmann, G. G.,** Influence of starvation and re-feeding on mucosal size and epithelial renewal in the rat small intestine, *Am. J. Anat.,* 133, 391, 1972.
32. **Hopper, A. F., Wannemacher, R. W., Jr., and McGovern, P. A.,** Cell population changes in the intestinal epithelium of the rat following starvation and protein-depletion. *Proc. Soc. Exp. Biol. Med.,* 128, 695, 1968.
33. **Hopper, A. F., Rose, P. M., and Wannemacher, R. W.,** Cell population changes in the intestinal mucosa of protein-depleted or starved rats. II. Changes in cellular migration rates, *J. Cell. Biol.,* 53, 225, 1972.
34. **Brown, H. O., Levine, M. L., and Lipkin, M.,** Inhibition of intestinal epithelial cell renewal and migration induced by starvation, *Am. J. Physiol.,* 205, 868, 1963.
35. **Clarke, R. M.,** The effect of growth and fasting on the number of villi and crypts in the small intestine of the albino rat, *J. Anat.,* 112, 227, 1972.
36. **Blair, D. G. P., Yakimets W., and Tuba, J.,** Rat intestinal sucrase. II. The effects of rat age and sex and of diet on sucrase activity, *Can. J. Biochem. Physiol.,* 41, 917, 1963.
37. **Deren, J. J., Broitman, S. A., and Zamcheck N.,** Effect of diet upon intestinal disaccharidases and disaccharide absorption, *J. Clin. Invest.,* 46, 186, 1967.
38. **McNeill, L. K. and Hamilton, J. R.,** The effect of fasting on disaccharidase activity in the rat small intestine, *Pediatrics,* 42, 65, 1971.
39. **Rosenweig, N. S. and Herman, R. H.,** Control of jejunal sucrase and maltase activity by dietary sucrose or fructose in man. A model for the study of enzyme regulation in man, *J. Clin. Invest.,* 47, 2253, 1968.
40. **Tepperman, J., Brobeck, J. R., and Long, C. N. H.,** The effects of hypothalamic hyperphagia and of alteration, in feeding habits on the metabolism of the albino rat, *Yale J. Biol. Med.,* 15, 855, 1943.
41. **Dowling, R. H.,** Compensatory changes in intestinal absorption, *Br. Med. Bull.,* 23, 275, 1967.
42. **Levine, G. M., Deren, G. G., Steiger, E., and Zinno, R.,** Role of oral intake in maintenance of gut mass and disaccharide activity, *Gastroenterology,* 67, 975, 1974.
43. **Feldman, E. J., Dowling, R. H., McNaughton, J., and Peters, T. J.,** The effects of oral versus intravenous nutrition on intestinal adaptation after small bowel resection in the dog, *Gastroenterology,* 70, 712, 1976.
44. **Gleeson, M. H., Cullen, J., and Dowling, R. H.,** Intestinal structure and function after small bowel bypass in the rat, *Clin Sci.,* 43, 731, 1972.
45. **Keren, D. F. and Elliot, H. L.,** A rapid development of mucosal atrophy in isolated (Thiry-Vella) ileal loops, *Fed. Proc.,* 32, 322, 1973.
46. **Keren, D. F., Elliott, H. L., Brown, G. D., and Yardley, J. H.,** Atrophy of villi with hypertrophy and hyperplasia of Paneth cells in isolated (Thiry-Vella) ileal loops in rabbits, *Gastroenterology,* 68, 83, 1975.
47. **Tompkins, R. K., Waisman, J., Watt, C. M. H., Corlin, R., and Keith, R.,** Absence of mucosal atrophy in the human small intestine after prolonged isolation, *Gastroenterology,* 73, 1406, 1977.
48. **Daly, G. M., Castro, G. A., Akhtar, M., and Dudrick, S. J.,** Morphologic and biochemical intestinal changes after jejuno-ileal bypass, *Gastroenterology,* 72, A 1042, 1977.
49. **Dowling, R. H. and Booth, C. C.,** Structural and functional changes following small intestinal resection in the rat, *Clin. Sci.,* 32, 139, 1967.
50. **Dowling, R. H. and Gleeson, M. H.,** Cell turnover following small bowel resection and bypass, *Digestion,* 8, 176, 1973.
51. **Levine, G. M., Deren, J. G., and Yezdimir, I. R.,** Small bowel resection: Oral intake is a stimulus for hyperplasia, *Am. Dig. Dis.,* 21, 542, 1976.
52. **Clarke, R. M.,** Luminal nutrition versus functional workload as controllers of mucosal morphology and epithelial replacement in the rat small intestine, *Digestion,* 15, 411, 1977.
53. **Altmann, G. L.,** Influence of bile and pancreatic secretions on the size of the intestinal villi in the rat, *Am. J. Anat.,* 132, 167, 1971.
54. **Philipson, B.,** Morphology in the rat ileal mucos following construction of an ileal reservoir or transposition of patches to different locations, *Scand. J. Gastroenterol.,* 10, 369, 1975.
55. **Roy, C. C., Laurendeau, G., Doyon, G., Chartrand, L., and Rivest, M. R.,** The effect of bile and sodium taurocholate on the epithelial cell dynamics of the rat small intestine, *Proc. Soc. Exp. Bio. Med.,* 149, 1000, 1975.
56. **Gronqvist, B., Engström, B., and Grimelius, L.,** Morphological studies of the rat small intestine after jejunoileal transposition, *Acta Chir. Scand.,* 141, 208, 1975.
57. **Weser, E., Heller, R., and Tawil, T.,** Stimulation of mucosal growth in the rat ileum by bile and pancreatic secretions after jejunal resection, *Gastroenterology,* 73, 524, 1977.
58. **Hughes, C., Bates, T., and Dowling, R. H.,** The trophic effect of cholecystokinin/secretin stimulated pancreatico-biliary secretions on dog intestine, *Eur. J. Clin Invest.,* 6, 320, 1976.

59. **Dworkin, L. D., Levine, G. M., Farber, N. J., and Spector, M. H.,** Small intestinal mass of the rat is partially determined by indirect effects of intraluminal nutrition, *Gastroenterology,* 71, 626, 1976.
60. **Touloukian, R. J. and Spencer, R. P.,** Ileal blood flow preceding compensatory intestinal hypertrophy, *Ann. Surg.,* 175, 320, 1972.
61. **Touloukian, R. J., Am-hajanian, G. K., and Roth, R. H.,** Adrenergic denervation of the hypertrophied gut remant, *Ann. Surg.,* 176, 633, 1972.
62. **Tutton, P. G. M. and Helme, R. O.,** The influence of adrenal-receptor activity on crypt cell proliferation in the rat jejunum, *Cell Tissue Kinet.,* 7, 125, 1974.
63. **Williamson, R. C. N.,** Intestinal adaptation. Structural, functional and cytokinetic changes, *N. Engl. J. Med.,* 298, 1393, 1978, 298, 1444, 1978.
64. **Weser, E.,** Role of gastrin in intestinal adaptation after small bowel resection, *Gastroenterology,* 75, 323, 1978.
65. **Abrams, G. D., Bauer, H., and Sprinz, H.,** Influence of the normal flora on mucosal morphology and cellular renewal in the ileum; a comparison of germ free and conventional mice, *Lab. Invest.,* 12, 355, 1962.
66. **Lesher, S., Walberg, A. G., and Sacher, G. A., Jr.,** Generation cycle in the duodenal crypt cells of germ free and conventional mice, *Nature,* 202, 884, 1965.
67. **Ryan, G. P., Dudrick, S. J., Copeland, E. M., and Johnson, L. R.,** Effects of various diets on colonic growth in rats, *Gastroenterology,* 77, 658, 1979.
68. **Jasper, D. K. and Bronk, J. R.,** Studies on the physiological and structural characteristics of rat intestinal mucosa. Mitochondrial structural changes during amino acid absorption, *J. Cell Biol.,* 38, 277, 1968.
69. **Nelson, L. M., Carmichael, H. A., Russell, R. I., and Lee, F. D.,** Small intestinal changes induced by an elemental diet (Vivonex) in normal rats, *Clin. Sci. Mol. Med.,* 55, 509, 1978.
70. **Nelson, L. M.,** Effects of Elemental Diet Feeding on Bile Acid Metabolism and Small Intestinal Structure and Function, Ph.D. Thesis, University of Glasgow, 1979, 97.
71. **Galjaard, H., van der Meer-Fieggen, W., and Giesen, J.,** Feedback control by functional villus cells on cell proliferation and maturation in intestinal epithelium, *Exp. Cell Res.,* 73, 197, 1972.
72. **Jacobs, L. R., Taylor, B. R., and Dowling, R. H.,** Effect of luminal nutrition on the intestinal adaptation following Thiry-Vella bypass in the dog (abstract), *Clin. Sci. Mol. Med.,* 49, 267, 1975.
73. **Young, E. A., Cioletti, L. A., and Weser, E.,** The effect of defined formula diets on mucosal mass of the small bowel in the rat, *Gastroenterology,* 74, A 1115, 1978.
74. **Ecknauer, R. E. R., Sircar, B., Lichtenberger, L. M., and Johnson, L. R.,** Role of food-bulk in maintaining mucosal morphology of rat small intestine, *Gastroenterology,* 74, A 1030, 1978.
75. **Ferguson, A., Logan, R. F. A., and MacDonald, T. T.,** Increased mucosal damage during parasite infection in mice fed on elemental diet, *Gut,* 21, 37, 1980.
76. **Hugon, J. S.,** Intestinal ultrastructure after prolonged use of an elemental diet, *Strahlentherapie,* 151, 541, 1976.
77. **Hugon, J. S., Maestracci, D., and Menard, D.,** Stimulation of glucose-6-phosphatase activity in the mucosal cells of the mouse intestine, *J. Hist. Chem., Cyt. Chem.,* 21, 426, 1973.
78. **Menard, D., Bertalood, A., and Hugon, J. S.,** Action of phenobarbitone on the ultrastructure and the enzymatic activity of the mouse intestine and the mouse liver, *Histochemistry,* 38, 241, 1974.
79. **Fenyo, G. and Hallberg, D.,** The influence of a chemical diet on the intestinal mucosa after jejuno-ileal bypass in the rat, *Acta Chir. Scand.,* 142, 270, 1976.
80. **Bounous, G., Hugon, J., and Gentile, J. M.,** Elemental diet in the management of the intestinal lesion produced by 5 flurourosil in the rat, *Can. J. Surg.,* 14, 298, 1971.
81. **Gardner, M. L. G. and Heading, R. C.,** Effects of elemental diets on absorptive and enzymic activities and in 5-fluorouracil toxicity in rat small intestine, *Clin. Sci.,* 56, 243, 1979.
82. **Gardner, M. L. G., Samson, R. R., and Heading, R. C.,** Changes in absorptive and peptide hydrolase activities in rat small intestine following administration of 5 fluorouracil, *Clin. Sci. Mol. Med.,* 54, 411, 1978.
83. **Reddy, B. S., Pleasants, J. R., and Wostmaun, B. S.,** Effect of dietary carbohydrate on intestinal disaccharidase in germ-free and conventional rats, *J. Nutr.,* 95, 413, 1968.
84. **Hietanen, E. and Hänninen, O.,** Comparison of mucosal metabolism in the small intestine of specific pathogen-free and conventional rats, *Scand. J. Gastroent.,* 6, 127, 1971.
85. **Nelson, L. M., Russell, P. I., and Lee, F. D.,** Elemental diet composition and the structure and function of rat small intestine: comparison of the effects of Vivonex and Flexical on morphology and in vivo absorption of water, *J. Parent. Ent. Nutr.,* in press, 1981.
86. **Davidson, R. E. and Leese, H. J.,** Sucrose absorption by rat small intestine in vivo and in vitro, *J. Physiol.,* 267, 237, 1977.
87. **Nelson, L. M.,** Effects of Elemental Diet Feeding on Bile Acid Metabolism and Small Intestinal Structure and Function, Ph.D thesis, University of Glasgow, 1979, 114.

88. **Moore, E. P., Copeland, E. M., Dudrick S. J., and Weisbrodt, N. W.,** Effect of an elemental diet on the electrical activity of the small intestine in dogs, *J. Surg. Res.*, 20, 533, 1976.
89. **Mosbach, E. H.,** Hepatic synthesis of bile acids, *Arch. Intern. Med.*, 130, 479, 1972.
90. **Myant, N. B. and Mitropoulos, K. A.,** Cholesterol 7α hydroxylase, *J. Lipid Res.*, 18, 135, 1977.
91. **Shefer, S., Hauser, S., Bekersky, I., and Mosbach, E. H.,** Feedback regulation of bile acid biosynthesis in the rat, *J. Lipid Res.*, 10, 646, 1969.
92. **Small, D. M., Dowling, R. H., and Redinger, R. N.,** The enterohepatic circulation of bile salts, *Arch. Intern. Med.*, 130, 552, 1972.
93. **Borgström, B., Lundh, G., and Hofmann, A.,** The site of absorption of conjugated bile salts in man, *Gastroenterology*, 45, 229, 1963.
94. **Dietschy, J. M.,** Mechanisms for the intestinal absorption of bile acids, *J. Lipid Res.*, 9, 297, 1968.
95. **Dowling, R. H.,** The enterohepatic circulation, *Gastroenterology*, 62, 122, 1972.
96. **Hill, M. J. and Drasar, B. S.,** Degradation of bile acids by intestinal bacteria, *Gut*, 9, 22, 1968.
97. **Lewis, R. and Gorbach, S.,** Modification of bile acids by intestinal bacteria, *Arch. Intern. Med.*, 130, 545, 1972.
98. **Meihoff, W. E. and Kern, F.,** Bile salt malabsorption in regional ileitis, ileal resection and mannatol-induced diarrhea, *J. Clin. Invest.*, 47, 261, 1968.
99. **Eastwood, M. A. and Boyd, G. S.,** The distribution of bile salts along the small intestine in rats, *Biochem. Biophys. Acta*, 137, 393, 1967.
100. **Dowling, R. H., Mack E., and Small, D. M.,** Effects of controlled interruption of the enterohepatic circulation of bile salts by biliary diversion and by ileal resection on bile salt secretion, synthesis, pool size in the Rhesus monkey, *J. Clin. Invest.*, 49, 232, 1970.
101. **Hofmann, A. F.,** Bile acid malabsorption caused by ileal resection, *Arch. Intern. Med.*, 130, 597, 1972.
102. **Dam, H.,** Nutritional factors in gallstone formation, in *Proceedings of the VIth International Congress of Nutrition*, Livingstone, Edinburgh, 1963, 6.
103. **Gustafsson, B. E. and Norman, A.,** Influence of the diet on the turnover of bile acids in germ free and conventional rats, *Br. J. Nutr.*, 23, 429, 1969.
104. **Portman, O. W. and Murphy, P.,** Excretion of bile acids and beta-hydroxysterols by rats, *Arch. Biochem. Biophys.*, 76, 367, 1958.
105. **Hellström, K., Sjövall, J., and Wigand, G.,** Influence of semi-synthetic diet and type of fat on the turnover of deoxycholic acid in the the rabbit, *J. Lipid Res.*, 3, 405, 1962.
106. **Antonis, A. and Bersohn, I.,** The influence of diet on faecal lipids in South African white and Bantu prisoners, *Am. Clin. Nutr.*, 11, 142, 1962.
107. **Sundaravalli, O. E., Shurpalekar, K. S., and Narayana, R.,** Effects of dietary cellulose supplements on the body composition and cholesterol metabolism on albino rats, *J. Agr. Gut Food Chem.*, 19, 116, 1971.
108. **Shurpalekar, K. S., Doraiswamy, T. R., Sundaravalli, O. E., and Narayana R.,** Effect of inclusion of cellulose in an atherogenic diet on the blood lipids of children, *Nature (London)*, 232, 544, 1971.
109. **Forman, D. T., Garvin, J. E., Forestner, J. E., and Taylor, C. B.,** Increased excretion of faecal bile acids by an oral hydrophylic colloid, *Proc. Soc. Exp. Biol. Med.*, 127, 1060, 1968.
110. **Beher, W. T. and Casazza, K. K.,** Effects of psyllium hydrocolloid on bile acid metabolism in normal and hypophysectomised rats, *Proc. Soc. Exp. Biol. Med.*, 136, 253, 1971.
111. **Stephens, R. V. and Randall, H. T.,** Use of concentrated balanced-liquid elemental diet for nutritional management of catabolic states, *Ann. Surg.*, 170, 164, 1969.
112. **Crowther, J. S., Drasar, B. S., Goddard, P., Hill, M. J., and Johnson K.,** The effect of a chemically defined diet on faecal flora and faecal steroid concentration, *Gut*, 14, 790, 1973.
113. **Perrault, J., Devroede, G., and Bounous, J.,** Effects of an elemental diet in healthy volunteers, *Gastroenterology*, 64, 569, 1973.
114. **Portman, O. W.,** Nutritional influences on the metabolism of bile acids, *Am. J. Clin. Nutr.*, 8, 462, 1960.
115. **Portman, O. W., Mann, G. B., and Wisocki, A. P.,** Bile acid excretion by the rats: nutrtional effects, *Arch. Biochem. Biophys.*, 59, 224, 1955.
116. **Panayiotides, T., Christofides, N., Bjornsson, O. G., Bloom, S. R., and Chadwick, V. S.,** Elemental diets, pancreaticobiliary secretions and gastrointestinal hormones, *Gut*, 20, A450, 1979.
117. **Nelson, L. M., Williamson, I., and Russell, R. I.,** Elemental diet composition—effect on bile acid metabolism and hepatic lipids, *Gut*, 1981, in press.
118. **Devereaux, D. F. and Baker, A. R.,** The effect of dietary fibre on stool bulk and gut transit time, *Gastroenterology*, 72, 1048, 1977.
119. **Madsen, D., Beaver, M., Chang, L., Bruckner-Kardoss, E., and Wostmann, B. S.,** Analysis of bile acids in conventional and germ-free rats, *J. Lipid Res.*, 17, 107, 1976.
120. **Lindstedt, S., Avigan, J., Goodman, D. S., Sjöall, J., and Steinberg, G.,** The effect of dietary fat on the turnover of cholic acid and on the composition of biliary bile acids in man, *J. Clin. Invest.*, 44, 1754, 1965.

121. **Nelson, L. M., Carmichael, H. A., Russell, R. I., and Atherton, S. T.,** Use of an elemental diet (Vivonex) in the management of bile acid-induced diarrhea, *Gut,* 18, 792, 1977.
122. **Hill, G. L., Main, W. S. J., Edwards, J. P., Morgan, D. B., and Goligher, J. C.,** Effect of a chemically defined liquid elemental diet on composition and volume of ileal fistula drainage, *Gastroenterology,* 68, 676, 1975.
123. **Hill, G. L., Main, W. S. J., Edwards, J. P., and Goligher, J. C.,** Decreased trypsin and bile acids in ileal fistula drainage during the administration of a chemically defined liquid elemental diet, *Br. J. Surg.,* 63, 133, 1976.
124. **Campbell, C. B., Spencer, J., and Dowling, R. H.,** Bile salt secretion and pool size in Rhesus monkeys with controlled interruption of the enterohepatic circulation, *Gut,* 10, 1050, 1969.
125. **Hepner, G.W.,** Effect of decreased gallbladder stimulation on enterohepatic cycling and kinetics of bile acids, *Gastroenterology,* 68, 1574, 1975.
126. **Attebery, H. P., Sutter, V. L., and Finegold, S. M.,** Effect of a partially chemically defined diet on normal human faecal flora, *Am. J. Clin. Nutr.,* 25, 1391, 1972.
127. **Preshaw, R. M. and Grossman, M. I.,** Stimulation of pancreatic secretion by extracts of the pyloric area of the stomach, *Gastroenterology,* 48, 36, 1965.
128. **Preshaw, R. M., Cooke, A. R., and Grossman, M. I.,** Stimulation of pancreatic secretion by a humoral agent from the pyloric gland area of the stomach, *Gastroenterology,* 49, 617, 1965.
129. **Wang, C. C. and Grossman, M. I.,** Physiological determination of release of secretin and pancreozymin from intestine of dogs with transplanted pancreas, *Am. J. Physiol.,* 164, 527, 1951.
130. **McClure, C. W.,** The exocrine functions of the pancreas, *Ann. Intern. Med.,* 10, 1848, 1937.
131. **Go, V. L. W., Hofmann, A. F., and Summerskill, W. H. J.,** Pancreozymin bioassay in man based on pancreatic enzyme secretion: potency of specific amino acids and other digestive products, *J. Clin. Invest.,* 49, 1558, 1970.
132. **Matthews, D. M. and Laster, L.,** Absorption of protein digestion products; a review, *Gut,* 6, 411, 1965.
133. **Mutt, V. and Jorpes, J. E.,** Structure of porcine cholecystokinin-pancreozymin. I. Cleavage with thrombin and with trypsin, *Eur. J. Biochem.,* 6, 156, 1968.
134. **Ertan, A., Brooks, F. P., Ostrow, J. D. Arvan, D. A. Williams, C. N., and Cerda, J. J.,** Effect of jejunal amino acid perfusion and exogenous cholecystokinin on the exocrine pancreatic and biliary secretions in man, *Gastroenterology,* 61, 686, 1971.
135. **Meyer, J. H. and Grossman, M. I.,** Comparison of d-and l-phenylalanine as pancreatic stimulants, *Am. J. Physiol.,* 222, 1058, 1972.
136. **Bounous, G. Sutherland, N. G., McArdle, A. H., and Gurd, F. N.,** The prophylactic use of an 'elemental' diet in experimental haemorrhagic shock and intestinal ischaemia, *Ann. Surg.,* 166, 312, 1967.
137. **Brown, R. A., Thompson, A. G., McArdle, A. H., and Gurd, F. N.,** Alteration of exocrine pancreatic storage enzymes by feeding on an elemental diet: a biochemical and ultrastructural study, *Surg. Forum,* 21, 391, 1970.
138. **McArdle, A. H., Brown, R. A., Echave, V., Rivilis, J., and Thompson A. G.,** Alterations in gastric and pancreatic secretion induced by an elemental diet., *Arch. Mal. Appar. Dig.,* 61, 115, 1972.
139. **Levenson, S., Kan, D., and Gruber, C.,** Haemolytic anaemia and pancreatic acinar atrophy and fibrosis conditioned by 'elemental' liquid diets and ordinary intestinal microflora, *Ann. Surg.,* 174, 469, 1971.
140. **Ragins, H., Levenson, S. M., Signer, R., Stamford, W., and Seifter, E.,** Intrajejunal administration of an elemental diet at neutral pH avoids pancreatic stimulation. Studies in dog and man, *Am. J. Surg.,* 126, 606, 1973.
141. **Konturek, S. J., Tasler, H., and Obtulowicz, W.,** Localisation of cholecystokinin release in intestine of the dog, *Am. J. Physiol.,* 16, 222, 1972.
142. **Wolfe, B. M., Keltner, P. M., and Kaminski, D. L.,** The effect of an intraduodenal diet on pancreatic secretion, *Surgery, Gynecol. Obstet.,* 140, 241, 1975.
143. **Cassim, M. M. and Allardyce, D. B.,** Pancreatic secretion in response to jejunal feeding of elemental diets, *Ann. Surg.,* 180, 228, 1974.
144. **Kerstein, M. D. and Neviackas, J. A.,** Histologic and ultrastructural studies of canine pancreas fed elemental diet, *Am. J. Gastroenterol.,* 66, 460, 1976.
145. **Kelly, G. A. and Nahrwold, D. L.,** Pancreatic secretion in response to an elemental diet and intravenous hyperalimentation, *Surgery, Gynecol. Obstet.,* 143, 87, 1976.
146. **Meyer, J. H. and Kelly, G. A.,** Canine pancreatic responses to intestinally perfused proteins and protein digests, *Am. J. Physiol.,* 231, 682, 1976.
147. **Kerstein, M. D. and Tonkens, R. M.,** Elemental diet and bile induced pancreatitis, *Surgery, Gynecol, Obstet.,* 143, 253, 1976.
148. **Neviackas, J. A. and Kerstein, M. D.,** Pancreatic enzyme response with an elemental diet, *Surgery, Gynecol. Obstet.,* 142, 71, 1976.

149. **Lewis, J. W. and Freeman, J. B.,** Canine pancreatic exocrine secretion in response to low and high fat elemental diets, *Gastroenterology,* 70, 907, 1976.
150. **Lewis, J. W. and Freeman, J. B.,** Canine pancreatic exocrine secretory response to low and high fat elemental diets, *Can. J. Surg.,* 20, 345, 1977.
151. **Vidon, N., Heckstsweiler, P., Butel, J., and Bernier, J. J.,** Effect of continuous jejunal perfusion of elemental and complex nutrition solutions on pancreatic enzyme secretion in human subjects, *Gut,* 19, 194, 1978.
152. **Atherton, S. T., Nelson, L. M., Robertson, E., and Russell, R. I.,** The effect of an elemental diet (Vivonex) on exocrine pancreatic secretion in man, *Scot. Med. J.,* 23, 115, 1978.
153. **McDonald, I.,** Effects of dietary glycerol on the serum glyceride levels of men and women, *Br. J. Nutr.,* 24, 537, 1970.
154. **McDonald, I.,** Effects of an amino acid-carbohydrate diet on fasting serum lipid levels in *Balanced Nutrition and Therapy,* Lang, K., Fekl, W., and Berg, G., Eds., Thieme, Stuttgart, 1971, 100.
155. **Young, D. E., Epley, J. A., and Goldman, P.,** Influence of a chemically defined diet on the composition of serum and urine, *Clin. Chem.,* 17, 765, 1971.
156. **Persson, B., Habte, D., and Sterky, G.,** Dietary effects in the early recovery phase of Kwashiorkor, *Acta Pediatr. Scand.,* 65, 329, 1976.
157. **Galant, S. P., Franz, M. L., Walker, P., Wells, I. D., and Lundak, R. L.,** A potential diagnostic method for food allergy: clinical application and immunogenicity evaluation of an elemental diet, *Am. J. Clin. Nutr.,* 30, 512, 1977.
158. **Eisen, H. N.,** *Immunology: An Introduction to Molecular and Cellular Principals of the Immune Responses,* Harper Row, New York, 1974, 386.
159. **Ferguson, A., Paul, G., and MacDonald, T. T.,** Immunodeficiency and fatty liver in mice reared on an elemental diet, *Arq. Gastroental. S. Paulo,* 15, 1, 1978.

Chapter 9

ELEMENTAL DIETS AND THE BACTERIAL FLORA OF THE GASTROINTESTINAL TRACT

M. J. Hudson, S. P. Borriello, and M. J. Hill

TABLE OF CONTENTS

I. INTRODUCTION

The bacterial flora of the human intestinal tract is an important part of the human environment and is in a favorable position to mediate between the host and his diet. The human intestinal flora is metabolically extremely active, and some of the interactions between dietary components and the flora have been discussed by Drasar and Hill.[1] In the normal person there is a wide variation in the bacterial flora at various sites along the digestive tract (Table 1). There is a rich flora in the mouth, which varies between the saliva, tongue, dental surface, etc., each representing a different ecological niche. The stomach contains a relatively sparse flora, as does the upper small intestine, but a rich flora is resident in the distal small intestine and in the large bowel.

There is a considerable person-to-person variation in the composition and distribution of the bacterial flora of the healthy digestive tract; further, in various disease states there are abnormalities evident in the flora. From these variations we can deduce some of the factors determining the composition and distribution of bacteria in the digestive tract.

Elemental diets may be used in preoperative bowel preparation and in the treatment of various diseases. It is important, therefore, that we understand the factors controlling the bacterial flora of the digestive tract in order to help us to formulate diets more effective in, for example, reducing the bulk of bacteria in the colon. We also need to understand the factors affecting the metabolic activity of the gut flora since, in general, it is these activities which concern the patient rather than the bacteria per se.

In this chapter we will first discuss the factors determining the composition and metabolic activity of the bacterial flora of the human digestive tract. We will then describe the effect of an elemental diet on the flora of various disease states such as obesity, inflammatory bowel disease, and in persons given the diet as preoperative bowel preparation. Finally we will describe the effect of elemental diets in some animal studies of interest.

II. FACTORS DETERMINING THE COMPOSITION AND ACTIVITY OF THE BACTERIAL FLORA

The factors affecting the composition and activity of the intestinal bacterial flora are summarized in Table 2. They can be divided into those related to the host physiology and pathology, those related to diet, and those classified as "bacterial interference".

A. Host Physiology and Pathology

1. pH and E_h

Most bacteria are killed by extremes of pH and only thrive at pH values between 7.5 and 5 (Table 3); within this range there are differences in the ability to cope with pH. The lactic acid bacteria (lactobacilli and streptococci), by virtue of their high yields of acid endproducts of fermentation, flourish at the expense of the putrefactive organisms (bacteroides, clostridia) as the environmental conditions become more acid. Between pH 4 and 5 bacteria are able to survive and multiply but, in general, are not very active metabolically. Thus, as a rough guide, it can be assumed that pH values above 8 and below 4 are bactericidal, but that bacteria only flourish between pH 5 and 7.5.

The majority of bacteria inhabiting the human GI tract produce enzymes to metabolize exogenous substrates with pH optima close to 7. Thus changes in the colonic pH may affect the activity of these enzymes. Redox potential (E_h) is a measure of the reducing conditions and is often, but not necessarily, related to the oxygen tension; most bacteria in the digestive tract are obligately anaerobic and are killed by oxygen. As illustrated in Table 4, anaerobic bacteria may be divided by their sensitivity to exposure to oxygen

Table 1
BACTERIAL FLORA OF THE HUMAN GI TRACT[1,63,64,65]

	Anaerobic bacteria				Aerobic bacteria			
	Bacteroides	**Gram nonsporing**	**Clostridia (spores)**	**Veillonella**	**Lactobacilli**	**Streptococci**	**Enterobacteria**	**Enterococci**
Saliva	4.7[a]	3.4	ND	—	4.5	7.3	ND	ND
Stomach	ND	ND	ND	ND	ND	ND	ND	ND
Small intestine								
jejunum	ND	ND	ND	—	2.4	2.4	ND	—
ileum	ND	ND	—	—	ND	ND	ND	—
distal ileum	5.7	5.8	ND	—	ND	2.5	3.3	2.2
Cecum	7.8	8.4	3.0	—	6.4	2.6	6.2	3.6
Feces	10.5	10.5	5	5	7	8	8	5

Note: ND = none detected (< 2.0); — = data not given.

[a] Log_{10} c.f.u. $m\ell^{-1}$ or gm^{-1}.

Table 2
FACTORS AFFECTING THE GI TRACT FLORA

1. Host–mediated factors		
		Secretions, e.g., immunoglobins, pH, bile salts, lysozyme, proteases
		Motility, e.g., speed, periodic stasis
		Water activity
		Physiology, e.g., compartmentalization
		Exfoliated cells, mucins, tissue exudate
2. Bacterial physiology		
		Adhesion
		Motility
		Nutritional flexibility
		Spores, capsules, and proteases
		Generation time
3. Bacterial interractions		
	Synergy	Metabolic cooperation
		Cofactor and vitamin excretion
		Alterations to E_h, pH, O_2 tension
	Antagonism	Fatty Acids, amines, phenols, bile acid production
		Alterations to E_h, pH, O_2 tension
		Antibiotic, colicin, phage production
		Proteases, lipases, etc.
4. Diet		
		Bile acids, steroids, and lipids
		Unabsorbed dietary excess
		Undigestible residues ("fiber")

Table 3
THE NUMBERS OF BACTERIA OF VARIOUS GENERA ISOLATED FROM GASTRIC JUICE OF VARIOUS pH VALUES

	pH <4	pH 4 to 5	pH >5
Number of specimens	30	5	20
Mean total anaerobic count[a]	<2	5.5	6.2
Total aerobic count	<2	4.9	5.7
Micrococci	<2	4.7	5.5
Streptococci	<2	4.0	3.8
Enterococci	<2	2.9	4.3
Lactobacilli	<2	2.7	2.4
Number of specimens with more than 10^5 organisms	1 (3%)	3 (60%)	18 (90%)
Number with more than 10^5 fecal streptococci	1 (3%)	1 (20%)	10 (50%)

[a] Counts expressed as $\log_{10}$ c.f.u. $m\ell^{-1}$.

in vitro and such groupings reflect the degree of difficulty encountered in the isolation and cultivation of particular groups of bacteria. At the extremes, the methanogenic bacteria require rigorous exclusion of oxygen during manipulation and cultivation from specimens, usually accomplished with techniques not usually available to most microbiology laboratories, whereas organisms such as *Clostridium tertium* and *C. carnis* will grow (albeit poorly) on blood agar incubated in air. Since the digestive tract contains

Table 4
OXYGEN SENSITIVITIES OF VARIOUS ANAEROBIC BACTERIA[a]

1. Extremely oxygen sensitive anaerobes
   Growth only at $pO_2 < 0.03\%$
   Methanogenic bacteria, e.g., *Methanobacterium ruminantium*

2. Strict anaerobes
   Growth maximal at $pO_2 < 0.5\%$
   Treponema denticola, T. oralis
   Selenomonas ruminantium, Butyrivibrio fibrisolvens
   Clostridium novyi type B, *Cl. haemolyticum*

3. Moderate anaerobes
   Growth maximal at $pO_2 < 3\%$
   Bacteroides fragilis, B. vulgatus
   B. oralis, B. melaninogenicus
   Clostridium novyi type A, *Cl. perfringens*
   Bifidobacterium infantis

4. Aerotolerant anaerobes
   Low pO_2 for maximal growth, but capable of aerobic growth on blood agar
   Cl. histolyticum, Cl. tertium, Cl. carnis

5. Microaerophiles
   Growth maximal between $pO_2 > 0.3\%$ and $< 20\%$ (air)
   Campylobacter fetus ss. fetus; *C. fetus* ss. jejuni

[a] Data from Ref. 66 and elsewhere.

a mixed flora of anaerobes and aerobes at all points it may be assumed that the aerobic organisms utilize any oxygen which enters the tract extremely rapidly, so protecting the anaerobic organisms.

2. Immune Systems

Although there is very little information on the role of humoral and cellular immunological processes in controlling the normal intestinal flora, it is likely that they are important, particularly in determining the sequence of establishment of the neonate flora by protection afforded in colostrum. The mucosa of the intestinal tract is rich in immunoglobulin (Ig) secreting cells and in lymphocytes and macrophages, and indeed there is every indication that since both IgA and IgM are secreted from the mucosa in a form which is resistant to proteolytic digestion (as secretory IgA and IgM), an immune suppression of particular components of the flora can be envisaged even in the intestinal lumen. More importantly, several groups of workers have shown that there is immune tolerance to the normal or indigenous flora, in animals at least, and may be due to shared antigenic determinants.[2-6] Such humoral accommodation of the commensal flora may explain pathological disturbances which may be sequelae to Ig deficiences, especially as regard to jejunal bacterial overgrowth.[7]

3. Secreted Enzymes

Many species of Gram-positive bacteria are sensitive to lysozyme, which is secreted in saliva and is present in intestinal secretions. Many of the proteolytic enzymes in intestinal secretions (e.g., pepsin in gastric secretions, trypsin in pancreatic secretions) affect bacterial growth and so might be expected to play a role in determining the composition of the proximal intestinal bacterial flora.

4. Digestive Secretions

Saliva is rich in lysozyme while gastric secretion is rich in acid and in pepsin, which have been discussed already. In addition, a wide range of bacterial species is sensitive to bile (Table 5); for example, most salivary organisms can be included in this group. Consequently bacteroides isolated from the upper digestive tract are usually bile-sensitive (e.g. *B. oralis* or *B. melaninogenicus*) while those found in the lower GI tract flora are bile-resistant (e.g., *B. vulgatus*). Pancreatic secretion is rich in enzymes which are able to affect bacterial growth.

5. Mucin

Apart from acting as a physical barrier to penetration of bacteria, mucin is a passive reservoir of immunoglobulins and also appears to dictate the establishment of particular components of the microflora. Some species are able to degrade mucins by specific enzymes, e.g., *Vibrio cholerae* and certain enterococci,[8] which may play a role in pathogenicity. Others, by virtue of their ability to cleave specific glycosides are favored by the presence of the particular glycoproteins of mucin dictated by the host antigenic make up as has been demonstrated by Hoskins and Boulding[9,10] for the mucin associated blood group "secretor" antigens.

B. Diet

Although it appears obvious that diet plays a major role in determining the composition of the bacterial flora of the GI tract, there is not a large body of evidence to support such a role. The diet may be considered in terms of its macronutrient composition, its "nonnutritive" components, and the availability of its nutrients.

The role of the macronutrients in determining the flora of the digestive tract has been particularly difficult to establish. Since the fats, proteins, and carbohydrates are present largely as macromolecules and since their residence time in the mouth is short, they would be expected to have little effect on the oral bacterial flora, and this appears to be so. In most healthy persons the flow of gastric acid is sufficient to maintain the stomach and small intestine in an almost sterile state; dietary macronutrients could only affect the flora in these regions if they inhibited gastric acid secretion. The macronutrients are readily digested and so are largely unavailable to the bacterial flora of the large bowel. Consequently, it is not surprising that diet appears to have little effect on the fecal flora (Table 6).

The "nonnutritive" or "unavailable" carbohydrates might be expected to be more influential in determining the flora by virtue of large amounts of such carbohydrate favoring saccharolytic organisms (e.g., lactobacilli and streptococci) at the expense of the putrefactive bacteria (e.g., bacteroides and clostridia). There is no evidence that this in fact happens, although data have only been obtained for the fecal flora while the changes would be expected to be more apparent in the cecum and proximal colon.

Where the diet contains a high proportion of monomers these may be immediately available to the bacterial flora even in the mouth, but this will only be so for nutrients whose utilization is controlled by constitutive enzymes. Many inducible enzymes are subject to glucose repression and for this reason sugars and sugar alcohols such as lactose, lactulose, xylitol, mannitol, and sorbitol are not utilized by the oral flora. Since all of the sugars listed are "unavailable" (i.e., are only poorly absorbed if at all from the small intestine) they reach the large bowel and are utilized by the colonic flora where there is no glucose present to repress the relevent enzymes. They will be fermented to yield short chain fatty acids with consequent reduction of the cecal pH; thus such sugars would be expected to affect the composition of the cecal flora both by supplying a nutrient more accessible to some organisms than to others and by modifying the pH. There are,

Table 5
BILE SENSITIVITY OF VARIOUS GENERA OF BACTERIA

Genus	Species sensitive to 10% bile	Species resistant to 10% bile
Streptococcus spp.	*S. pyogenes,*	Enterococci
	S. viridans	
	S. salivarius	
	S. mutans	
Staphylococcus spp.	All species	None
Micrococcus spp.	All species	None
Neisseria spp.	All species	None
Enterobacteriaceae	None	*Escherichia* spp.
		Salmonella spp.
		Shigella spp.
		Proteus spp.
		Klebsiella spp.
Bacteroides spp.	*B. oralis*	*B. fragilis*
	B. melaninogenicus	*B. vulgatus*
Lactobacillus spp.	Most species	*L. acidophilus*
	L. lactis	*L. fermentum*
	L. casei	*L. bulgaricus*
Clostridium spp.	*C. tetani*	*C. perfingens*
	C. haemolyticum	*C. paraputrificum*
		C. difficile

Table 6
FECAL BACTERIAL FLORA OF PERSONS LIVING ON VARIOUS DIETS

Dietary type	Duration	Type of population	Effect on fecal flora (compared with that on a normal western diet)
Bran supplement	3 Weeks	Volunteers	No effect
Bagasse supplement	12 Weeks	Volunteers	No effect
Pectin supplement	3 Weeks	Volunteers	No effect
High meat	4 Weeks	Volunteers	No effect
Matoke (boiled mashed banana)	Lifetime	Ugandan	Decreased bacteroides, increased enterobacteria
Rice-based diet	Lifetime	Indian	No effect
Low protein, low fat High vegetable diet	Lifetime	Japan	Very high enterobacteria

unfortunately, no data on the effect of sugar alcohols or lactulose on the cecal flora of humans.

It is assumed that the human colonic flora is maintained as a complex, metabolically interactive consortium of microorganisms competing for available nutrients. As has been found in the bovine and ovine rumen microflora, such consortia are comprised of a chain of species, each living off the metabolism of each other. Thus broadly proteolytic, lipolytic, or saccharolytic types provide less complex nutrients for their neighbors to metabolize, and so on. Salyers[11] has described the ability of a range of bacterial species from the human intestine able to degrade various complex carbohydrates. Monosaccharides and partially degraded polysaccharides are then released for the use of other components of the flora. In addition, the fatty acid end-products (lactate, succinate, acetate, and other short chain fatty acids) can be used as sole carbon sources by other bacteria. Ultimately, carbon dioxide and hydrogen liberated by fermentations may be fixed by methanogenic bacteria to form methane. Similarly, protein is ultimately degraded to amino acids, ammonia, amines, and fatty acids. The interested reader is referred to recent reviews by Smith and Bryant,[12] and Miller and Wolin[13] for introductions to the complexities of bacterial nutritional cooperation in man and other mammals.

C. Bacterial Interference

Bacteria compete for ecological niches by producing antibacterial substances active against their competitors; these may be antibiotic substances (active against organisms of other species or genera), or bacteriocines and bacteriophage (active against organisms of the same species or genus), or normal metabolic end-products (such as volative fatty acids, amines, or phenols). Such mechanisms are poorly understood in man but certainly exist in experimental infections of animals. One serotype of *Escherichia coli* will hinder the proliferation of other serotypes. The normal microflora will hinder the establishment of pathogens such as *Shigella flexneri* in mice[14] and *Salmonella* spp. in chicks.[15,16] The stability of such interferences is easily disrupted, for instance by antimicrobial agents and this can either hinder normal clearance of pathogens (thus extending the "carrier" state) as has been demonstrated in food-poisoning salmonellosis, or may allow drastic overgrowth with such pathogens as *Staphylococcus aureus, Candida albicans* or *Clostridium perfringens (welchii).* It is widely thought that the overgrowth of toxigenic *Cl. difficile* seen in pseudomembranous colitis is a result of decimation of the normal flora by such antibiotics as ampicillin and lincomycin.[17,18]

D. Environmental Pathology

The environmental pathology plays a major role in determining the local bacterial flora; consequently, in the mouth, there are differences in the flora of the saliva, tongue surface, tooth surface, etc. The greatest differences observed are between the mucosal surface of the GI tract and the lumen at the same point in the tract. This has been documented for the mouth,[19] jejunum,[20] and large bowel.[21] Organisms that are not intimately associated with epithelial surfaces can be removed mechanically by peristalsis. Indeed, many people believe intestinal motility to be one of the more important methods of controlling bacterial establishment and proliferation within the small intestine.[22] Disruption of active peristalsis may result in disruption of GI function and bacterial establishment and proliferation as is manifest in the blind loop syndrome.[23,24] Overgrowths by the intestinal flora resulting from various gastric or small intestinal surgical procedures are discussed by Drasar and Hill.[1]

E. Role of an Elemental Diet

The factors affecting the flora at various subsites in the GI tract are listed in Table 7. An elemental diet will affect the flora of the mouth because its nutrients are more available to the bacteria. An elemental diet is known to affect gastric, pancreatic, and biliary secretions and so will affect the flora of the stomach and small intestine. It is residue-free and so should be very efficiently absorbed and should permit maximum recovery of bile salts and cholesterol; this should have an effect on the large intestinal flora. These effects will now be discussed in more detail.

III. EFFECT BY SUBSITE IN HEALTHY PERSONS OF ELEMENTAL DIETS

Although almost all of the studies of the effects of elemental diets on the GI flora have concerned the fecal bacteria, there are some data on the oral flora. We can make some deductions of the effects on the gastric and small bowel flora.

Table 7
FACTORS CONTROLLING THE MICROFLORA AT VARIOUS SUBSITES WITHIN THE GASTROINTESTINAL TRACT

Subsite	Factors controlling the microflora
Mouth	Nutrient availability (time, complexity)
	salivary excretions (lysozyme, immunoglobulins)
Stomach	Gastric acid (low pH)
	Mucus barrier
	Nutrient availability (time, complexity)
Small intestine	Biliary and pancreatic secretions
	"seeding" flora from mouth
	Rapid peristalsis
	Mucus, immunoglobulins
Large intestine	Nutrient availability
	Bacterial interference and cooperation
	pH, E_h
	Bile acids, fatty acids
	Water content
	Transit time

A. Oral Bacterial Flora

In a small pilot study the oral bacterial flora of three persons consuming an elemental diet (the "Howard" diet) was compared with that of the same persons consuming a normal diet (Table 8). Total anaerobic and aerobic counts both showed a tendency to increase during the elemental diet period, as did counts of *Streptococcus salivarius* and *Veillonella* spp. Other species showed variable responses to changes in diet. The proportion of the flora able to reduce nitrate increased greatly during the elemental diet period, a finding somewhat difficult to explain in view of the extremely low nitrate level of this diet (prepared in distilled water) and must represent an increase in those components of the flora which are constitutive for nitrate reductase.

The normal diet of humans is macromolecular and the proportion of the total diet available to the oral bacterial flora is small. In contrast the elemental diet is almost entirely available to the oral bacteria and consequently it is not surprising that the bacteria thrive on this diet.

B. Gastric Bacterial Flora

The normal human stomach is effectively sterilized by the gastric hydrochloric acid. There is evidence that an elemental diet has the effect of reducing the amount of gastric acid secreted,[25-27] and the lack of a solid particulate component to the diet might be expected to affect its buffering capacity. Thus, although there are no data available, we might expect the reduced rate of acid secretion, the increased buffering effect of an elemental diet, and the greater load of bacteria present in the saliva to result in an increased normal gastric flora during the consumption of a meal.

C. The Small Intestinal Bacterial Flora

One of the major factors controlling the small bowel bacterial flora is the bile salt concentration, since bile salts are bactericidal to most salivary and gastric organisms. Perault et al.[28] showed that, while the bile salt secretion in response to aminosol stimulation in persons consuming an elemental diet is similar to that in persons eating a normal control diet, the secretion in response to pancreozymin is reduced. Further,

Table 8
THE BACTERIAL FLORA OF SALIVA OF THREE PERSONS CONSUMING A CONTROL (NORMAL) DIET AND AN ELEMENTAL DIET

		Aerobes			Anaerobes		
Person	Diet	Total	Strep. salivarius	Micrococci	Total	Veillonellae	Lactobacilli
A	Control	7.8	7.4	7.4	8.0	6.4	3.4
	Elemental	8.4	8.1	7.6	8.8	7.7	<2
B	Control	8.4	7.9	7.5	8.2	6.8	4.7
	Elemental	8.4	7.9	7.2	8.5	7.4	<2
C	Control	8.1	7.7	7.5	7.5	6.7	4.4
	Elemental	8.4	7.9	7.3	8.5	7.8	4.9

Note: Expressed as $\log_{10}$ c.f.u. $m\ell^{-1}$.

pancreatic secretion of lipase is also reduced on an elemental diet. Thus in persons consuming an elemental diet we might expect bacteria swallowed with food and which survive transit through the stomach to be able to more readily survive the lethal effects of the bile and pancreatic secretions. There are at present few data to confirm or refute this expectation. This is despite the observations that it appears that this is one region of the GI tract that may be influenced from a microbiological point of view by dietary means.

Dickman et al.[29] monitored the small bowel flora, pre- and post-treatment with the elemental diet Vivonex®, of a patient with an ileoproctostomy for ulcerative colitis. This patient exhibited bacterial overgrowth in the small bowel and symptoms of chronic diarrhea. Microbiological analysis of samples obtained at the ligament of Treitz before the diet and on the 11th day of the diet showed a reduction in the microbial flora from 10^7 to 10^5 c.f.u.$m\ell^{-1}$ concommitant with a reduction in "stool" frequency from about 20 per day to 5 to 7 per day. Reductions in the flora were evident in the numbers of *Enterobacteriaceae*, streptococci, staphylococci, yeasts, *Veillonella* spp and fusobacteria isolated.

Axelsson and Justessen[30] demonstrated that Vivasorb® "normalized" an abnormal duodenal flora of 4 of 6 patients. They also showed that administration of the diet in 17 patients was associated with a decrease in the total number of organisms recoverable in 11 patients, an increase in 5, and no change in 1. The patient that exhibited no change failed to yield recoverable organisms during the trial. The complexity of the flora in terms of variety of organisms that could be cultivated decreased when the patient was receiving the diet in ten cases and increased in complexity in four cases. In four of the cases where there was both a qualitative and quantitative decrease in the flora present when on the diet, the numbers of microorganisms present were reduced to levels that were not recoverable by the methods used in the study. The results of a limited number of studies imply that an elemental diet can be used to reduce the small bowel flora from both a qualitative and quantitative point of view and that elemental dietary intervention may be a useful adjunct in the treatment of small bowel overgrowth and does not carry the risk of antibiotic-associated diarrhea or the emergence of antibiotic–resistant bacteria, that may be associated with antimicrobial therapy. The use of elemental diets in conjunction with carefully chosen antimicrobial regimens deserves further study, as do the mechanisms by which such diets are able to bring about reductions and simplifications in the contaminated small bowel syndromes. It is tempting to speculate that the improvement in nutritional status of the patient may increase the competence of local immune clearance mechanisms in the bowel.

D. The Large Bowel Bacterial Flora

The first study of the effect of elemental diets on the composition of the fecal bacterial flora was by Winitz et al.[31] who studied the effect of an elemental diet containing glucose as the main energy source. Their principal findings were that within 6 days the number of bacteria per gram of feces was reduced by 10^5 and that after 13 days only three types of bacteria remained (*Bacteroides* spp., enterococci, and coliforms), none at levels of more than 10^3/g. The flora returned to its normal complexity with respect both to numbers of types of organisms and numbers of organisms per gram feces within 4 days of resuming a normal diet. Not only was the number of organisms per gram of feces greatly reduced by the elemental diet, but also the number of grams of feces passed per day was also greatly reduced; this indicated that the bacterial flora of the large bowel had been reduced to a very low level and suggested a major role for elemental diets in, for example, preoperative bowel preparation.

When the energy source was changed from glucose to sucrose the effect was less dramatic, but nevertheless the number of organisms per gram of feces was still reduced by a factor of 10 to 100 fold.[31] Although the number of bacteroides remained high and no consistent trend was seen with the coliforms, enterococci totally disappeared from the stools of 4/8 volunteers (and were greatly reduced in numbers in an additional three persons) while lactobacilli and yeasts completely disappeared.

These were very dramatic observations and provoked a flood of attempts to verify them (Table 9). Most of these were considered to be unsuccessful and there were two major reasons for this. The first was that the most dramatic effects had been obtained using a glucose based elemental diet which was never marketed (since it gave rise in some persons to severe rebound hypoglycemia); the effects of commercial elemental diets were nevertheless compared with the glucose-based diet rather than those based on sucrose. The second reason was that most attention was centered on the effects of the elemental diet on the number of organisms per gram of feces rather than on the number of bacteria excreted in feces per day. Thus Attebury et al.,[32] Crowther et al.,[33] Bounous and Devroede,[34] and Koumans[35] all reported little or no effect on the numbers of bacteria per gram of feces. All reported that the consumption of an elemental diet resulted in a decrease in the numbers of enterococci per gram of feces and there were also reports of decreases in the numbers of lactobacilli and in the highly oxygen-sensitive anaerobes. All noted that the stool frequency was greatly reduced and it is a common observation that elemental diets also greatly reduce the mean daily stool weight; thus, it is clear that there is qualitative support for the observation by Winitz et al.[31] that elemental diets reduce the bacterial population of the large bowel but there has been no support for their results on the magnitude of the decrease.

Although most studies have revealed little change in the total number of bacteria per gram of feces they have usually shown that the composition of the flora is modified (Table 9). Attebury et al.[32] studied three volunteers; in all three there was an observed increase in the total number of aerobic organisms per gram, no change in the total number of anaerobic organisms, but a total elimination of what they refer to as the "extremely oxygen sensitive" anaerobes (e.g., *Eubacterium rectale, Peptococcus* spp. and *Butyrivibrio fibrisolvens*) while *Bifidobacterium* spp. were eliminated from the flora of two persons and the numbers of *Clostridium perfringens* per gram was greatly reduced in two of the three persons. The increase in total aerobes was due to an increase in coliforms; the number of lactobacilli was reduced in two of the three subjects. Bounous and Devroede[34] studied 14 persons and observed no changes in the composition of the fecal flora except for a decrease in the number of enterococci; they did not study the "very oxygen-sensitive" group of anaerobes and so could not comment on the observation by Attebury et al.[32] Crowther et al.[33] studied the flora of three healthy volunteers and

Table 9
THE EFFECT OF AN ELEMENTAL DIET ON THE COMPOSITION OF THE FLORA IN HEALTHY PERSONS

			Effect on the fecal flora		
Diet	Time on diet	Number of persons	Total no. of bacteria/gm	Specific organisms	Refs.
CDD6 (glucose)	2 Weeks	8	Marked decrease	Marked decrease in all organisms	31
CDD7 (sucrose)	2 Weeks	8	Decrease	Marked decrease in enterococci and lactobacilli	
CDD6[a]	8—10 Days	3	None	Decrease in enterococci and "extremely oxygen-sensitive" anaerobes	32
CDD6[a]	14 Days	3	None	Decrease in enterococci and lactobacilli	33
3200AS	12 Days	14	None	Decrease in enterococci	34
Howard diet	7 Days	6	None	Decrease in enterococci, veillonellae and lactobacilli	—

[a] Oligosaccharide based diets.

observed little change in the total number of anaerobes or the total number of aerobic organisms per gram of feces, but they noted that the numbers of *Streptococcus viridans,* enterococci, and lactobacilli were reduced. Koumans[35] studied three patients with various GI diseases and observed a decrease in the total number of bacteria and in particular, a decrease in the number of enterococci. Bornside and Cohn[35] studied ten healthy volunteers and found no effect either on the total number of bacteria per gram of feces or on the composition of the fecal flora. Uphill[37] studied baboons and found no change in the total number of organisms per gram of feces but a decrease in the numbers of *Cl. perfringens* and of lactobacilli (and, interestingly, an increase in the number of coliforms). Thus, although there is no real agreement on any specific change in the flora, four of the seven groups reported a reduction in the number of enterococci and 4/7 reported a decrease in the number of lactobacilli; 2/7 noted a decrease in *Cl. perfringens* 2/7 an increase in coliforms. Our own results on six healthy volunteers are illustrated in Table 10 and demonstrate that although some individuals showed marked reduction in enterococci, clostridia, and lactobacilli, such trends were inconsistent in the group as a whole.

When we try to rationalize these changes, the lack of uniformity in the reports clearly presents difficulties. Winitz et al.[31] suggested that the lack of residue in the diet meant that the amount of nutrient available to the flora was dramatically reduced; this could provide an explanation for the reduction in the total number of organisms only if the diet is, directly, the main source of nutrient. The major nutrients entering the large bowel include the undigested residue of the diet together with mucus and dead intestinal mucosal cells which slough off into the gut lumen; there is no clear information on the relative contribution made by these components, but it should be noted that the rate of turnover of the small intestinal mucosa is diet dependent and so the effect of the elemental diet could be secondary to this effect on the rate of desquamation of mucosal cells. We know that most of the "indigestible" residue of the diet is digested by the gut bacteria and that an increase in the amount of dietary residue leads to an increase in the total number of bacteria excreted in feces per day.[38,39] If this were the cause of the decrease

Table 10

Subject	Total aerobes		Total anaerobes		Clostridia		Veillonellae		Bifidobacteria		Bacteroides		Lactobacilli		Enterococci	
A	6.6[a]	6.9[b]	10.1	9.3	7.1	5.2	5.1	2.9	8.0	6.6	9.4	8.7	5.8	2.9	ND	7.8
B	7.0	7.9	9.1	9.8	5.6	4.4	5.6	3.3	7.6	7.5	8.4	9.9	5.4	3.9	6.2	6.1
C	3.9	5.9	8.9	9.9	5.9	7.2	ND	ND	3.7	6.3	8.4	9.2	ND	5.4	—	—
D	9.1	8.0	9.7	9.8	5.0	5.6	6.7	2.0	7.9	7.5	9.6	9.5	5.6	4.4	8.5	ND
E	9.3	12.0	9.2	12.0	2.8	4.5	ND	ND	4.9	ND	9.1	11.4	4.5	ND	—	—
F	7.2	8.2	9.4	10.2	5.3	5.4	2.7	1.6	6.1	5.1	9.0	9.7	3.9	3.1	6.1	ND

Note: Counts expressed as $\log_{10}$ No/gm wet weight of stool; ND is none detected.

[a] Normal diet.
[b] After 7 days elemental diet.

in total numbers of organisms we would expect the decrease to be greatest in the saccharolytic organisms (since these would be expected to thrive selectively in an environment where the main source of nutrient was dietary fiber); if, however, the effect was secondary to an effect on the rate of mucosal cell desquamation then this might be expected to affect the proteolytic organisms more. In fact, the effect is mixed, being mainly directed at the saccharolytic streptococci and lactobacilli in some reports and against the putrefactive *Cl. perfingens* in others.

It is known that one of the major effects of an elemental diet on the colonic physiology is to bring about a large reduction in the colonic bile acid and cholesterol concentration[33] and this has been used as the rationale for the successful treatment of cholerrheic diarrhea using an elemental diet.[40] Some of our unpublished results on the effect of an elemental diet on fecal steroid concentration are given in Table 11. It has been suggested that the colonic bile acid concentration might be important in determining the relative proportions of the strict anaerobes in the flora; since in vitro the bacteroides group of organisms are stimulated by bile salts. There have been no published reports that an elemental diet results in a decrease in the numbers of *Bacteroides* spp. and a compensating increase in the numbers of Gram positive anaerobes.

E. The Effect of An Elemental Diet on the Biochemical Activity of the Gut Bacterial Flora

There are few data on the effects of an elemental diet on the metabolism of colonic substrates by the gut bacteria; there is information only on the metabolism of bile pigments, bile acids, cholesterol, and tyrosine. The first observation was by Winitz et al.[31] who noted that the stools of persons consuming an elemental diet based on glucose were green. The major pigments in feces are derived from bilirubin which is secreted in the bile and which is itself derived from hemoglobin and heme-containing enzymes. Bilirubin is metabolized by the flora via a series of reductive steps yielding a range of colored and colorless products. A precursor of bilirubin is biliverdin which is colored green and the observation by Winitz et al.[31] indicated that, when consuming an elemental diet with glucose as the energy source, the gut flora were virtually totally inactive in these reductive reactions as would be expected if the flora had been decreased to the extent claimed by Winitz et al.[31] These effects on bile pigment metabolism have not been reported by other groups (who used elemental diets based on energy sources other than glucose) and were not observed by us in any of our studies.

Crowther et al.[33] reported that persons consuming an elemental diet had relatively low fecal concentrations of neutral steroids and that these were mainly in the form of undegraded cholesterol. Cholesterol is normally extensively degraded by the gut bacterial flora, with more than 80% of the fecal neutral steroids being in the form of the bacterial metabolites coprostanol, coprostanone, and cholestenone. In the volunteers studied by Crowther et al.[33] this was reduced to less than 20%; Table 11 illustrates some of our unpublished results of the effect of an elemental diet in obese persons (where the diet was also used as a means of caloric control). These studies were carried out in collaboration with Dr. I. M. Baird of the West Middlesex Hospital, London. Crowther et al.[33] noted that the decrease in the proportion of neutral steroid metabolized decreased with the number of enterococci per gram of feces but concluded that this was a coincidental observation. The decrease in metabolism is probably related to a decrease in the total number of bacteria in the colon.

The gall bladder is virtually unstimulated by elemental diets[40] and consequently relatively little bile acid enters the small intestine. Because the diet contains no residue for the bile salt to adsorb to, there is virtually no hindrance to the recovery of bile salts from the terminal ileum and consequently the amount of bile salt entering the colon is

Table 11
THE EFFECT OF AN ELEMENTAL DIET ON THE FECAL STEROID CONCENTRATION/ (mg/g DRY WEIGHT)

Subject	Diet	Number of days on diet	Neutral steroids: Total	Neutral steroids: % as bacterial[a] metabolites	Total acid steroids
A	Control	—	11.1	81	6.8
	Elemental	1	14.8	—	6.6
		2	12.5	71	4.2
		6	7.6	41	3.1
		28	5.0	10	—
		56	4.1	24	4.2
B	Control	—	13.0	68	12.0
	Elemental	3	9.6	35	5.6
		7	8.1	12	4.0
		12	7.6	8	4.0
		25	5.2	10	4.5
C	Control	—	12.4	73	6.3
	Elemental	1	15.7	69	6.3
		8	6.8	15	4.7
		21	3.7	24	2.9
		29	6.0	26	3.8

[a] $\% \text{ Bacterial metabolites} = \frac{\text{coprostanol} + \text{coprostanone}}{\text{cholesterol} + \text{coprostanol}} + \text{coprostanone}^{\times 100}$

very small in persons on an elemental diet in comparison with those consuming a normal diet, as illustrated in Table 12. The extent of dehydroxylation of these bile acids is also much lower than in persons on a normal diet, with monosubstituted bile acids accounting for less that 20% of the total (compared with 40 to 50% of the fecal bile acids of persons on a normal diet[41]). Again, this is probably due to the overall reduction in the total number of bacteria in the colon of persons consuming an elemental diet. The effect of elemental diets on bile acid metabolism is further discussed in Chapter 8.

The aromatic amino acids tyrosine and phenylalanine are metabolized by the gut bacteria to yield a range of volatile phenols (reviewed by Drasar and Hill[1]), the major of which are phenol and *p*-cresol, and these are absorbed from the colon and excreted in the urine. Normal human urine contains 50 to 100 mg volatile phenols per day of which 80 to 90% is usually *p*-cresol and the remainder is phenol.[42] Persons consuming an elemental diet excreted only 30% of the normal amount of urinary volatile phenols; it is likely that urinary indican levels are similarly reduced. All of these changes in the metabolic activity of the gut flora can be explained by the overall reduction in the total colonic bacterial flora rather than to the effect of an elemental diet on any particular species or group of organisms.

IV. EFFECT OF ELEMENTAL DIETS ON INTESTINAL FLORA IN DISEASE

Despite the many clinical studies of the use of elemental diets in human disease, very few data are available concerning the effects of such treatments on the intestinal flora.

Table 12
FECAL BILE ACID EXCRETION IN PERSONS CONSUMING AN ELEMENTAL DIET COMPARED WITH A CONTROL DIET

	Control diet			Elemental diet		
Person	Daily fecal dry wieght (g)	Mean FBA conc (mg/g dry wt)	Daily FBA (mg/day)	Daily fecal dry weight (g)	Mean FBA conc (mg/g dry wt)	Daily FBA (mg/day)
1	75	4.8	358	23	2.1	47
2	31	5.3	165	16	2.2	35
3	30	6.5	194	17	1.5	25

There is much need for biochemical and bacteriological studies on the intestinal flora in conditions which appear to respond to elemental dietary intervention, if only to exclude the intestinal flora of a role in the etiology of the disease.

A. Preoperative Bowel Preparation

In preoperative bowel preparation patients treated with an elemental diet should be compared with those given an alternative preoperative bowel preparation rather than a normal diet. Very few such studies have been published, although the efficacy of elemental diets in producing a clean colon have been well documented.

Arabi et al.[43] studied the effect of an elemental diet in preoperative bowel preparation, in comparison with a regime based on magnesium sulfate, enemas and wash-out and with one based on whole bowel irrigation, on the luminal bacterial flora. The results showed that the elemental diet left fewer bacteria per gram contents, both aerobic and anaerobic, than either of the two alternative methods; addition of antibiotics (neomycin and metronidazole) to all three regimes resulted in a massive reduction in bacterial counts, with all three regimes giving essentially similar results.

In our own study of the fecal flora of patients treated with a short period of elemental diet prior to surgery for nonobstructive colorectal carcinoma (Table 13), we found that no overall changes occurred in the fecal flora after 5 days elemental diet; this is, of course, consistent with the results presented on the fecal flora of healthy volunteers (Table 10).

A review of the large numbers of studies conducted for the comparison of various antimicrobial agents given pre- or postoperatively is not the purpose of this chapter but it is perhaps pertinent to draw attention to the growing number of reports suggesting that preoperative bowel sterilization with poorly absorbed antimicrobial agents is not necessarily the best method of preventing postoperative sepsis but may disrupt the flora to a degree which permits overgrowth with enteric pathogens such as *Staphylococcus aureus* and *Clostridium difficile* (see Section II.C of this chapter). The most effective regimens appear to be those based upon the use of antimicrobials, such as metronidazole, which are active against anaerobes — the most commonly encountered causes of postoperative abdominal sepsis and wound infection — and achieve high levels in the tissue when given peri- and postoperatively. In a study by Marks et al.[43] it was shown that although a combination of mechanical bowel preparation and a nonabsorbed sulfonamide (phthalylsulfathiazole) resulted in a reduction of the fecal bulk and microbial flora, the flora attached to the mucosa was unaffected; it is not difficult to envisage that it is this flora which acts as the reservoir for tissue infection, anastomosis breakdown, etc., and thus an effective policy of reducing fecal soiling during surgery by dietary or mechanical reduction of intestinal contents and the use of adequate doses of appropriate antimicrobials would appear to be the most logical method for reducing sepsis.

Table 13
EFFECTS OF ELEMENTAL DIET ON FECAL FLORA DURING PREOPERATIVE BOWEL PREPARATION

	Aerobes			Anaerobes			
			Gram + ve			Clostridia	
Subject	Total	Coliforms	cocci	Total	Bacteroides	lec+	lec−
A	7.8	7.4	7.6	10.2	9.0	5.8	7.1
A[a]	7.6	6.9	7.6	9.2	9.1	6.1	7.7
B	8.7	8.5	7.7	10.3	9.5	3.0	7.0
B[a]	7.3	7.3	ND	9.3	8.7	2.7	5.7
C	8.4	7.2	8.4	9.0	8.4	3.1	6.1
C[a]	8.2	7.5	8.0	9.0	9.0	ND	3.0
D	6.9	6.9	ND	8.3	8.3	ND	6.0
D[a]	7.9	7.9	ND	8.8	8.1	3.9	5.9
E	7.5	7.5	ND	8.8	8.2	2.9	7.0
E[a]	7.9	7.9	ND	8.4	7.8	ND	5.7
F	8.3	8.1	7.8	9.4	8.6	3.2	7.2
F[a]	8.7	8.5	8.2	10.5	9.7	4.2	6.0

Note: ND = none detected; other results are for normal diet.

[a] Denotes sample taken at operation, i.e., after 5 days of diet.

B. Inflammatory Bowel Disease

In an investigation involving seven patients with active Crohn's disease, Barclay and O'Morain (personal communication) studied the effect of an elemental diet (Vivonex®), consumed for one month, on the aerobic bacterial flora of the feces. Despite a marked clinical improvement, the only consistent finding at the end of the diet period was a 5- to 500-fold *increase* in *E. coli* per gram of feces. In view of the results reported by others of the effect of an elemental diet on enterococci in normal healthy persons a special study was carried out using a range of selective media to try to detect some similar effect in these Crohn's patients, but no such effect was apparent.

It is possible that the looser stools and relatively rapid transit of colonic contents which characterize Crohn's disease patients in comparison with healthy persons might be responsible for the failure of the colonic flora to react "normally" to an elemental diet. However, it is more likely that the Crohn's disease lesion, which affects mainly the small intestine and in particular the ileum, might result in impaired absorption so that an elemental diet, far from depriving the colonic flora, actually enriches their supply of nutrients. We have been unable to find any reports of the microbiological effects of the use of elemental diets as an adjunct to the treatment of ulcerative colitis.

C. Soluble Diets and Experimental Colon Cancer in Rodents

The observations of Laqueur et al.[45] of a high incidence of colon adenocarcinoma in rats fed a diet rich in cycad meal have led to the development of an animal model of colon carcinogenesis. The carcinogen contained in cycad meal is produced by the action of bacterial β-glycosidase or cycasin and is thought to be azoxymethanol (AOM). Dimethylhydrazine (DMH), given subcutaneously to rodents, is metabolized in the liver to yield AOM,[46] a carcinogen which is sufficiently organotrophic to give a similar high incidence of colon cancer to that of feeding with cycad meal. Although far removed from the postulated etiology of human colon cancer (discussed by Hill[47]) this remains a convenient and well-defined animal model of colon carcinogenesis in which to study the effects of dietary manipulation, immunological data, etc.

Bacteriological studies are conspicuous by their absence in this model and we must make assumptions that bacterial metabolism is an important promotor of DMH-induced colon cancer from the observations of Reddy et al.[48] These workers demonstrated that given DMH, only 21% of germ-free rats developed colon cancer compared to 93% of conventional rats. An obvious explanation of the relative resistance of germ-free animals is that a proportion of the DMH is excreted in the bile unchanged or as conjugated noncarcinogens and is passed in the feces. In the conventional rat colon, bacterial secondary metabolism and deconjugation might be expected to occur with the local release of AOM. This is supported by the observation of these workers that intrarectal administration of AOM resulted in colon tumors in 93% and 60% of germ-free and conventional rats, respectively. The authors speculate that some protective metabolism of AOM by the conventional GI microflora might be occurring and reducing local availability of the carcinogen.

Given that dietary modifications have many effects on both host and microflora, it is difficult to assess the significance of observations of enhanced carcinogenesis by DMH on high fat[49] and high protein[50] diets.

Perhaps the most interesting experiments are those in which dietary fiber of various kinds is either excluded or supplements a defined soluble diet. In such studies it has become obvious that experimental design must be carefully examined to exclude gross alterations in the growth rates on different regimens (as experienced by Fleiszer et al.[51]) and of protective effects of soluble diets such as Vivonex® on DMH-induced hepatic toxicity.[52] The latter author showed that Vivonex®-fed rats were far less susceptible to the carcinogenic effects of DMH than those fed a standard rat chow, even when supplemented with any of a variety of "stool bulking" supplements. A similar low incidence of tumors was noted by Fleiszer et al.[51] using Flexical® as the elemental diet. These workers claimed that supplementation of bran resulted in a very much reduced tumor incidence but this may reflect the severe growth retardation seen in the rats on this diet (50% of the control weights after 28 weeks). A protective role for dietary fiber has been noted in this model by Freeman et al.[53] and Barbolt and Abraham[54] but unsupported by Cruse et al.[55] The latter workers supported Castleden's observation and in subsequent studies have shown that the protective effect of elemental diet against DMH–induced carcinogenesis is abolished by supplementation with cholesterol.[56] Such a supplement might be expected to increase bile acid secretion into the colon and bacterial bile acid metabolites might then exert a promoting effect on chemically induced carcinogenesis as has been shown to occur.[57] Elemental diets, in this model, have provoked the most interesting observations on dietary modification of carcinogenesis. However, not until further studies are made on the effects of dietary modification of DMH carcinogenesis in conventional rats with fecal steroid analyses and bacteriological investigations or in comparison with germ-free or gnotobiotic rats, will we be able to assess the usefulness of this model in the study of the genesis of human colon cancer.

D. Elemental Diet in the Treatment of Pneumatosis Cystoides Intestinalis (PCI)

Although the etiology of PCI remains unclear, the demonstration of a high percentage of hydrogen (H_2— not a normal metabolite of mammalian tissues) in the gas-filled cysts suggests an involvement of bacterial metabolism in or near the intestinal mucosa. High breath H_2 excretion[58] in PCI patients supports this theory and at least two animal models of similar conditions exist.[59,60] Treatment with antibiotics is sometimes effective[58] as is intermittent oxygen-breathing therapy, although the latter does not appear to be due to the elimination of anaerobic flora of either mucosa or lumen.[61] Although neither therapy can be relied upon to elicit permanent remission, they can be envisaged as methods for temporary suppression of anaerobic microbial fermentation within the intestine, perhaps by an abnormal flora or one unbalanced toward excess gas production. It is interesting to note that the simple model of Meyer and Simon[60] involves both a gas-producing bacterium *E. coli* lodged in the GI tract and an artificially elicited hyperimmunity to the same organism. Perhaps bacteria, immune response, and availability of nutrients are all involved in a complex etiology for PCI.

Van der Linden and Marsell[62] treated a patient with PCI confined to the colon and associated with a high fasting breath H_2 excretion, with an elemental diet (Vivasorb®) for 2 weeks. During this time, breath H_2 fell from approximately 170 ppm to approximately 55 ppm, diarrhea stopped and these was radiological evidence of cyst regression. After 4 months of normal diet PCI recurred. The authors speculate that the breath H_2 never fell to normal values (15 ppm) and relapse with normal diet was probably inevitable The data represent more evidence for a bacterial etiology for PCI which resolved when the colonic flora was limited for fermentable carbohydrate, since that present in the elemental diet would be rapidly absorbed from the small intestine. Elemental dietary modification of PCI might be a useful alternative, or adjunct to, oxygen or antibiotic therapy.

V. CONCLUSIONS

In this chapter we have briefly summarized the composition of the microflora throughout the GI tract and the various exogenous and endogenous factors which appear to control it, with particular reference to the effects of dietary components. Elemental diets do not have a profound effect on the types of bacteria present, but do reduce the overall bacterial mass present in intestinal contents. Limited data show that the metabolites of the microflora are greatly reduced during elemental diet treatment and it is important that future studies on the effects of such diets on various diseases should examine these metabolites in greater detail.

With a greater understanding of the role played by modification of the intestinal flora during treatment of disease with elemental diets we can look forward to a greater understanding of both the etiology of a number of human GI disorders and of the factors controlling the microbial ecology of the human gut. With such data it may be possible to predict other disorders which might benefit from treatment with elemental diet.

REFERENCES

1. **Drasar, B. S. and Hill, M. J.,** *Human Intestinal Flora,* Academic Press, London, 1974.
2. **Carter, P. B. and Pollard, M.,** Host responses to normal microbial flora in the germ-free mouse, *J. Reticuloendothelial Soc.,* 9, 580, 1971.
3. **Foo, M. C. and Lee., A.,** Immunological response of mice to members of the autochthonous intestinal microflora, *Infect. Immun.,* 6, 525, 1972.
4. **Foo, M. C. and Lee. A.,** Antigenic cross-reaction between mouse-intestine and a member of the autochthonous microflora, *Infect. Immun.,* 9, 1066, 1974.
5. **Foo, M. C., Lee, A., and Cooper, G. N.,** Natural antibodies and the intestinal flora of rodents, *Aust. J. Exp. Biol. Med. Sci.,* 52, 321, 1974.
6. **Berg, R. D. and Savage, D. C.,** Immunological responses and micro-organisms indigenous to the gastrointestinal tract, *Am. J. Clin. Nutr.,* 25, 1364, 1972.
7. **Hersch, T., Floch, M. H., Binder, H. J., Conn, H. O., Prizont, R., and Sprio, H. M.,** Disturbance of the jejunal and colonic bacterial flora in immunoglobulin deficiences, *Am. J. Clin. Nutr.,* 23, 1595, 1970.
8. **Van der Wiel-Korstanje, J. A. A. and Winkler, K. C.,** The faecal flora in ulcerative colitis, *J. Med., Microbiol.,* 8, 491, 1975.

9. **Hoskins, L. C. and Boulding, E. T.,** Degradation of blood group antigens in human colon ecosystems: I. *In vitro* production of ABH blood group-degrading enzymes by enteric bacteria, *J. Clin. Invest.*, 57, 63, 1976.
10. **Hoskins, L. C. and Boulding, E. T.,** Degradation of blood group antigens in human colon ecosystems: II. A gene interaction in man that affects the fecal population diversity of certain enteric bacteria, *J. Clin. Invest.*, 57, 74, 1976.
11. **Salyers, A. A.,** Energy sources of major intestinal fermentative anaerobes, *Am. J. Clin. Nutr.*, 132, 158, 1979.
12. **Smith, C. J. and Bryant, M. P.,** Introduction to metabolic activities of intestinal bacteria, *Am. J. Clin. Nutr.*, 32, 149, 1979.
13. **Miller, T. L. and Wolin, M. J.,** Fermentations by saccharolytic intestinal bacteria. *Am. J. Clin. Nutr.*, 32, 164, 1979.
14. **Maier, B. R., Onderdonk, A. B., Baskett, R. C., and Hentges, D. J.,** *Shigella*, indigenous flora interactions in mice, *Am. J. Clin. Nutr.*, 25, 1433, 1972.
15. **Nurmi, E. and Rantala, M.,** New aspects of *Salmonella* infection in broiler production, *Nature (London)*, 241, 210, 1973.
16. **Barnes, E. M., Impey, C. S., and Cooper, D. M.,** Competitive exclusion of salmonellas from the newly hatched chick, *Vet. Rec.*, 106, 61, 1980.
17. **George, W. L., Rolfe, R. D., Sutter, V. L., and Finegold, S. M.,** Diarrhoea and colitis associated with antimicrobial therapy in man and animals, *Am. J. Clin. Nutr.*, 32, 251, 1979.
18. **Borriello, S. P.,** *Clostridium difficile* and its toxin in the gastrointestinal tract in health and disease, *Res. Clin. Forums*, 1, 33, 1979.
19. **Hardie, J. M. and Bowden, G. H.,** The normal microbial flora of the mouth, in *The Normal Microbial Flora of Man*, Skinner, F. A. and Carr, J. G., Eds., Academic Press, New York, 1974, 47.
20. **Tomkins, A., Drasar, B. S., and James, W. P. T.,** Bacterial colonisation of jejunal mucosa in acute tropical sprue, *Lancet*, 1, 59, 1975.
21. **Peach, S. L., Drasar, B. S., Hawley, P. R., Hill, M. J., and Marks, C. G.,** Mucosal flora of the human colon, *Gut*, 16, 824, 1975.
22. **Dack, G. M. and Petran E.,** Bacterial activity in different levels of intestine and in isolated segments of small and large bowel in monkeys and in dogs, *J. Infect. Dis.*, 54, 204, 1934.
23. **Reilly, R. W. and Kirsner, J. B.,** Blind Loop Syndrome, *Gastroenterology*, 37, 491, 1959.
24. **Gracey, M.,** The contaminated small bowel syndrome: pathogenesis, diagnosis and treatment, *Am. J. Clin. Nutr.*, 32, 234, 1979.
25. **McArdle, A. H., Brown, R. A., Echave, V., Rivilis, J., and Thompson, A. G.,** Alterations in gastric and pancreatic secretion induced by feeding of an elemental diet, *Arch. Mal. Appar. Dig. Nutr.*, 61, 115c, 1972.
26. **Rivilis, J., McArdle, H., Wlodek, G. K., and Gurd, F. N.,** The effect of an elemental diet on gastric secretion, *Ann. Coll. Surg., Canada*, 5, 57, 1972.
27. **Bury, K. D. and Jambunathan, G.,** Effects of elemental diets on gastric emptying and gastric secretion in man, *Am. J. Surg.*, 127, 59, 1974.
28. **Perault, J., Devroede, G., and Bounous, G.,** Effects of an elemental diet in healthy volunteers, *Gastroenterology*, 64, 569, 1973.
29. **Dickman, M. D., Chappelka, A. R., and Schaedler, R. W.,** Evaluation of gut microflora during administration of an elemental diet in a patient with an ileoproctostomy, *Dig. Dis.*, 20, 377, 1975.
30. **Axelsson, C. K. and Justessen, T.,** Studies of the duodenal and fecal flora in gastrointestinal disorders during treatment with an elemental diet, *Gastroenterology*, 72, 397, 1977.
31. **Winitz, M., Adams, R. F., Seedman, D. A., Davis, P. N., Jayko, L. G., and Hamilton, J. A.,** Studies in metabolic nutrition emplying chemically defined diets. II. Effects on gut microflora populations, *Am. J. Clin. Nutr.*, 23, 546, 1970.
32. **Attebury, H. R., Sutter, V. L., and Finegold, S. M.,** Effect of a partially chemically defined diet on normal human fecal flora, *Am. J. Clin. Nutr.*, 25, 1391 1972.
33. **Crowther, J. S., Drasar, B. S., Goddard, P., Hill, M. J., and Johnson, K.,** The effect of a chemically defined diet on the faecal flora and faecal steroid concentration, *Gut*, 14, 790, 1973.
34. **Bounous, G. and Devroede, G.,** Effects of an elemental diet on human faecal flora, *Gastroenterology*, 66, 210, 1974.
35. **Koumans, R. K. J.,** Ruimtevaartdieet en darmchirurgie, *Ned. Tijdschr. Geneesk.*, 116, 1040, 1972.
36. **Bornside, G. H. and Cohn, I.,** Stability of normal human faecal flora during a chemically defined, low liquid diet, *Ann. Surg.*, 181, 58, 1975.
37. **Uphill, P. F.,** A quantitative comparsion of the fecal microflora of baboons fed a natural diet or a synthetic diet complete or deficient in pyridoxine or riboflavine, *J. Appl. Bacteriol.*, 36, 501, 1973.

38. **Stephen, A. M. and Cummings, J. H.,** The microbial contribution to human faecal mass, *J. Med. Microbiol.*, 13, 45, 1980.
39. **Stephen, A. M. and Cummings, J. H.,** Mechanism of action of dietary fibre in the human colon, *Nature*, 284, 283, 1980.
40. **Nelson, L. M., Carmichael, H. A., Russell, R. I., and Atherton, S. T.,** The use of an elemental diet (Vivonex) in the management of bile acid-induced diarrhoea, *Gut*, 18, 792, 1977.
41. **Hill, M. J. and Aries, V.,** Faecal steroid composition and its relationship to cancer of the large bowel, *J. Pathol.*, 104, 129, 1971.
42. **Bone, E., Tamm, A., and Hill, M. J.,** The production of urinary phenols by gut bacteria and their possible role in the causation of large bowel cancer, *Am. J. Clin. Nutr.*, 29, 1448, 1976.
43. **Arabi, Y., Dimock, F., Burdon, D. W., Alexander-Williams, J., and Keighley, M. R. B.,** Influence of bowel preparation and antimicrobials on colonic microflora, *Br. J. Surg.*, 65, 55, 1978.
44. **Marks, C. G., Hawley, P. R., Peach, S. L., Drasar, B. S., and Hill, M. J.,** The effects of phthalylsulphathiazole on the bacteria of the colonic mucosa and intestinal contents as revealed by the examination of surgical samples, *Scand. J. Gastroenterol.*, 14, 891, 1979.
45. **Laqueur, G. L., Mickelson, O., Whiting, M. G., and Kurland, T.,** Carcinogenic properties of nuts from *Cycas circinalis* L. indigenous to Guam, *J. Natl. Cancer Inst.*, 31, 919, 1963.
46. **Fiala, E. S.,** Investigations into the metabolism and mode of action of the colon carcinogen. 1,2-dimethylhydrazine, *Cancer (Philadelphia)*, 36, 2407, 1975.
47. **Hill, M. J.,** Carcinogenesis of gastrointestinal cancer, *Front. Gastrointest. Res.*, 4, 1, 1979.
48. **Reddy, B. S., Narisawa, T., Wright, P., Vukusich, D., Weisburger, J. H., and Wynder, E. L.,** Colon carcinogenesis with azoxymethane and dimethylhydrazine in germ-free rats, *Cancer Res.*, 35, 287, 1975.
49. **Reddy, B. S., Mangat, S., Sheinfil, A., Weisburger, J. H., and Wynder, E. L.,** Effect of type and amount of dietary fat and 1,2-dimethylhydrazine on biliary bile acids, fecal bile acids and neutral sterols in rats, *Cancer Res.*, 37, 2132, 1977.
50. **Reddy, B. S., Narisawa, T., and Weisburger, J. H.,** Effect of a diet with high levels of protein and fat on colon carcinogenesis in F344 rats treated with 1,2-dimethylhydrazine, *J. Natl. Cancer Inst.*, 57, 576, 1976.
51. **Fleiszer, D., Murray, D., MacFarlane, J., and Brown, R. A.,** Protective effect of dietary fibre against chemically induced bowel tumours in rats, *Lancet*, ii, 552, 1978.
52. **Castleden, W. M.,** Prolonged survival and decrease in intestinal tumours in dimethylhydrazine treated rats fed a chemically defined diet, *Br. J. Cancer*, 35, 491, 1977.
53. **Freeman, H. J., Spiller, G. A, and Kim, Y. S.,** A double blind study on the effect of purified cellulose dietary fiber on 1,2-dimethylhydrazine-induced rat colonic neoplasia, *Cancer Res.*, 38, 2912, 1978.
54. **Barbolt, T. A., and Abraham, R.,** The effect of diet on dimethylhydrazine-induced colon carcinogenesis in the rat, *Proc. Soc. Exp. Biol. Med.*, 157, 656, 1978.
55. **Cruse, J. P., Lewin, M. R., and Clark, C. G.,** Failure of bran to protect against experimental colon cancer in rats, *Lancet*, ii, 1278, 1978.
56. **Cruse, J. P., Lewin, M. R., Ferulano, P., and Clark, C. G.,** Co-carcinogenic effects of dietary cholesterol in experimental colon cancer. *Nature (London)*, 276, 822, 1978.
57. **Reddy, B. S.,** Role of bile metabolites in colon carcinogenesis; Animal Models, *Cancer (Philadelphia)*, 36, 2401, 1975.
58. **Gillon, J., Tadesse, K., Logan, R. F. A., Holt, S., and Sircus, W.,** Breath hydrogen in pneumatosis cystoides intestinalis, *Gut*, 19, A973, 1978.
59. **Yale, C. E., Balish, E., and Wu, J. P.,** The bacterial etiology of pneumatosis cystoides intestinalis, *Arch. Surg.*, 109, 89, 1974.
60. **Meyer, R. C. and Simon, J.,** Intestinal emphysema (pneumatosis cystoides intestinalis) in a gnotobiotic pig, *Can. J. Comp. Med. Vet., Sci.*, 41, 302, 1977.
61. **Holt, S. and Heading, R. C.,** Observations on the treatment of primary pneumatosis coli, *Gut*, 19, A976, 1978.
62. **Van der Linden, W. and Marsell, R.,** Pneumatosis cystoides coli associated with high H_2 excretion: Treatment with an elemental diet, *Scand. J. Gastroenterol.*, 14, 173, 1979.
63. **Hill, M. J. and Drasar, B. S.,** The normal colonic bacterial flora, *Gut*, 16, 318, 1975.
64. **Bartholomew, B. A., Hill, M. J., Hudson, M. J., Riddell, W. S. J., and Walters, C. L.,** Gastric bacteria, nitrate, nitrite and nitrosamines in patients with pernicious anaemia and in patients trieated with cimetidine, Proc. 6th Meet. N-nitroso Compounds, WHO/IARC Conf. 1979, Budapest, October.
65. **Hill, M. J., Drasar, B. S., Aries, V. C., Crowther J. S., Hawksworth, G. M., and Williams, R. E. O.,** Bacteria and the etiology of cancer of the large bowel, *Lancet*, i, 95, 1971.
66. **Loesche, W. J.,** Oxygen sensitivity of various anaerobic bacteria, *Appl. Microbiol.*, 18, 723, 1969.

SECTION III

CLINICAL USES OF ELEMENTAL DIETS

Chapter 10

INTRODUCTION

R. I. Russell

Elemental diets have been suggested as being of value in the management of a wide range of conditions. The purpose of this section is to consider the indications for their use, critically assessing their value in each disease state.

The two principal properties of elemental diets which can be utilized in various clinical situations are

1. The provision of nutritional support.
2. Application of their specific metabolic effects on the normal or diseased gastrointestinal tract.

Elemental diets were introduced as a means of oral nutritional support in patients who were nutritionally deficient. They are effective in maintaining nutritional status in normal individuals over a period of time. It is more contentious, however, if elemental diets have major specific importance in correcting nutritional deficiency in patients with chronic and severe disease processes. As such, they require to be compared with other nutritional aids such as intravenous nutrition and other forms of enteral nutrition such as blenderized food, standard tube feeds, or other more recently developed forms of enteral nutritional support such as complete oral liquid diets. Few controlled data are available comparing elemental diets with other methods of improving nutritional status. Although elemental diets are of value in improving nutritional insufficiency, they are no better than complete oral liquid diets in this respect. It should be stated that any patient with severe nutritional deficiency or with nutritional deficiency associated with alimentary failure may be considered a candidate for i.v. nutrition rather than any form of enteral nutritional support. When the alimentary tract is functional and nutritional deficiency is not severe, some form of enteral nutrition should be considered. The relative merits of the various nutritional support methods are considered in Chapter 20.

A further principal indication for the use of elemental diets relates to their composition, and the application of their metabolic effects on the normal or diseased GI tract. The effect of the various components of diet on GI structure and physiological functions is an important subject, and the different formulations of elemental diets reflects these effects. The influence of these various diet formulations on GI physiology and their more widespread metabolic effects are described in Section II. Elemental diets are charcterized by their minimal digestive requirements, low residue nature, and low allergenicity, and these properties may all be of specific value in certain disease states.

A number of reviews of the clinical uses of elemental diets have appeared over the past 15 years and these are specified in the reference list at the end of this Chapter.[1-20] It is interesting and instructive to assess the evolution of views regarding the uses of elemental diets in the light of increasing knowledge of nutrition and its management, and the development of other forms of enteral nutritional support.

This section consists of chapters on the potential clinical uses of elemental diets in the following disease groups, considering in each case their value in the provision of nutritional support, and the application of their specific metabolic effects on the GI tract.

These are as follows:

- Elemental diets in surgical practice
- Maldigestion and malabsorption states
- Inflammatory bowel disease
- Cancer
- Burns
- Pediatrics
- Other uses, including colonic preparation, allergies and immunological problems, phenylketonuria and mental deficiency, Kwashiorkor, obesity, hepatic disease, and renal disease.

The final chapter in this section describes the techniques and problems of administration of elemental diets, and the potential hazards of their use.

REFERENCES

1. **Winitz, M., Graff, J., Gallagher, N., Narkin, A., and Seedman, D. A.,** Evaluation of chemical diets as nutrition for man in space, *Nature (London)*, 205, 741, 1965.
2. **Winitz, M. and Adams, R. F.,** Chemically defined diets — a new approach to metabolic nutrition in *Balanced Nutrition and Therapy*, Lang, K., Fekl, W., and Berg, G., Eds., Thieme, Stuttgart, 1971, 46.
3. **Glotzer, D. J.,** Space diets: comment, *Gastroenterology*, 61, 405, 1971.
4. **Beigler, M. A.,** The elemental diet: a new concept in nutritional support of a debilitated patient, *Surg. Dig.*, 18, 1971.
5. **Kark, R. M.,** Liquid formula and chemically defined diets, *J. Am. Diet. Assoc.*, 64, 476, 1974.
6. **Bury, K. D., Stephens, R. V., Cha, C., and Randall, H. T.,** Chemically defined diets, *Can. J. Surg.*, 17, 124, 1974.
7. **Russell, R. I.,** Elemental diets, *Gut*, 16, 68, 1975.
8. **Voitk, A. J.,** The place of elemental diet in clinical nutrition, 5BrJ. Clin. Pract., 29, 55, 1975.
9. Editorial, Elemental diets, *Lancet*, 2, 68, 1975.
10. **Freeman, J. B., Egan, M. C., and Millis, B. J.,** The elemental diet, *Surg. Gynecol. Obstet.*, 142, 925, 1976.
11. **Bury, K. D.,** The use of elemental diets, in *Current Concepts in Parenteral Nutrition*, Greep, J. M., Soeters, P. B., Wesdorp, R. I. C., Phaf, C. W. R., and Fischer, J. E., Eds., Martinus Nijhoff, The Hague, 1976, 243.
12. **Kaminski, M. V.,** Enteral hyperalimentation, *Surg. Gynecol. Obstet.*, 143, 12, 1976.
13. Elemental diets, *Drug Therapeut. Bull.*, 14, 23, 1976.
14. **Shils, M. E.,** Enteral nutrition by tube, *Cancer Res.*, 37, 2432, 1977.
15. **Fowell, E., Lee, H. A., and Dickerson, J. W. T.,** Intragastric tube feeds and elemental diets, in *Nutrition in the Clinical Management of Disease*, Edward Arnold, London, 1978, 332.
16. **Russell, R. I. and Hall, M. J.,** The practical value of elemental diets, *Practitioner*, 222, 631, 1979.
17. **Russell, R. I.,** Elemental diets, in *Practical Nutritional Support*, Karran, S. J. and J. G. M. M., Alberti, Eds., Pitman Medical, London, 1980, 227.
18. **Koretz, R. L. and Mayer, J. H.,** Elemental diets — fact and fantasies, *Gastroenterology*, 78, 393, 1980.
19. **Russell, R. I.,** Intravenous nutrition and elemental diets, in *Scientific Foundations of Gastroenterology*, Sircus, W., and Smith, A. N., Eds., Heinemann, London, 1980, 130.
20. **Russell, R. I.,** Enteral nutrition in *Recent Advances in Clinical Nutrition.*, Vol. 1, I., McLean, B. and Howard, A. N., Eds., John Libbey, London, 1981.

Chapter 11

ELEMENTAL DIETS IN SURGICAL PRACTICE

A. J. Rich and Ivan D. A. Johnston

TABLE OF CONTENTS

I. INTRODUCTION

When it was first announced in 1957, the concept of the elemental diet was of considerable interest to surgeons. The idea of being able to provide full nutritional support through a short, diseased, or malfunctioning gut was inherently attractive, particularly with the difficulties which were then being experienced with the complications of parenteral nutrition. In addition, the almost complete absence of residue implied that it might be a useful adjunct in the treatment of fistulas or in the preparation of the colon for surgery. This chapter will examine the current place of elemental diets in surgery in the light of these early hopes.

II. BASIC PROPERTIES IN RELATION TO SURGERY

The surgical interest in the properties of elemental diets lies first and foremost in their nutritional content. Their effects on GI function and their low residue are perhaps more secondary properties.

A. Nutrition

Undernutrition is now recognized as a frequent occurrence in surgical wards[1] and in the pre- and postoperative periods.[2] Nutritional care is now assuming increasing importance in the management of patients but it is not clear if this is simply because of increased awareness of the problem or whether advances in other surgical support techniques have enabled surgery to be performed and survival to occur in circumstances where nutrition would not previously have been a limiting factor.

There is no doubt that elemental diets are capable of providing complete nutritional support for long periods in individuals with an intact gut,[3] with as little as 4 cm of jejunum[4] or in chronic inflammatory bowel disease.[5] However, it is not entirely clear whether they have any inherent advantage over other methods of feeding, and in particular, parenteral nutrition, beyond ease of administration. Studies[6-9] comparing nitrogen balance in the postoperative period in patients fed similar diets either in an elemental form or parenterally have reached opposing conclusions and it seems that if there is any one method that has an inherent superiority, then this will be so small as to require large numbers of subjects in a carefully controlled study to obtain incontrovertible proof.

B. GI Function

Elemental diets have been used for feeding purposes in obstructed[10,11] or postoperative[12,13] bowel and to reduce the volume of intestinal fluid to enable fistulas to heal.[14-16] In such situations their efficacy is said to be due to their reduction in gastric[17,18] and pancreatic[19,20] secretions and their reduction in stool bulk.[3] Reduction in gastric secretion is almost certainly due to a reduction in the cephalic phase[21] which results from the unpalatability and unpleasant smell of most elemental diets. It has been suggested that there is also a reduction in the local stimulatory effects on gastric mucosa due to the predigestion of the elemental diet.[22] However, protein digestion products, but not intact proteins, stimulate oxyntic cell secretion, an effect that is enhanced by simultaneous distension of the stomach.[23] Stevens et al.[24] have also demonstrated that neither the carbohydrate source nor the osmolarity of liquid diets affects the rate of gastric emptying. Indeed, Ragins et al.[20] showed that intragastric infusion of elemental diets in the intact dog stomach produced marked secretory stimulation.

Pancreatic secretions are stimulated less by elemental diets at a neutral pH than with a normal meal in both experimental animals[20] and man.[25] Panayiotides and colleagues[26] compared the response in normal volunteers to a nonneutralized elemental diet or an isocaloric, isonitrogenous normal meal which had been liquidized. Using a duodenal perfusion technique they found a 26% reduction in trypsin and 12% reductions in bile acid and duodenal fluid output with elemental diet. Hill et al.[27] studied ten patients with established ileostomies as a model for intestinal fistulas. Mean daily ileostomy volume fell by only 17% during 10 days administration of an elemental diet but in two patients there was an increase of 4 to 6%. This and other studies[28] have failed to confirm the drastic reduction of small bowel output and fistula drainage reported in clinical reports of fistulas' treatment.[16,29] Voitk[29] has suggested that the nature of fistula drainage rather than the volume is more important for healing and it is possible that the moderate reduction in pancreaticobiliary secretion[26] and the reduction in exogenous fecal residue[30] would support this observation.

C. Fecal Residue and Flora

Early reports of elemental diets reported marked reductions in the amount of fecal volume[3] and in the concentration and types of large bowel microorganisms.[31] However, other investigators[32,33] have failed to confirm the reduction in microorganisms. Although the total number of bacteria in the feces was reduced, the concentration remained the same and the reported reduction in numbers merely resulted from the reduction in fecal volume.

From a surgical point of view, interest lies in the possible "cleansing" action of elemental diets for bowel preparation prior to surgery. Although this will be discussed in detail below, it seems likely that a purging action may be achieved by excessive ingestion of elemental diets,[34] resulting in the dumping of ileal fluid into the colon at a rate which overwhelms its absorptive capacity. Even in the absence of a purging dose of elemental diet, since a considerable proportion of dry stool weight is contributed endogenously from desquamated cells and stool bacteria,[23] some residue is bound to remain. Low-residue diets in general have a prolonged large-bowel transit time[23] and the increased time thus available for fluid absorption by the colon may account for the reduced fecal bulk presenting in the rectum.

III. HEAD AND NECK SURGERY

Patients presenting for head and neck surgery are frequently undernourished because of anorexia, pain, or dysphagia.[35] Apart from their local disease, however, they usually have an intact GI tract which is perfectly capable of absorbing nutrients provided they can reach it. Their poorly nourished state makes them poor candidates for any major surgical procedures which may be undertaken. Skin flaps and anastomoses are liable to break down and respiratory problems assume greater significance.[36] Multiple operations are often required to complete an excisional procedure so that eating may be impossible for several weeks during the reconstructive stage. Obviously, further starvation will seriously deplete already low sources of protein which are required for recovery.

Such patients, then, would seem ideal candidates for feeding by the enteral route. However, the lesion preventing adequate voluntary intake may also pose problems in obtaining nonoperative access to the GI tract. Sip feeding may be impossible because of abnormal or distorted anatomy which also prevents the passage of a feeding tube. Anorexia, altered taste sensation,[37] or previous unpleasant experiences with liquid diet also make sip feeding unlikely to succeed. Tube feeding, if it is possible to thread a catheter past the obstruction, is a possible alternative, as are the construction of various feeding ostomies. But the decision as to whether the enteral or parenteral routes are most suitable for an individual patient depends on potential complications, safety and cost, and duration of treatment. Copeland[38] has suggested that enteral nutrition cannot adequately meet the increased nutritional needs of patients undergoing head and neck surgery, but this view is not borne out by other workers reviewed below.

A. Nasogastric Tube Feeding

Standard polyethylene or rubber gastric aspiration tubes may be used for feeding purposes, but small-caliber flexible Silastic tubes are soft and better tolerated by most patients. They allow swallowing to continue so that patients can take sip-feeds or drink beverages, as well as being fed through the tube. Because of their flexibility they are prone to expulsion by regurgitation or coughing but the risk of this can be reduced by weighting the end of the tube with a small mercury-filled bag.

The fine-bore tube has undoubted advantages in terms of patient comfort over the standard Ryle's tube but the fluid diet to be used with it must be chosen with care since not all are sufficiently liquid to pass. It is not necessary to resort to commercially produced liquid diets, however. Fallis and Baron[39] used a feed of their own manufacture based on milk, eggs, and casein hydrolysate. They found no difficulties in maintaining tube patency in 150 patients. Several patients with large nitrogen losses were successfully kept in positive nitrogen balance with this feed. Another paper[40] reports a milk-based liquid diet which was fed by a small-bore tube to patients with advanced cancer of the head and neck. Many recovered their appetite sufficienly to "eat round" the tube, gained weight, and showed conversion of their nitrogen balances from negative to positive

Tweedle and colleagues[41] compared the efficacy of nasogastric tube feeding with i.v. feeding following major surgery for head and neck cancer. Intake by both routes was related to body surface area. I.v. feeding was provided by aminoacid solutions, fat emulsion, and glucose and the nasogastric feed was based on a bovine protein hydrolysate and a glucose polymer. Mean energy and nitrogen intakes in the two groups were similar and both regimens were given continuoulsly over 24 hr. The two groups of patients differed in the period of their feeding and in the type of surgery performed and their nutritional status is not clear. However, there was no difference in the clinical outcome between the two groups, although the daily nitrogen balance in the enterally fed group was significantly greater. Nausea and diarrhea occurred in 4 out of the 15 patients being fed enterally and responded to slowing of the infusion and codeine phosphate. No complications were seen in the six patients fed by the i.v. route but the average daily cost for parenteral nutrients was £32 compared with £6 for the nasogastric feeds.

In this study, abnormal liver function tests were noted in the majority of patients in both groups, in some cases of sufficient magnitude to cause the authors to terminate the feeding regimen. They comment that abnormal liver function tests have been recorded previously during parenteral feeding but not in enteral feeding. However, disordered liver function might be expected in many patients fed artificially because of their tendency to be undernourished, septic, and to have undergone surgery and anesthesia. It is thus difficult to attribute such abnormalities with certainty to the feeding regimen. One obvious difference between natural and artificial nutrition is the tendency for the latter to be given continuously throughout the 24 hr. This will presumably result in continuing stimulation of gut, pancreas, and liver which may deplete an organ already functioning inefficiently because of previous undernutrition and intercurrent sepsis. However, it will be necessary to repeat these studies in a more closely controlled group of patients with evidence of previously normal liver function and to exclude other causes for alterations in liver function before accepting unequivocally that nutritional support is culpable.

B. Esophagostomy

If long-term feeding is contemplated in patients with head and neck cancer, esophagostomy or pharyngostomy offer suitable alternatives to nasogastric tube feeding. These procedures eliminate the social problem faced by a patient who has to walk around with a tube issuing from his nose, and are simpler to perform than a gastrostomy, the other alternative.

Both pharyngostomy[42] and esophagostomy[43] require esophagal intubation and if large-bore tubes are used the longterm risk of esophagitis and stricture need to be taken into account. Such risks may be somewhat exaggerated, however. Banfield and Hurwitz[44] reviewed 2000 patients with esophagal stricture and concluded that the structure was related to esophagal intubation in only 3.

In general, esophagostomy or pharyngostomy have been used in patients with inoperable head and neck cancer or where a reconstructive operation has been impossible, but several studies[40,45] have demonstrated that long-term survival is perfectly compatible with such feeding. Hartwell[45] reviewed 104 patients with esophagostomies of which over half had head and neck cancer. In the 13-year period under review only 38 deaths had occurred and he recorded no complications of the technique, which used blenderized standard food down the relatively large-bore tube.

Royster et al.[46] described a simple technique of cervical pharyngostomy where a polyethylene feeding tube was brought out through the pyriform fossa onto the neck, the distal end being positioned in the stomach. The authors described the results obtained in feeding 55 patients who had undergone maxillo-facial surgery. Forty-nine were for malignancy and the remainder for neurological disorders with dysphagia. Patients were fed with gastrostomy feeds or blenderized food for up to 374 days, usually until they could take food orally. After the tube had been *in situ* for 1 week a granulation-lined track remained and it was possible to change and clean tubes so that several patients were able to manage their feeding at home. A particular advantage claimed for this method was that patients were able to conceal the tubing beneath clothing and did not need to undress in order to use it. The only complication noted was occasional inflammation around the tube.

Noone and Graham[47] reviewed nutritional support techniques for extensive head and neck surgery and suggested that cervical pharyngostomy or esophagostomy were the routes of choice for long-term nutrition. Nasogastric intubation was particularly criticized because of its increased incidence of pulmonary complications and possible trauma to pharyngeal suture lines. The authors reviewed 80 percutaneous pharyngostomies carried out over a 6-year period for carcinoma of the head and neck. A blenderized diet of standard foods was given through a 14- or 16-gauge tube and was capable of providing up to 4500 calories daily in 3 liters. Complications related to the tube were rare but in one case the external jugular vein was damaged during placement. Complications related to the feed were confined to occasional diarrhea and it was suggested that it was preferable to stimulate peristalsis by bolus feeding rather than administer the feed by continuous drip.

C. Gastrostomy

It is unlikely that the construction of a feeding gastrostomy is part of today's armamentarium in the nutrutional support of head and neck cancer. Indeed, gastrostomy was commonly associated with early postoperative death[48] usually because of the extreme debility and cachexia of such patients. If it is impossible to pass a feeding tube into the stomach from above the alternatives lie between parenteral feeding and a jejunostomy. Unless the needle type of jejunostomy, as described by Delany[49] is contemplated, it would seem that any other operative procedure would be of equal magnitude to a gastrostomy, and hence, equally hazardous. However, if it is possible to negotiate an esophageal malignancy a pull-through feeding tube of the Celestin type would seem to be a humane palliative procedure, since gastrostomy does not in itself prolong life.

Established gastrostomies usually have wide stomata or wide-bore catheters *in situ* so that insertion of feeds is no problem. It seems more logical in such cases to use a blenderized diet rather than an expensive proprietary preparation.

D. Jejunostomy

Formal jejunostomy is occasionally performed at the time of surgery when a GI obstruction is present at a higher level. More recently the technique for fine needle jejunostomy has been described.[49] However, this technique seems best reserved for relatively short-term feeding because of the potential complications[13] and it will be discussed under the heading of pre- and postoperative care.

Boles and Zollinger[50] fed 103 patients homogenized milk with added starch and protein hydrolysate. All had undergone major upper GI surgery and had suffered a preoperative weight loss of more than 20 lb. The feed was found to be of "great value" in one quarter of all cases, but 15 patients were unable to tolerate the feeding because of distension and abdominal pain.

In another study,[51] 34 patients with inoperable esophageal lesions were fed a milk-based diet of between 2000 and 3000 calories through a formal jejunostomy. Nitrogen excretion studies on some of the patients confirmed the maintenance of a positive nitrogen balance in the face of measured daily losses of 16 g of nitrogen or more. However, hyperglycaemia was found frequently and in five patients a jejunostomy prolapse occurred.

Allerdyce and Groves[52] reported the results of feeding a heterogenous group of patients by either a jejunostomy stoma or intravenously. Six of the group fed elemental diets had undergone esophageal surgery. The enterally fed group received considerably larger quantities of both nitrogen and energy than the parenteral group and had improved nitrogen balances and made obvious weight gains. The authors comment that an elemental diet fed through a jejunostomy achieved results comparable to the parenteral route without the septic complications.

Most types of liquid feed have been reported to give rise to frequent episodes of dumping when used as jejunostomy feeds. Allerdyce and Groves[52] found it in all their patients. This is a not unexpected effect of instilling a hyperosmolar load into a jejunum that has effectively lost its "gastric umbrella" and can be minimized by the usual methods of slow introduction by continuous pumped infusion. We have found that warming the feed close to body temperature appears to reduce dumping, but this gives rise to difficulties in preventing bacteria multiplication. It has been suggested[53] that jejunal feeding may result in inadequate mixing of the diet with pancreatic juice and bile so that digestion is depressed. If, indeed, this occurs then this would be a clear indication for the use of an elemental diet which may be absorbed without pancreatic enzymes or bile.

The use of enteral feeding in the patient with head and neck lesions is of great value, particularly in the patient suffering from starvation and hypermetabolism. A fine-bore nasogastric tube is probably most suitable for repletion prior to surgery or for maintenance during radiotherapy. In the postoperative period, especially if long-term feeding is likely, an "ostomy" into the upper GI tract, particularly a pharyngostomy, is probably most satisfactory. Reasonable clinical results have been achieved with a variety of liquid diets but it is possible that jejunostomy feeds will be more adequately absorbed if given in an elemental form. Because of the particular intraoral disorders associated with head and neck cancer.[35] and the preference of cancer patients for milk-based products,[54] it is unlikely that oral feeding of elemental diets has any part to play in nutritional support.

IV. FISTULA MANAGEMENT

It is in the area of fistula management that elemental diets have been used most enthusiastically by surgeons. Fistulas constitute one of the more serious complications of intestinal surgical procedures and a review of the literature in 1960 of almost 1400 cases found that less than half the patients who developed such a complication survived.

Clearly, a fistula poses two problems to a patient; the local problem of skin excoriation with the infected tract and the surrounding inflamed tissues; and the steady loss of body cell mass because of a combination of catabolism, inability to eat and, in some cases, inability to absorb. Chapman and colleagues[56] studied the factors contributing to successful fistula management and found suboptimal nutrition to be the single most important item contributing to mortality. In a series of 58 cases a mortality of 58% was noted in those who did not receive positive nutritional support, whereas those whose nutrition was optimal had a mortality rate of 16%. Roback and Nicoloff[57] in a series of 55 small bowel fistulas concluded that the nutritional status was intimately associated with the success obtained in healing a fistula. Preexisting undernutrition, equally, is a potent cause of anastomotic leakage and hence, fistula formation.[15]

Nutritional support has been used to aid fistula closure since at least 1945 when Brunschwig et al.[58] used i.v. feeding as part of their management of small bowel fistulas. Smith and Lee[15] seem to have been the first to use a liquid diet which they provided through an intrajejunal tube distal to the fistula. All 11 of their patients with duodenal fistulas survived on a drip feed of high protein, high calorie solutions. The fistulas closed spontaneously in from 7 to 28 days.

Bury and colleagues[14] reported the use of an elemental diet in fistula management. Their 13 patients had lesions ranging from esophageal to colonic fistulas and averaged a fluid drainage of 800 mℓ/day. All patients received elemental diets administered by a pump, sometimes with food or nonelemental diets. The feeds were given via a nasogastric tube in six cases, orally in two, and by a gastrostomy or a jejunostomy in the remainder. Seven fistulas closed spontaneously and these had averaged an output of 835 mℓ/day which fell to 193 mℓ/day once feeding with elemental diets had been established. Four fistulas, gastric, pancreatic, ileal, and colonic, became chronic and in two of these persisted due to inflammatory bowel disease. Half of the patients gained weight on the feeding regimen and serum proteins rose. This paper, together with others,[56] emphasizes the importance of a specific plan of management to maintain control of the patient and the fistula. All too often, the patient is left unfed for several days in the hope that the fistula will close spontaneously.

Voitk et al.[29] gave elemental diets alone through a nasogastric or an enterostomy tube in 29 patients, 4 with metastatic cancer. The two esophageal and three gastroduodenal fistulas healed spontaneously. Seven out of eight colonic fistulas and five out of six pancreaticobiliary fistulas did the same. Small bowel fistulas did less well, only just over half closing spontaneously. There was an overall mortality rate of 16%. The authors noted that the change to an elemental diet altered the character of the fistula effluent so that it became inoffensive and no longer appeared to have a corrosive effect on the skin. Although fistula volume diminished this was not invariable. However, the authors considered the content of fistula fluid was of more importance than its volume in allowing the fistula to heal.

Elemental diets, with or without parenteral nutrition, were also used successfully by Rocchio and colleagues[16] in 37 patients over a 3½-year period. One third of the patients had inflammatory bowel disease and in a further third a malignant lesion was directly associated with the fistula. Elemental diets were fed via a nasogastric tube, gastrostomy, or jejunostomy using a pump. Thirteen patients received only the elemental diet and the remainder had a high-calorie i.v. feeding regimen followed by elemental diet. Fistula drainage diminished significantly in 78% of cases and increased in 5%. Operative closure was required in only six patients, all with high or midgut fistulas, and spontaneous closure occurred in the remainder, including six with malignancy and seven with inflammatory bowel disease. The paper emphasizes the care that must be taken with elemental diets in order to avoid dumping and recommends that both concentration and volume should be gradually increased over a four- to five-day period. The authors thought that their successful treatment of fistulas associated with inflammatory bowel disease was due largely to the elemental diets. Their minimal fat content was felt to be useful because of its low level of stimulation of biliary secretion.

In an evaluation of enteral or i.v. feeding[52] in the treatment of fistulas, problems were found with both routes of therapy. The two patient groups were not matched and did not contain equal numbers of fistulas, more being present in the enterally fed group. I.v. feeding was used mainly in patients with ileus or distal obstruction, and was given into peripheral veins unless these had all become thrombosed, when a central line was used. The enterally fed group received an elemental diet containing fat and averaging 4000 kcal and 14 g of nitrogen by a variety of routes. The parenteral group received a protein hydrolysate, fructose, alcohol, and fat mixture averaging 2700 kcal and 9 g N per day. Clinical results are not reported in this paper but one patient in the elemental group and two in the parenteral group died. The high concentrations of elemental diet given (up to 55% weight for volume) led to complications apart from the expected diarrhea. Gastric retention, hyperkalemia and hyperchloremic acidosis were seen in several patients. Hyperglycemia severe enough to require insulin on a regular basis developed in two patients. In the i.v. group there was only one episode of catheter-related sepsis and the remaining complications seem to be related to the low-calorie, low-nitrogen and high-water content of the regimen used, and could be traced to the use of peripheral veins. The authors concluded that an elemental diet via a jejunal stoma was the most effective means of providing extended nutritional support during fistula care.

Although it is apparent from the work reviewed above that many fistulas close spontaneously during treatment with elemental diet, those associated with hypermetabolism and sepsis frequently require parenteral nutrition to provide adequate amounts of energy and nitrogen and to replace electrolyte losses until the fistula can be brought under control. Later it may be possible to switch to elemental diet alone. Early aggressive surgery without nutritional support is associated with a high mortality rate[59] and, except to control sepsis, should not be attempted in patients in negative nitrogen balance. A conservative approach along these lines may allow a fistula to close spontaneously and if it does not, will allow a reasonable chance of success at a later, planned, operation.

There is no doubt that liquid tube feed diets have been a significant advance in the management of fistulas, allowing the maintenance or repletion of the nutritional status in the postacute stage without the necessity for the very detailed care needed for continuing parenteral nutrition. However, does the feed need to be truly "elemental" in terms of nonresidue, low fat, amino acids, and glucose? Smith and Lee[15] obtained excellent results using a feed based on partially hydrolysed milk protein with glucose and alcohol. Celestin[60] reported that a whole-protein liquid diet is as effective as an elemental diet and has suggested that it is the nutritional value rather than the relative lack of residue that is effective in the closure of the fistula. This is also borne out by the observation of Voitk et al.[29] that the volume of fistula fluid was less important than its nature. In one study[59] of fistula output in relation to mortality rate, no increased risk was demonstrated with higher volumes and in several of the studies reviewed above elemental diets have been associated with increases in fistula output.

Do elemental diets reduce bile and pancreatic secretions to a greater extent that other liquid diets? Studies in dogs[20] suggested that the stomach and duodenum had to be bypassed in order to avoid the stimulatory effects of amino acids on the duodenum. In clinical studies, however, there appeared to be no differences in the closure rates whether feeding was carried out intragastrically or via jejunostomy. The early elemental diets were almost fat-free but the stimulus to bile and pancreatic secretion was not entirely eliminated[25] although Voitk[29] observed a biliary fistula draining. unchanged amounts of bile with an elemental diet and the results obtained by direct intubation of the duodenum in normal volunteers sipping elemental diets showed reductions of only 12% from normal.[26] More recent formulations of elemental diets (Flexical®, Mead Johnson) contain up to one third of their energy content as fat and might therefore be expected to promote the flow of bile and pancreatic juice to a greater extent.[23] However, this formulation seems to be equally as effective as low-fat elemental diets in the management of fistulas[52] and it is possible that the small reduction in secretion achieved by elemental diets may be irrelevant.

One observation repeatedly made[27,29] is that of fistula or ileostomy drainage becoming inoffensive and odor-free on an elemental diet. This would appear to be a function of the exogenous residue and the endogenous bowel flora, possibly contaminated by unusual overgrowth in the case of fistulas. Any low residue diet, including a diet of specially selected common foods,[61] will reduce fecal output and may result in alterations to bowel flora. Although it is not suggested that a diet of normal food would be effective in the management of fistulas it would seem that there is a reasonable case to be made for a trial of high-calorie, high-nitrogen liquid feeds based on whole protein.

V. TRAUMA

Patients suffering from severe multiple trauma may suffer from direct injury to the GI tract, or from temporary reduction in gut function due to ileus, peritonism, or sepsis. Lesser degrees of trauma, and particularly those involving the head and maxillofacial areas, form another group of patients suffering from effective intestinal insufficiency because of their inability to eat. Both of these groups where nutrition may be impossible because of lack of volition to eat for an extended period of time may be suitable for enteral feeding. Indeed, lack of suitable sites for an i.v. catheter or the patient's mental state may make i.v. feeding well nigh impossible, so that the enteral route is preferable.

Although undoubtedly many injured patients, particularly those in coma, are fed enterally for prolonged periods, little has appeared in the literature on the results of such nutritional support. Liffmann and Randall[62] report a technique for making a feeding jejunostomy together with a case report on an 18-year-old girl suffering from severe cerebral trauma. They felt that jejunostomy offered significant advantages over a feeding gastrostomy, chiefly because of the safety factor for aspiration of gastric contents. In this case an elemental diet was used with apparently successful results.

Nealon et al.[63] report a "malnourished" patient with facial fractures and thoracic injuries among a series of several cases supported with elemental diets. This patient was fed successfully for a 40-week period with more than 4000 kcal/day and the authors suggested that the high-energy, high-nitrogen content of elemental diets is particularly suitable for patients in the postinjury phase.

Woolfson and colleagues[64] used a tube-feed derived from protein-hydrolysate and a glucose polymer with various additives in six patients with severe injuries. The feed was administered by continuous drip through an eight-gauge nasogastric tube for up to 41 days. No gross nutritional changes were seen and the patients were said to be maintained in good nutritional state. Diarrhea was not a problem and the authors felt that this was due to the continuous drip feeding and to the glucose polymer which allowed the feed to remain close to serum osmolarity. The mixing of the feed described from basic ingredients in a hospital diet kitchen considerably reduced costs and permitted flexibility in composition. These factors alone were considered to provide superiority over elemental diets and the feed was recommended for use on intensive care units.

Recently we have carried out a comparative study of elemental and whole protein liquid diets in unconscious male head injury patients.[65] Fifty patients who had sustained severe head injuries and who were judged by an independent clinician to be likely to remain unconscious for at least 10 days were allocated randomly to one of five groups (Table 1). The groups were well-matched in terms of age, degree of injury as judged by Injury Severity Scoring, and nutritional status, as judged by anthropometric measurements (Table 2). Three groups were fed elemental diets (groups V, F, and AC) and two, whole protein diets (groups C, T) for 12 days. Feeding began on the day following admission and was given through a wide-bore nasogastric tube passed into the stomach, either by bolus or continuous drip, depending upon which method was best tolerated by each patient. Feeds were given at one third strength on day one, two thirds strength on days two and three, then at full strength. No other oral or i.v. nutrition was given. At the beginning and end of the study the nutritional status of the patients was assessed using standard anthropometric methods (Table 2) and daily urinary nitrogen excretion was estimated using the Kjeldahl method of 24-hour urine collections.

Although it was planned to provide isonitrogenous diets for the patients in each group at a level of 0.2 g N/kg body weight in three liters of fluid this target was not reached easily. In all groups, because of the need to introduce the feeds gradually, only comparatively small amounts were given in the first 4 days. In the elemental groups V, F, and AC, gastric dilatation, delayed gastric emptying, regurgitation, and ileus frequently caused the feed to be lost, or required feed dilution. The net effect of these difficulties was that the elemental groups all received significantly less nitrogen than the whole-protein groups (Table 3). Energy intake, except for group AC which had a larger mean intake, did not differ significantly between the groups in spite of the wide differences in their nitrogen to calorie ratios. This was probably because the higher nitrogen to calorie ratios of the elemental diets made up, in terms of energy intake, for the reduced amounts of feed that had been given. Mean nitrogen balance remained negative in all the elemental groups (Figure 1). Whole-protein groups C and T achieved positive balances from day 7 or 8 but only group T had a mean positive nitrogen balance for the 12-day period as a whole. The differences in mean nitrogen balance between the elemental groups and the whole-protein groups were significant.

All the patients in the study lost weight and body fat, as measured by triceps skinfold thickness. Arm muscle circumference increased in group C, but fell in all the other groups (Table 2). However, there were no significant alterations either within or between the groups.

The study points up the general difficulties encountered in administering an enteral feed in a catabolic patient. The need to introduce the feed at a reduced strength means an inevitable deficit in the nutritional intake. If additional nutrition has to be provided by the i.v. route as a supplement it may be necessary to balance the extra risks involved in running two drip feeding systems against the additional risk of sepsis entailed in keeping an already existing parenteral feeding line running. It seems reasonable to suggest that if total nutritional needs cannot be provided enterally for short-term feeding, i.e., less than 12 days, then the parenteral route may be preferable. If feeding is likely to be needed for longer than this, tandem feeding using both enteral and parenteral

Table 1
COMPOSITION AND COSTS OF THE DIETS USED

	Vivonex® standard	Flexical®	Albumaid® plus Caloreen®	Clinifeed® 400	Triosorbon® MCT
Nitrogen (g)	12	12	12	12	12
Energy (kcal)	3500	3360	3320	2000	1850
% Fat contribution to total energy	1.3	30.5	14.0	30.0	36.3
Nitrogen: calorie ratio	1:292	1:280	1:277	1:167	1:154
Cost per day[a]	£6.60	£7.20	£3.10	£3.66	£2.81

Note: Figures are calculated for an intake of 0.2 g N/kg for a 60-kg man.

[a] Based on hospital pharmacy costings at July, 1979.

Table 2
PATIENT DETAILS BEFORE AND AFTER THE STUDY PERIOD

	Vivonex® standard	Flexical®	Albumaid® plus Caloreen®	Clinifeed® 400	Triosorbon® MCT
Day 1					
Median age (years)	37	42	43	38	58
Mean injury score	32.4 ± 9.3	32.1 ± 7.9	30.5 ± 6.1	29.7 ± 6.0	33.0 ± 8.6
Mean weight (kg)	61.6 ± 4.3	61.7 ± 3.4	64.5 ± 2.9	63.2 ± 5.1	61.2 ± 7.1
Mean arm muscle circumference (cms)	23.9 ± 3.0	24.8 ± 2.56	23.2 ± 2.9	22.3 ± 3.3	23.0 ± 2.9
Mean triceps skinfold thickness (mms)	17.1 ± 10.0	17.6 ± 8.8	19.2 ± 6.5	21.7 ± 8.4	15.3 ± 6.5
Day 12					
Mean weight (kg)	58.5 ± 3.3	59.0 ± 3.9	61.3 ± 3.1	61.5 ± 5.0	58.6 ± 6.1
Mean arm muscle circumference (cms)	23.9 ± 2.6	24.2 ± 3.3	23.2 ± 3.6	22.6 ± 2.9	23.0 ± 3.6
Mean triceps skinfold thickness (mms)	15.0 ± 8.4	15.1 ± 8.4	16.2 ± 4.5	18.1 ± 8.2	13.0 ± 4.9

Note: Figures shown are mean values ± sd.

routes is acceptable, perhaps using a peripheral i.v. infusion site. With care, the dangers of running two drip systems are small and the i.v. line may be removed when full nutritional needs are being met enterally.

Apart from these considerations, this study indicates that whole protein diets offer a distinct advantage over elemental diets in terms of patient tolerance and ease of administration. The whole protein diets achieved nitrogen balance at an earlier stage and were associated with considerably fewer complications. These advantages undoubtedly outweigh any theoretical benefits attributable to possibly improved GI absorption.

Table 3
MEAN DAILY ENERGY INTAKE AND NITROGEN BALANCE

	Vivonex® standard	Flexical®	Albumaid® plus Caloreen®	Clinifeed® 400	Triosorbon® MCT	Significant *p* values
Mean daily energy intake (kcal/kg)	25.1 ± 1.8	27.0 ± 3.6	30.3 ± 10.1	24.3 ± 4.3	20.7 ± 2.2	AC:T = 0.034
Mean daily nitrogen intake (g/kg)	0.085 ± 0.006	0.099 ± 0.013	0.099 ± 0.030	0.148 ± 0.025	0.135 ± 0.015	C:V, F, AC ≤ 0.003 T:V, F, AC ≤ 0.009
Mean daily urinary nitrogen excretion (g/kg)	0.161 ± 0.009	0.156 ± 0.066	0.144 ± 0.007	0.181 ± 0.016	0.131 ± 0.006	T:V, F, C ≤ 0.015
Mean daily nitrogen balance (g/kg)	− 0.080 ± 0.014	− 0.060 ± 0.012	− 0.056 ± 0.009	− 0.003 ± 0.020	+ 0.005 ± 0.018	T:V, F, AC ≤ 0.01

Note: Figures are mean values ± 1 sd.

It is possible that some of the complications noted in this study and others[16,29] might have been reduced by using a feeding catheter placed within the duodenum or jejunum. However, other studies[13] have reported similar difficulties with this technique and it seems that the single most effective preventative measure is an iso-osmolar solution.

Whole protein liquid diets are also considerably cheaper than elemental diets. This is a particularly important consideration in trauma patients such as burns when nutritional support may be needed for many weeks. If the two varieties of liquid feed are equally as effective, the cheaper preparation must be the obvious choice. A feed derived from blenderized whole food of equal nutritional quality might be provided at still lower cost and be equally efficacious. Bondy and colleagues,[66] compared an elemental and a whole protein diet with one derived from common low-residue foods. All diets were fed to normal volunteers by the oral route for 1-week period. The common food diet was the only one to maintain the subjects in a positive nitrogen balance and was associated with fewest upper GI symptoms. In our own hospital, the diet kitchens have been able to produce a liquid feed of adequate quality from blenderized standard food that will pass down a fine-bore (1-mm diameter) nasogastric tube without blockage. The relative merits of a common food diet have still to be determined in clinical studies but if results similar to those obtained above are found then they should replace elemental diets and perhaps compete directly with commercially produced whole protein liquid diets on the basis of other factors, such as sterility.

One word of caution should be sounded in the early use of tube feeds in patients with head injuries. Bouzarth[67] reviewed five recent reports of intracranial insertion of nasogastric tubes. All had occurred in patients who had suffered massive frontal impacts to the skull and the tubes had been inserted for the purposes of gastric emptying. The possibility of similarly misplaced nasogastric feeding tubes, particularly of the fine-bore variety, would seem very real in multiple head trauma and can only be guarded against by postprocedure radiography. Aspiration of the tube is no guarantee of correct placement since in several of the reports fluid was successfully aspirated and assumed to be gastric in origin.

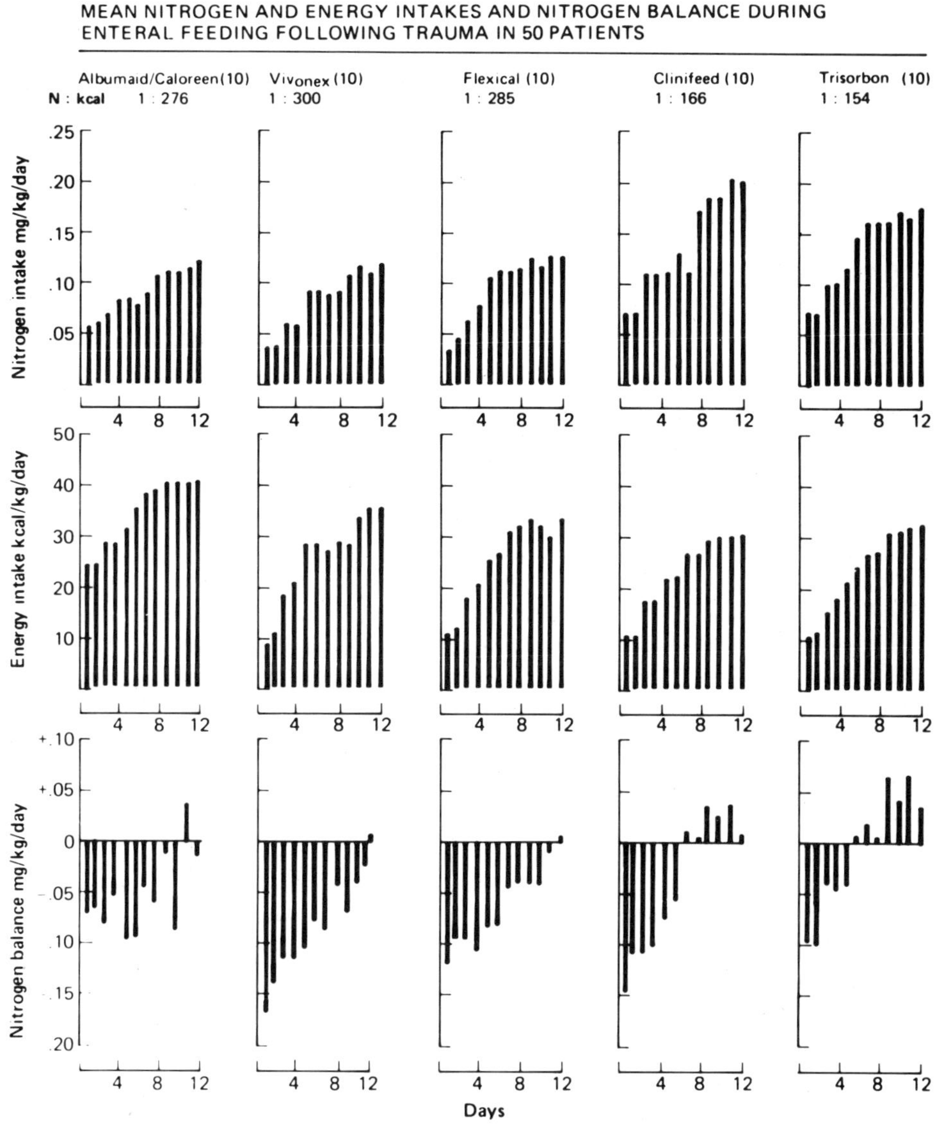

FIGURE 1. Mean nitrogen and energy intakes and nitrogen balance during enteral feeding following trauma in 50 patients.

Inhalation of vomited gastric contents is another possible complication of enteral feeding, particularly in the unconscious patient. It can be avoided by regular gastric aspiration between feeds.[64] which ensures that gastric stasis and dilatation do not occur.

VI. PRE- AND POSTOPERATIVE CARE

Poor nutrition before surgery and deteriorating nutritional state after complicated operative procedures are potent factors in surgical morbidity and morality. In the past, nutritional support has often been provided by the parenteral route, particularly when intestinal surgery is involved. This is based on the false supposition that the GI tract is nonfunctional because of ileus or obstruction. Recent studies, outlined below, have suggested that this view is somewhat simplistic and that the enteral route may be entirely suitable for feeding purposes under certain circumstances.

A. Preoperative Preparation of the Undernourished

A number of studies[1,2,68] have confirmed that preoperative undernutrition is relatively common in surgical wards and becomes more so in the postoperative period. A poor nutritional state is associated with an increased surgical risk[69] and there is little doubt that replacement of fluid, electrolytes, plasma protein, and blood, and a conversion to a positive nitrogen balance will help maintain body protein and hence, improve the operative risk. Nutrition may play an important part in such a regimen, particularly if it is used in a catabolic, underweight patient requiring investigation or stabilization prior to surgery.

Nealon and colleagues[63] used an elemental diet to provide up to 4000 kcal and 28 g N in 11 apparently undernourished patients prior to surgery. The patients encompassed a wide range of pathology and were fed for up to 16 weeks, usually by an intragastric drip. All the patients gained weight and had an increase in their serum albumin. All underwent definitive treatment which ranged from wound debridement to laryngectomy with esophagectomy and right colonic interposition. No complications were reported and all wounds healed by first intention.

Goode et al.[5] reported using elemental diets for up to 360 days as nutritional support in eight patients with Crohn's disease whose mean weight loss was 30%. Three preoperative patients who had been unable to maintain their weight on a normal diet were shown to restore up to 10% of their lean tissue mass per month as indicated by whole body potassium measurements.

Liquid diets have even been used in intestinal obstruction, and in those patients in a poor nutritional state a period of intestinal decompression with concomitant nutritional repletion may considerably improve the ability to withstand definitive surgery. Johnston[70] suggested that simple intestinal obstruction could be decompressed with a 10-foot long small bowel tube, similar to that later described by Cantor.[71] Johnston suggested that with low intestinal obstructions the decompression tube could also be used to maintain "nutrition, fluid, and salt balance without resort to parenteral fluids". It was recommended that the diet used was low in fiber. The paper also reports a series of 63 cases of simple intestinal obstruction treated by this method of decompression and feeding with a mortality rate of 19%. Unfortunately, it is not clear to what extent nutritional support was provided in these patients.

More recently, Carlton et al.[11] reported 11 cases treated by distal decompression of small bowel using a long tube with simultaneous intragastric feeding. The patients studied appeared to be of normal weight, or slightly below normal, and all had small bowel obstruction. In six cases this was due to irradiation damage and in three to inflammatory bowel disease. Decompression was first begun by allowing a long sump-drainage tube to pass into small bowel to the most distal point possible. After decompression for up to three days, during which time i.v. fluids were given, a small nasogastric feeding tube was passed and an elemental diet infused at gradually increasing rates until the limits of gastric tolerance were reached. Elemental diet was then continued until discharge or operation. The authors considered that the patients fell into two groups; six patients who were treated expectantly in the hope the obstruction would resolve; and five where it was hoped to reverse catabolism prior to surgery for the obstruction. Five out of the six patients treated expectantly resolved with elemental feeding of an average of 1859 kcal and 12 g N per day. One case did not resolve and required surgery. This case, and the five given preoperative nutrition, survived surgery. All patients maintained their body weight and three gained weight during the period of elemental feeding.

The authors caution that this method of treating small bowel obstruction should only be used in radiation enteritis, acute exacerbations of inflammatory bowel disease, an intraabdominal inflammatory mass, or a local transient motility abnormality. Continuing abdominal evaluation is necessary to ensure that bowel viability is not becoming threatened and total parenteral nutrition should be used if nutritional maintenance or repletion is not being achieved. Early surgical intervention is still the correct treatment for patients with acute mechanical obstruction or in chronic obstruction with doubtful bowel viability.

B. Early Postoperative Feeding

Several investigators[6,72-74] have shown that the administration of amino acids and energy in the immediate postoperative period, especially in the undernourished patient, can reduce the negative nitrogen balance resulting from surgical stress. Oral feeding in the early postoperative period is not popular because of delayed gastric emptying[75] which may cause vomiting. Postoperative ileus is often thought to preclude feeding. However, Shields[76] has shown that the absorptive capacity of small bowel is impaired only if intraluminal pressure is raised and Bunch and Shields[77] demonstrated unimpaired functional capacity of the small bowel in the immediate postoperative period. Shoemaker and Wright[78] demonstrated that the postoperative jejunum would tolerate a pumped infusion rate of 2 mℓ of water per min without untoward symptoms.

In clinical practice enteral feeding, usually bypassing the stomach by one means or another, has proved successful. In a controlled comparison of similar levels of i.v. and transnasal intraduodenal nonelemental feeding after a standard operation in patients matched for age and weight, Hindmarsh and Clarke[8] reported the best nitrogen economy in the enterally fed group. The intravenously fed group did better than a control group who were unfed for theee days postoperatively. Hindmarsh and Clarke suggested that nutrients were probably utilized more efficiently when given by the intraduodenal route, possibly because their diet was derived from whole protein.

The same authors describe a liquid diet[79] which they used as a postoperative gastrostomy feed in seven patients. It was based on milk with added ground-nut oil and glucose, but difficulty was experienced in passing it through a standard gastrostomy catheter. Fecal losses of fat and nitrogen were normal even though some bulky stools were passed. In another group of patients with intestinal fistulas steatorrhea was noted. This was attributed to the high fat content of the feed and the loss of pancreatic enzymes and bile in the fistula drainage.

The effect of oral or i.v. feeding on the strength of a standard colonic anastomosis was studied by Daly et al.[80] The same solutions of dextrose and amino acids were given either orally or parenterally to groups of rats matched for weight over a 7-day period postoperatively. Whether fed orally or intravenously the dextrose and amino acid groups had significantly greater anastomotic strengths than similar groups of animals unfed or fed dextrose alone. There were no significant differences between the enterally and parenterally fed groups in any parameter measured but hepatic morphology was more disordered in the parenterally fed group. It was suggested that the changes seen might have been due to the hypertonic dextrose solution used.

Delany[49] described a technique for insertion of a fine-bore catheter into the jejunum for feeding purposes at the completion of surgery. His method, which was a modification of an earlier techinique, used a hollow needle down which the fine-bore tube was led. Delany recommended the technique for use in the debilitated patient requiring complicated surgery and suggested that it was a simple procedure to carry out at the end of an operation. It was contraindicated in bowel distension and inflammatory bowel disease. Both elemental and standard diets could be passed down the 16-gauge tube which was removed at the end of feeding by simple traction.

In a subsequent report[81] the authors described the results achieved in 110 patients using their technique. The patients ranged from head and neck surgery to penetrating abdominal injuries. The catheter was inserted into the jejunum on a prophylactic basis in all cases but was only used for feeding purposes in 19. Eight of these had had major esophageal or upper GI surgery for carcinoma and were possibly undernourished, although this is not stated. Varying amounts of elemental diet were given via the fine-bore tube from 6 to 55 days. The complications noted were diarrhea, mild abdominal distension both of which responded to reduction of the rate of flow; and hyperglycemia which required management with insulin. In two patients the catheter fell out and in one case elemental diet was infused into the peritoneal cavity. This required drainage. In another case the catheter fell inside the peritoneal cavity and required surgical removal. Two deaths occurred, both in multiple trauma patients.

Yeung and colleagues[13] carried out a controlled trial of needle catheter jejunostomy with the aim of assessing the technique and determining the effect of the feeding on nutritional status and clinical outcome. Changes in body composition and plasma proteins in 20 patients fed by jejunostomy after major colo-rectal surgery were compared with those of matched controls who did not have nutritional support. Both groups had lost about 8% of their body weight prior to admission. The needle jejunostomy group was fed for an average of 10 days a fat-containing elemental diet using an infusion pump. Feeding began 48 to 72 hr postoperatively and was given in increasing concentrations up to 2000 to 3500 kcal per day, according to estimated patient requirements. Patients were also allowed free oral intake. The control group was treated postoperatively in the conventional manner with nutritional supplementation of a normal diet. The group fed elemental diets lost less body weight and lean body mass (as measured by total body potassium) and their serum prealbumin levels fell less than the control group. There was no difference in postoperative morbidity or length of stay in hospital. The authors concluded that the technique of needle catheter insertion and management was safe, but the delivery of the liquid diet gave rise to complications. In over one quarter of 43 patients in whom the technique was used feeding had to be temporarily or permanently stopped because of abdominal distension, vomiting, or other GI symptoms. Two deaths occurred, one due to aspiration pneumonia, but this could not be definitely attributed to the elemental diet. Needle catheter jejunostomy is not indicated after routine colo-rectal surgery but should be reserved for patients who have considerable preoperative weight loss and in whom complications or delay in oral intake can be anticipated in the postoperative period. Gastroesophageal surgery is a good example of such indications.

Sagar et al.[12] carried out a similar controlled trial using a double lumen nasogastric tube rather than a jejunostomy. Their fed and control groups underwent a variety of major surgical procedures and appeared to be reasonably well matched. The fed group was given a fat-containing elemental diet infused through one lumen of the double tube beginning on the first postoperative day, initially at a reduced strength and increasing over a 5-day period prior to removal on the 6th day. An average of 1600 kcal were being delivered by the fifth day as compared with an average voluntary intake of 700 kcal in the unfed control group. The group fed elemental diet maintained body weight and had a significantly shorter hospital stay, a median of 14 days as compared to 19 days for the control group. No severe complications associated with feeding were noted, nausea and diarrhea in two patients being attributed to inadequate dilution of the feeds in the early stages of the feeding regimen. Sagar and his colleagues comment that their double-lumen tube offered distinct advantages over fine-needle jejunostomy feeding because of the reduced risk of complications associated with the technique of tube insertion. Fine-needle jejunostomy certainly has its risk, Delany[81] noting five patients in a series of 110 with catheter displacement. Yeung[13] had fewer complications, but nasogastric intubation with a soft tube still remains relatively free of serious complications and would seem to be the route of choice if enteral feeding is contemplated.

The contrast in findings between the two well-designed studies reviewed above is of interest. They may perhaps be explained in terms of regimens used. The nasogastric patients were fed immediately postoperatively so that on the first postoperative day they received an average of 600 kcal. The jejunal group was not fed until the 3rd or 4th day by which time the nasogastric group was receiving a mean of 1300 kcal — it is impossible to estimate nitrogen intake from the data given. In many of the patients in both these series the major catabolic response would take place in the first 3 or 4 postoperative days and it has been shown elsewhere[73] that nutritional support in this period improves nitrogen balance. This early boost received by the nasogastric group but not by the jejunal group toward maintaining energy and protein requirements might well be sufficient to account for the differences in clinical outcome between these two reports.

It can be concluded that enteral nutrition is of value in maintaining nutritional status in both pre- and postoperative patients. The method of choice is probably by a double-lumen nasogastric tube. Most studies have used elemental diets but considerable difficulties appear to have been associated with their administration. Controlled trials of whole protein liquid diets and elemental diets in the postoperative period have not yet appeared although some case reports[60,82] suggest that they may be as effective nutritionally as elemental diets. It seems possible that whole protein diets may give rise to similar difficulties in administration as elemental diets, but comparative studies are awaited.

VII. BOWEL PREPARATION

From a surgeon's point of view two types of bowel preparation are required. For large bowel surgery the lumen should be clear of feces and bacteriologically "clean" even if not sterile. For an adequate view of the lower bowel and for anal and perianal surgery the relevant area should be free of both liquid and solid feces but no more than "socially" clean.

A. Large Bowel Surgery

Conventional bowel preparation aims to reduce the number of intestinal bacteria with appropriate antibodies and to remove feces by mechanical means, either by enemata and/or aperients. The results of different techniques are usually judged on clinical grounds by the rates of septic complications or anastomotic leakage, but since these obviously depend, at least partly, on other factors such as surgical technique or the nutrition of a patient, truly controlled studies are difficult to achieve.

Conventional bowel preparation may fail for a number of reasons. The antibiotics used may be ineffective against at least some of the organisms present, and may allow overgrowth of one species to occur. Mechanical methods of clearance are ineffective and may be contraindicated in the presence of total or partial bowel obstruction.

Elemental diets seemed to offer some solutions to these problems as a result of the initial studies of Winitz et al.[31] who reported both a reduction in fecal bulk and in the concentrations of fecal bacteria in normal volunteers fed an elemental diet. An additional advantage of elemental diets was said to be that they aided in maintaining nutritional status in the patient awaiting surgery.

Glotzer and colleagues[83] were the first group to report on the use of elemental diets as part of a mechanical bowel preparation. In addition to ingesting an elemental diet for five days, patients were given twice daily magnesium sulfate and regular enemas until the day before operation. Only nine patients were studied. No controls were used. No change was found in fecal bacterial counts or in the spectrum of fecal flora and the authors concluded that there was no clear evidence than an elemental diet provided superior intestinal preparation to any other regimen. In fact, the regimen described above differs so little from the "standard" U.K. bowel preparation described by Arabi et al.[84] of magnesium sulfate, enemata, and a low-residue diet, it is doubtful if the elemental diet in Glotzer's regimen would be expected to have any noticeable effect.

A similar study[85] compared a group of patients prepared using an elemental diet with a control group eating normal ward food. Both groups had no other preparation except an enema 24 hr preoperatively. Wound infection or anastomotic leakage were considered to be evidence of failure of the preparation and the quality of preparation was judged at operation which was in all cases for elective colonic surgery. Stool specimens were taken during preparation and from the bowel lumen at surgery. Although the elemental diet resulted in an acceptable preparation as judged at operation, no change in colonic microflora occurred and sepsis rates were unchanged from the controls.

Simple mechanical preparation is undoubtedly an important part of bowel cleansing. In clinical studies[86,87] where postoperative sepsis was used as an indication of the efficacy of bowel preparation, fecal loading and the absence of adequate mechanical preparation were found to be among the causative factors of postoperative sepsis. However, the addition of oral neomycin and metronidazole to a mechanical preparation for 48 hr preoperatively reduced significantly the numbers of colonic bacteria.[84] No difference was seen whether the mechanical preparation was conventional (oral low residue diet, magnesium sulfate and enemata for 3 days), an elemental diet for 5 days, or whole bowel irrigation with normal saline for 30 min on the preoperative day.

Further studies from the same group[88] conducted on a multicenter basis produced similar results. Conventional bowel preparation was as effective as preparation with an elemental diet and oral neomycin and metromidazole. Both regimens reduced significantly the rates of wound sepsis, septicemia, and anastomotic dehiscence. However, the elemental diet patients had a significantly longer hospital stay (25 days) than those having conventional bowel preparation (17 days).

It has been suggested that elemental diets are particularly suitable for bowel preparation where a stenosing lesion of the bowel is present.[89] on the grounds that the stool is able to pass the obstruction easily and the purging effect of magnesiun sulfate is avoided. However, Arabi et al.[84] studied the effect of narrowing of the bowel lumen at the site of the lesion on fecal bacterial counts with various bowel preparations. Reduction in the luminal diameter did not significantly affect the bacterial count, irrespective of the method of mechanical preparation (conventional, elemental diet, or whole bowel irrigation), whether or not oral antibiotics were used.

The other claimed advantage for elemental diets as a bowel preparation is that starvation is avoided in the possibly undernourished patient awaiting bowel surgery.[83] Glotzer's patients[83] all maintained their weight during their 5-day preoperative preparation with elemental diet, but all the seven patients whose weight is recorded appear to be normal or overweight. In a small study [90] of a 4-day preparation with elemental diet in rats undergoing standard colonic anastomoses, weight loss occurred to a similar extent as in groups given either clear fluids or antibiotics as a bowel preparation. It must therefore be doubted if this theoretical advatage is real. There are several practical difficulties in persuading patients to take an elemental diet for 5-day period and several of the studies[83,89] comment on strong patient resistance. Furthermore, one can hardly expect a significant impact to be made on weeks or months of undernutrition by a few days of an elemental diet. If nutrition is a significant limiting factor for an individual patient about to undergo surgery then formally defined nutritional support should be provided and, if necessary, operation and preoperative preparation delayed. It seems clear that elemental diets offer no advantages over the considerably cheaper mechanical methods of bowel preparation.

B. Bowel Preparation for Minor Surgery and Endoscopy

In a number of procedures the surgeon requires a bowel lumen free of fecal material so that an adequate view of eithter the mucosa or of an operative field can be obtained. Elemental diets have also been tried as a bowel preparation for such procedures.

Tomlinson et al.[91] compared an elemental diet and a fluid diet, both with distal luminal washouts, prior to intraperitoneal colostomy closure. There was no difference in wound sepsis, postoperative weight loss, or length of hospital stay between the groups.

Rosser[92] used an elemental diet as preoperative preparation for hemorrhoidectomy on the grounds that it would reduce fecal bulk postoperatively and hence, diminish the discomfort associated with postoperative bowel movement. Patients were given either elemental diet alone for 3 days before and 4 days after hemorrhoidectomy, or were given routein hemorrhoid preparation with a fluid diet on the pre operative day and normal diet postoperatively. At operation only 5 of the 12 control patients were judged to be adequately prepared, whereas all 10 in the elemental group were satisfactory. The control group had more bowel movements and more postoperative pain and bleeding, as judged by the investigator. Only one third of the elemental diet group had experienced a bowel movement by the fourth postoperative day implying that in most patients in the elemental diet group defecation was delayed until some primary tissue repair had taken place.

Elemental diets have also been used to prepare the large bowel prior to colonoscopy. Teague et al.[93] randomly assigned 30 patients to two treatment groups, one given an elemental diet for 5 days and the other a liquid low residue diet prepared by a dietitian. Both diets were equally as effective in producing a reasonably clean bowel for total colonoscopy. Celestin,[60] however, suggests that it takes 3 or more days for the residue of a normal diet to be evacuated before a low residue diet begins to have an effect, and comments that elemental diets are an ineffective method of clearing the bowel when a simple wash-out can accomplish the same objective in 30 min. Celestin also discussed the role of commercially prepared whole-protein liquid diets as a bowel preparation and concludes that in his experience such diets are also unsatisfactory because small fecal pellets are produced.

It seems reasonable to conclude, again, that elemental diets show no advantage over conventional method of bowel preparation in minor surgery and endoscopy procedures. However, the possibility of using an elemental diet as a method of relieving some of the post hemorrhoidectomy pain is interesting and deserves further study.

VIII. CONCLUSIONS

Elemental diets have not fulfilled their earlier promise in surgery, at least. Cheaper whole protein or blenderized standard diets seem able to maintain nutrition equally as effectively and probably with a slightly smaller incidence of unpleasant side-effects in surgical patients. The unique position of elemental diets in pre- and postoperative care is now being seriously questioned and it seems likely that similar doubts can be expressed on their role in fistula management. It is quite clear that they offer no advantage as a preoperative bowel preparation.

Their greatest use has probably been in drawing attention away from the unquestioning use of the i.v. route as the "normal" way for providing nutritional support, toward the realization that an intact gut is the right and proper route for feeding.

REFERENCES

1. **Bistrian, B. R., Blackburn, G. L., Hallowell, E., Heddle, R.,** The protein status of general surgical patients, *JAMA,* 230, 858, 1974.
2. **Hill, G. L., Pickford, I., Young, G. A., Schorah, C. J., Blackett, R. L., Burkinshaw, L., Warren, J. V., and Morgan, D. B.,** Malnutrition in surgical patients, *Lancet,* 1, 689, 1977.
3. **Winitz, M., Seedman, D. A., and Graff, J.,** Studies in metabolic nutrition employing chemically defined diets. I. Extended feeding of normal human adult males, *Am. J. Clin. Nutr.,* 23, 525, 1970.
4. **Thompson, W. R., Stephens, R. V., Randall, H. T., and Bowen, J. R.,** Use of the 'Space Diet' in the management of a patient with extreme short bowel syndrome, *Am. J. Surg.,* 117, 449, 1969.
5. **Goode, A. W., Hawkins, T., Feggetter, J. W. G., and Johnston, I. D. A.,** Use of an elemental diet for long-term nutritional support in Crohn's disease, *Lancet,* 1, 122, 1976.
6. **Koop, C. E., Reigel, C., Grigger, R. P., and Barnes, M. T.,** A study of protein hydrolysates, ossein gelatin and glucose in parenteral nutrition, *Surg. Gynecol. Obstet.,* 84, 1065, 1947.
7. **Abbott, W. E. and Albertsen, K.,** Intravenous protein alimentation, *Nutr. Dieta,* 5, 339, 1963.
8. **Hindmarsh, J. T. and Clarke, R. G.,** The effects of intravenous and intraduodenal feeding on nitrogen balance after surgery, *Br. J. Surg.,* 60, 589, 1973.
9. **Bethel, R. A., Jansen, R. D., Heymsfield, S. B., Ansley, J. D., and Rudman, D.,** Nasogastric hyperalimentation through a polyethylene catheter: an alternative to central venous hyperalimentation, *Am. J. Clin. Nutr.,* 31, 698, 1978.
10. **Cantor, M. D., Kennedy, C., and Reynolds, R.,** Use and abuse of intestinal decompression tube, *Am. J. Surg.,* 73, 437, 1947.
11. **Carlton, P. K., Page, C. P., Haff, R. C., and Bickley, C. J.,** Distal decompression and proximal feeding for nutritional support during bowel obstruction, *J. Parent Ent. Nutr.,* 2, 658, 1978.
12. **Sagar, S., Harland, P., and Shields, R.,** Early postoperative feeding with elemental diet, *Br. Med. J.,* 1, 293, 1979.
13. **Yeung, C. K., Young, G. A., Hackett, A. F., and Hill, G. L.,** Fine needle catheter jejunostomy — an assessment of a new method of nutritional support after major gastrointestinal surgery, *Br. J. Surg.,* 66, 727, 1979.
14. **Bury, K. D., Stephens, R. V., and Randall, H. T.,** Use of a chemically-defined, liquid, elemental diet for nutritional management of fistulas of the alimentary tract, *Am. J. Surg.,* 121, 174, 1971.
15. **Smith, D. W. and Lee, R. M.,** Nutritional management in duodenal fistulas, *Surg. Gynecol. Obstet.,* 103, 666, 1956.
16. **Rocchio, M. A., Cha, C. M., Haas, K. F., and Randall, H. T.,** Use of chemically-defined diets in the management of patients with high output gastrocutaneous fistulas, *Am. J. Surg.,* 127, 148, 1974.
17. **Rivilis, J., McArdle, H., Wlodek, G. K., and Gurd, F. N.,** The effect of an elemental diet on gastric secretion, *Ann. R. Coll. Surg. Can.,* 5, 57, 1972.
18. **Bury, K. D. and Jambunathan, G.,** Effects of elemental diets on gastric emptying and gastric secretion in man, *Am. J. Surg.,* 127, 59, 1974.
19. **Brown, R. A., Thompson, A. G., McArdle, A. H., and Gurd, F. N.,** Alteration of exocrine pancreatic storage enzymes by feeding an elemental diet: a biochemical and ultrastructure study, *Surg. Forum,* 21, 391, 1970.
20. **Ragins, H., Levenson, S. M., Signer, R., Stamford, W., and Seifter, E.,** Intrajejunal administration of an elemental diet at neutral pH avoids pancreatic stimulation: studies in dog and man, *Am. J. Surg.,* 126, 606, 1973.
21. **Janowitz, H. O.,** A quantitative study of the gastric secretory response to sham feeding in a human subject, *Gastroenterology,* 16, 104, 1950.
22. **Russell, R. I.,** Elemental diets, *Gut,* 16, 68, 1975.
23. **Davenport, H. W.,** *Physiology of the Digestive Tract,* Year book, 4th ed., Yearbook Medical Publishers, Chicago, 1977, chap. 12.
24. **Stevens, C. Costill, D. L., and Maxwell, B.,** Impact of carbohydrate source and osmolality on gastric emptying rates of liquid, *J. Parent. Ent. Nutr.,* 3, 32, 1979.
25. **McArdle, A. H., Brown, R. A., Echave, V., Rivilis, J., and Thompson, A. G.,** Alterations in gastric and pancreatic secretion induced by the feeding of an elemental diet, *Arch. Mal. Appar. Dig.,* 61, 1152, 1972.
26. **Panayiotides, T., Cristofides, N., Bjornsson, O. G., Bloom, S. R., and Chadwick, V. S.,** Elemental diets, pancreaticobiliary secretions and gastrointestinal hormones, *Gut,* 20, A450, 1979.
27. **Hill, G. L., Mair, W. S. J., Edwards, J. P., Morgan, D. B., and Goligher, J.,** Effect of a chemically-defined liquid elemental diet on the composition and volume of ileal fistula drainage, *Gastroenterology,* 68, 676, 1975.
28. **Wolfe, B. M., Keltner, R. M., and Willman, V. L.,** Intestinal fistula output in regular elemental and intravenous alimentation, *Am. J. Surg.,* 124, 803, 1972.

29. **Voitk, A. J., Echave, V., Brown, R. A., McArdle, A. P., and Gurd, F. N.,** Elemental diet in the treatment of fistulas of the alimentary tract, *Surg. Gynecol. Obstet.*, 137, 68, 1973.
30. **Morgan, A., Filler, R. M., and Moore, F. D.,** Surgical nutrition, *Med. Clin. N. Am.*, 54, 1367, 1970.
31. **Winitz, M., Adams, R. F., Seedman, D. A., Davis, P. N., Jayko, L. G., and Hamilton, J. A.,** Studies in metabolic nutrition employing chemically-defined diets. II. Effects on gut microflora populations, *Am. J. Clin. Nutr.*, 23, 546, 1970.
32. **Attebery, H. R., Sutter, V. L., and Finegold, S. M.,** Effect of a partially chemically defined diet on normal faecal flora, *Am. J. Clin. Nutr.*, 25, 1391, 1972.
33. **Crowther, J. S., Drasar, B. S., Goddard, P., Hill, M. J., and Johnson, K.,** The effects of a chemically-defined diet on the faecal flora and faecal steroid concentration, *Gut,* 14, 790, 1973.
34. **Kaminski, M. V.,** Elemental hyperalimentation, *Surg. Gynecol. Obstet.*, 143, 12, 1976.
35. **Dwyer, J. T.,** Dietetic assessment of cancer patients, *Cancer,* 43, 2077, 1979.
36. **Keys, A., Brozek, J., Henschel, A., Mickelsen, O., and Taylor, H. L.,** in *The Biology of Human Starvation,* vol. 2, Minnesota Press, Minneapolis, 1950, chap. 46.
37. **deWys, W. D. and Walters, K.,** Abnormalities of taste sensation in cancer patients, *Cancer,* 36, 1888, 1975.
38. **Copeland, E. M., MacFadten, B.V., MacComb, W. S., Guillamondequi, C., Jesse, R. H., and Dudrick, S. J.,** Intravenous hyperalimentation in patients with head and neck cancer, *Cancer,* 35, 606, 1975.
39. **Fallis, L. S. and Baron, J.,** Gastric and jejunal alimentation with fine polyethylene tubes, *Arch. Surg.*, 65, 373, 1952.
40. **Pereira, M. D., Conrad, E. J., Hicks, W., and Elman, R.,** Clinical responses and changes in nitrogen balance, body weight, plasma proteins and hemoglobin following tube feeding in cancer cachexia, *Cancer,* 8, 803, 1955.
41. **Tweedle, D. E. F., Skidmore, F. D., Gleave, E. N., Knass, D. A., and Gowland, E.,** Nutritional support for patients undergoing surgery for cancer of the head and neck, *Res. Clin. Forums,* 1, 59, 1979.
42. **Graham, W. P., and Royster, H. P.,** Simplified cervical oesophagostomy for long-term feeding, *Surg. Gynecol. Obstet.*, 125, 127, 1967.
43. **Ketcham, A. S. and Smith, R. R.,** Elective oesophagostomy, *Am. J. Surg.*, 104, 682, 1962.
44. **Banfield, W. J. and Hurwitz, A. C.,** Oesophageal strictures associated with nasogastric intubation, *Arch Intern. Med.*, 134, 1083, 1974.
45. **Hartwell, S. W.,** Oesophagostomy for feeding, *Clin. Plast. Surg.*, 3, 459, 1976.
46. **Royster, H. P., Noone, R. B., Graham, W. P., and Theogaraj, S. D.,** Cervical pharyngostomy for feeding after maxillo-facial surgery, *Am. J. Surg.*, 116, 610, 1968.
47. **Noone, R. B. and Graham, W. P.,** Nutritional care after head and neck surgery, *Postgrad. Med.*, 53, 80, 1973.
48. **Johnson, H. D.,** Gastrostomy, in *Operative Surgery,* Vol. 4, Part 1, 2nd ed., Rob, H., Smith, R., and Morgan, C. N., Eds., Butterworth, London, 1969, 62.
49. **Delany, H. M. and Garvey J. W.,** Jejunostomy by a needle catheter technique, *Surgery,* 73, 786, 1973.
50. **Boles, T. and Zollinger, R. M.,** Critical evaluation of jejunostomy, *Arch. Surg.*, 65, 358, 1952.
51. **Britnall, E. S., Daum, K., and Womack, N. A.,** Maydl jejunostomy, *Arch. Surg.*, 65, 367, 1952.
52. **Allerdyce, D. B. and Groves, A. C.,** A comparison of nutritional gains resulting from intravenous and enteral feeding, *Surg. Gynecol. Obstet.*, 139, 179, 1974.
53. **Shils, M. E.,** Enteral nutrition by tube, *Cancer Res.*, 37, 2432, 1977.
54. **deWys, W. D. and Herbst, S. H.,** Oral feeding in the nutritional management of the cancer patient, *Cancer Res.*, 37, 2429, 1977.
55. **Edmunds, L. H., Williams, G. M., and Welch, C. E.,** External fistulas arising from the gastrointestinal tract, *Ann. Surg.*, 152, 445, 1960.
56. **Chapman, R., Foran, R., and Dumphy, J. E.,** Management of intestinal fistulas, *Am. J. Surg.*, 108, 157, 1964.
57. **Roback, S. A. and Nicoloff, D. M.,** High output enterocutaneous fistulas of the small bowel, *Am. J. Surg.*, 123, 317, 1972.
58. **Brunschwig, A., Bigelow, R. R., and Nicholls, S.,** Intravenous nutrition for eight weeks: partial enterectomy, recovery, *JAMA,* 129, 441, 1945.
59. **Himal, H. S., Allard, J. R., Nadeau, J. E., Freeman, J. B., and McLean, L. D.,** The importance of adequate nutrition in closure of small intestinal fistulas, *Br. J. Surg.*, 61, 724, 1974.
60. **Celstin, L. R.,** Residue — sense and nonsense, *Res. Clin. For.*, 1, 91, 1979.
61. **Beyer, P. L. and Flynn, M. A.,** Effects of high and low fibre diets on human faeces, *J. Am. Diet. Assoc.*, 72, 271, 1978.
62. **Liffmann, K. E. and Randall, H. T.,** A modified technique for creating a jejunostomy, *Surg. Gynecol. Obstet.*, 134, 663, 1972.
63. **Nealon, T. F., Grossi, C. E., and Steier, M.,** Use of elemental diets to correct catabolic states prior to surgery, *Ann. Surg.*, 180, 9, 1974.

64. **Woolfson, A. M. J., Saour, J. N., Ricketts, C. R., Pollard, B. J., Hardy, S. M., and Allison, S. P.,** Prolonged nasogastric tube feeding in critically ill and surgical patients, *Postgrad. Med. J.*, 52, 178, 1976.
65. **Jones, D. C., Rich, A. J., Wright, P. D., and Johnston, I. D. A.,** A comparison of proprietary elemental and whole protein diets, *Br. Med. J.*, 280, 1493, 1980.
66. **Bondy, R. A., Beyer, P. L., and Rhodes, J. B.,** Comparison of two commercial low residue diets and a low residue diet of common foods, *J. Parent. Ent. Nutr.*, 3, 226, 1979.
67. **Bouzarth, W. F.,** Intracranial nasogastric tube insertion, *J. Trauma*, 18, 818, 1978.
68. **Bollet, A. J. and Owen, S.,** Evaluation of the nutritional status of selected hospitalized patients, *Am. J. Clin. Nutr.*, 26, 931, 1973.
69. **Studley, H. O.,** Percentage of weight loss: a basic indication of surgical risk in patients with chronic peptic ulcer, *JAMA*, 106, 458, 1938.
70. **Johnston, C. C.,** Decompression in the treatment of intestinal obstruction, *Surg. Gynecol. Obstet.*, 86, 647, 1948.
71. **Cantor, M. O.,** New simplified intestinal decompression tube, *Am. J. Surg.*, 72, 137, 1946.
72. **Lee, H. A.,** Intravenous nutrition, *Br. J. Hosp. Med.*, 11, 719, 1974.
73. **Craig, R. P., Davidson, H. A., Tweedle, D. E. F., and Johnston, I. D. A.,** Intravenous glucose, aminoacids and fat in the postoperative period, *Lancet*, 2, 8, 1977.
74. **Collins, J. P., Oxby, C. B., and Hill, G. L.,** Intravenous aminoacids and intravenous hyperalimentation as protein-sparing therapy after major surgery, *Lancet*, 1, 788, 1978.
75. **Wells, C. A.,** Ileus and postoperative intestinal motility, *Lancet*, 2, 136, 1961.
76. **Shields, R.,** The absorption and secretion of fluid and electrolytes by the obstructed bowel, *Br. J. Surg.*, 52, 774, 1965.
77. **Bunch, G. A. and Shields, R.,** Absorption of water and electrolytes by human small intestine after surgical operations, *Br. J. Surg.*, 56, 708, 1969.
78. **Shoemaker, C. P. and Wright, H. K.,** Rates of water and sodium absorption from the jejunum after abdominal surgery, *Am. J. Surg.*, 119, 62, 1970.
79. **Hindmarsh, J. T. and Clarke, R. G.,** New jejunostomy feed, *Br. Med. J.*, 3, 609, 1973.
80. **Daly, J. M., Steiger, E., Vars, H. M., and Dudrick, S. J.,** Postoperative oral and intravenous nutrition, *Ann. Surg*, 180, 709, 1974.
81. **Delany, H. M., Carnevale, N., Garvey, J. W., and Moss, C. M.,** Postoperative nutritional support using needle catheter feeding jejunostomy, *Ann Surg.*, 186, 165, 1977.
82. **Allison, S. P., Walford, S., Todorovic, V., and Elliot, E. T.,** Practical aspects of nutritional support, *Res. Clin. For.*, 1, 49, 1979.
83. **Glotzer, D. J., Boyle, P. L., and Silen, W.,** Preoperative preparation of the colon with an elemental diet, *Surgery*, 74, 703, 1973.
84. **Arabi, Y., Dimock, F., Burdon, D. W., Alexander-Williams, J., and Keighley, M. R. B.,** Influence of bowel preparation and antimicrobials on colonic microflora, *Br. J. Surg.*, 65, 555, 1978.
85. **Gurry, J. F. and Ellis-Pegler, R. B.,** An elemental diet as preoperative preparation of the colon, *Br. J. Surg.*, 63, 969, 1976.
86. **Rosenberg, I. L., Graham, N. G., de Dombal, F. T., and Goligher, J. C.,** Preparation of the intestine in patients undergoing major large bowel surgery, mainly for neoplasms of the colon and rectum, *Br. J. Surg.*, 58, 266, 1971.
87. **Barker, K., Graham, N. G., Mason, M. C., de Dombal, F. T., and Goligher, J.C.,** The relative significance of preoperative antibiotics, mechanical bowel preparation and preoperative peritoneal contamination in the avoidance of sepsis after radical surgery for ulcerative colitis and Crohn's disease of the large bowel, *Br. J. Surg.*, 58, 270, 1971.
88. **Matheson, D. M., Arabi, Y., Baxter-Smith, D., Alexander-Williams, J., and Keighley, M. R. B.,** Randomized multicentre trial of oral bowel preparation and antimicrobials for elective colorectal operations, *Br. J. Surg.*, 65, 567, 1978.
89. **Johnson, W. C.,** Oral elemental diet, *Arch. Surg.*, 108, 32, 1974.
90. **Cooney, D. R., Wassner, J. D., Grosfeld, J. L., and Jesseph, J. E.,** Are elemental diets useful in bowel preparation?, *Arch. Surg.*, 109, 205, 1974.
91. **Tomlinson, R. J. R., Newman, B. M., and Schofield, P. F.,** Is colostomy closure a hazardous procedure? A comparison of an elemental diet and a routine bowel preparation, *Br. J. Surg.*, 63, 799, 1976.
92. **Rosser, R. G.,** Dietary preparation for haemorrhoidectomy. Advantages of a nutritionally complete chemically-defined low residue diet, *Am. J. Surg.*, 130, 78, 1975.
93. **Teague, R. H., Salmon, P. R., and Read, A. E.,** Fibreoptic examination of the colon: a review of 255 cases, *Gut*, 14, 139, 1973.

Chapter 12

MALDIGESTION AND MALABSORPTION STATES

R. I. Russell

TABLE OF CONTENTS

I. INTRODUCTION

Elemental diets are absorbed in the small intestine with minimal digestive requirements and have low residue. They have thus been suggested as being of value in a number of conditions associated with maldigestion and malabsorption. In this chapter the use of elemental diets in maldigestion and malabsorption states is considered and the evidence for their use in such conditions reviewed. Their value will be assessed in chronic pancreatic insufficiency and other pancreatic diseases, the short bowel syndrome, coeliac disease and other malabsorption states, and in bile acid-induced diarrhea.

II. CHRONIC PANCREATIC INSUFFICIENCY AND OTHER PANCREATIC DISEASES

A. Chronic Pancreatic Insufficiency

As chemically defined diets require little or no digestion in the upper alimentary tract they are absorbed adequately in the presence of reduced pancreatic exocrine secretions. They are thus of potential value in maintaining adequate nutritional status when pancreatic exocrine secretions are reduced by disease as in chronic pancreatic insufficiency. It has been considered from early studies of elemental diets that their use may be associated with reduced pancreatic exocrine secretion, and the evidence for this has been reviewed in Chapter 8. There are a number of animal and some human studies on the subject and the results, especially in studies on normal human volunteers, suggest that the elemental diets Vivonex® and Flexical® do stimulate exocrine pancreatic secretion to about the same extent as would be expected from the ingestion of food containing equivalent amounts of amino acids. Some modification of response may occur with Vivonex® due to its high glucose content or, if introduced directly in the stomach, this elemental diet may alter gastric emptying so as to reduce or modify exocrine pancreatic secretion. Thus, although further studies are required both in normal human subjects and in patients with pancreatic insufficiency, the evidence does suggest that elemental diets do stimulate exocrine pancreatic secretion. Their principal value in the presence of chronic pancreatic insufficiency may thus lie in allowing effective absorption of nutrients in the absence of normal pancreatic enzyme secretory function. This property may be of value in various diseases associated with pancreatic insufficiency.

Vivonex® was used successfully in the management of seven of eight patients with chronic pancreatic insufficiency by Pincus et al.[1] These patients presented with marked steatorrhea, weight loss and weakness, and had not improved with pancreatic supplements. The use of the elemental diet, either as the sole source of nutrition or as a supplement to normal food, was successful in improving the nutritional status of seven of the eight patients. In this study, therefore, the elemental diet was used as nutritional support in patients with chronic pancreatic insufficiency who were nutritionally depleted. Adequate absorption could be achieved by the nutritional support administered in this way.

B. Pancreatic Fistula

The use of the elemental diet Flexical® has been successfully reported in the management of patients with pancreatic fistulas,[2,3] and the same elemental diet was used effectively as the sole source of nutrition in six patients with chronic pancreatic insufficiency associated with development of pancreatic pseudocysts and pancreatic fistulas.[4] These patients were unable to eat normally and were considered to be unsuitable for intravenous nutrition. The patients were not able to tolerate normal oral intake and responded to each attempt at feeding by the development of abdominal pain associated with a rise of serum amylase and clinical deterioration. They tolerated the elemental diet well and five of the six recovered completely. A positive nitrogen balance, weight gain, resolution of sepsis, and spontaneous closure of the pancreatic fistulas were reported in five of the six patients. The authors considered that the principal beneficial effect of the elemental diet in these patients was its nonstimulatory effect on the pancreas. It seems likely, however, in the light of later studies, that the main benefit may well have been to improve the nutritional state of the patients by providing adequate oral nutritional support. The low residue nature of the elemental diets would also be helpful in the management of the pancreatic fistulas. Controlled studies comparing the use of different formulations of elemental diets in patients with chronic pancreatic insufficiency and pancreatic fistulas have not been performed.

C. Acute Pancreatitis

Although there were early suggestions that chemically defined diets may be of value in the management of acute pancreatitis on the basis of the supposed reduced pancreatic stimulation which may favorably alter the course of the disease,[4] there is no convincing data in the literature to support this contention. Indeed, in a study using dogs in which the elemental diet, Vivonex®, was investigated as both a prophylactic and therapeutic agent in experimental canine pancreatitis induced by the operative injection of bile-saline solution under pressure into the main pancreatic duct, no marked benefit was detected in the Vivonex®-treated group.[5] There was no ultrastructural evidence for the modification of zymogen granules when the elemental diet was given prior to the induction of pancreatitis, nor were differences evident histologically or ultrastructurally in the severity of pancreatitis between the groups given Vivonex® and those not given the elemental diet. The mortality figures demonstrated no efficacy of the elemental diet in the pretreatment prophylaxis of actue pancreatitis in this experimental animal model. There are several other uncontrolled reports of an elemental diet being used in acute pancreatitis. One reports a patient who was unable to ingest a low-fat diet, but could take an elemental diet and was able to return to normal food after 4 weeks. Another study reported good results in 11 of 13 patients with acute pancreatitis who were given combinations of enteral and i.v. nutrition.[6] These authors considered that there is no strong evidence for reduced pancreatic secretion with amino acids compared with whole protein. On a basis of the published data, however, there is no indication for the use of elemental diets in the management of patients with acute pancreatitis.

D. Pancreatic Abscess

An elemental diet has also been reported to be helpful in maintaining nutrition in seven patients with pancreatic abscess following acute pancreatitis without the presence of pancreatic pseudocyst.[7] These patients all developed nutritional deficiency due to the presence of the abscess following pancreatitis. The abscess was drained surgically and the elemental diet fed through a jejunostomy with subsequent clinical improvement in these patients.

E. Cystic Fibrosis

An elemental diet may also be of value in the management of pancreatic insufficiency associated with cystic fibrosis. The importance of nutritional support has been well recognized in children with cystic fibrosis, in which pancreatic insufficiency is an important feature. Nutritional supplementation was reported to improve patients with cystic fibrosis,[8-10] although in another study the use of a diet containing glucose polymers and a protein hydrolysate led to little nutritional improvement.[11] In a controlled study of 43 children treated with the elemental diet Flexical® over 1 year, 10 (36%) gained marked benefit in relation to height, weight, bone age, and skinfold thickness.[12] Because of palatability problems and some side effects, these authors concluded that chemically defined diets would only be of value in a few selected patients with cystic fibrosis

F. Conclusions

Nutritional deficiency may be a feature of chronic pancreatic insufficiency, cystic fibrosis, pancreatic fistula, and abscesses. Occasionally, nutritional insufficiency may be severe, requiring i.v. feeding, but in most patients enteral nutritional support is adequate. Elemental diets are absorbed effectively in the presence of reduced pancreatic secretions and thereby may be of value in the management of some patients with chronic pancreatic insufficiency or cystic fibrosis associated with chronic pancreatic insufficiency, when nutritional support is required and a poor response has been obtained by the use of standard pancreatic supplementation. As these patients may also have diabetes mellitus, the additional glucose load supplied by the elemental diet Vivonex® may complicate diabetic control and may necessitate an adjustment of insulin dosage in some patients.

Elemental diets may also be helpful in improving the nutritional status of patients with a pancreatic fistula or pancreatic abscess. Their low residue nature makes them potentially valuable in allowing healing of a pancreatic fistula. Elemental diets have no part to play in the management of acute pancreatitis.

III. MASSIVE SMALL INTESTINAL RESECTION — THE SHORT BOWEL SYNDROME

An important indication for the use of elemental diets has been considered to be the provision of nutritional support and the induction of adaptive changes in the intestine following massive small bowel resection. The purpose of this section is to consider the evidence for the use of elemental diets in the management of patients with the short bowel syndrome.

The factors involved in maintaining normal small intestinal structure and function, together with a consideration of the effect of elemental diets on the structure and function of the small intestine, have been considered in Chapter 8. There is considerable evidence favoring luminal nutrition as an important factor in maintaining adequate small intestinal structure and function.

Massive small intestinal resection may follow an acute vascular episode or be associated with volvulus or tumors of the small intestine. Following resection, patients develop severe diarrhea, steatorrhea, fluid and electrolyte imbalance, marked weight loss, negative nitrogen balance with the subsequent development of a wide range of deficiencies including minerals and vitamins.[13] Patients in whom up to 75% of the small intestine has been resected may remain in reasonably good health but those with more extensive resections may die without adequate nutritional support. With good nutritional support much better results are obtained, and long-term survival has been reported in a patient in whom only 6 inches of intestine remained after resection,[14] and in a patient who had undergone resection of the entire jejunum, ileum, and ascending colon.[15] The position is complicated in these patients as they may be in a poor nutritional state prior to surgery due to the basic disease process which has led to the resection. This, together with the catabolic state associated with surgery, results in the patient being in a bad nutrtional state by the time resection is performed. After the resection, the remaining gut undergoes adaptation with lengthening of villi, thickening of the wall, dilatation, and a slowing of motility.[16] Following adaptation, transit time is lengthened, steatorrhea and diarrhea reduced, and nutrient absorption improved.[17] During this period of adaptation good nutritional support is required to correct the nutritional deficiency associated with the basic disease process followed by surgery. The importance of nutritional support during this period was shown in a study in dogs which reported increased survival rate after massive small bowel resection in animals given i.v. nutrition during the postoperative phase.[18] Although i.v. nutrition is frequently required before and after surgery in patients with massive small intestinal resection in order to maintain the nutritional status of the patient, there is now much evidence to suggest that luminal nutrition speeds the adaptive process. The factors associated with intestinal adaptation have been discussed in Chapter 8. After surgery of this kind, conventional food may be inadequately tolerated by the patient and it is in this situation that elemental diets have been considered to be of value. They supply luminal nutrition which may help to speed up the adaptive changes in the intestine, are absorbed effectively in small lengths of intestine, and at the same time provide an easily assimilable source of nutrition which may allow nutrients to be absorbed rapidly and effectively by the remaining gut. Other forms of enteral nutrition have not been adequately studied in this situation to date, and little information is available on the speed and effectiveness of absorption of elemental and other forms of enteral nutrition.

A. Animal Studies

Some studies in animals have investigated the effect of elemental diets in inducing adaptive changes after intestinal resection. In one study using rats, the elemental diet Flexical® was compared with normal rat food after resection of 85% of the intestine.[19] It was demonstrated that the elemental diet could support the rats nutritionally following this operation but offered no advantages over normal food in bringing about the adaptive changes. The elemental diet, however, was considered to be inferior to normal food in providing adequate nutrition.

In another study, rats undergoing jejuno-ileal bypass surgery excluding 85% of the small intestine were studied with the elemental diet Vivonex®, and compared with standard rat food.[20] In both diet groups hypertrophy of the functioning part of the small intestine and atrophy of the blind loop occurred with significantly changed villus heights compared with controls. The results suggested that the chemically defined diet was capable of stimulating the mucosa of the small intestine to develop compensatory adaptive changes in the rat under the conditions of that study. It was noted in this study that animals on normal food had a higher calorie intake and consequently a higher body weight than those taking the elemental diet. The morphological adaptive changes in the normally fed animals were of the same order as those induced by Vivonex®. This fact was also emphasized in another study in which the growth and nutrition of rats were investigated after small bowel resection and treatment with an elemental diet.[21] It would thus appear that, although luminal nutrition is important, the elemental diet in these animal studies did not induce adaptive changes any more effectively than normal food. However, it may be more effectively absorbed in the remaining small intestine.

Luminal nutrition appears to play an important role, particularly in the ileum, which receives a greater nutrient load after proximal resection or bypass.[22] Adaptive changes take time to occur and thus luminal nutrition would require to be continued for several weeks to allow adequate changes to occur. One recent study in monkeys and in man investigated the effectiveness of amino acid-based and hydrolysate-based elemental diets in inducing gastrointestinal (GI) changes as reflected by the alteration of fecal composition and output.[23] Several days of treatment were required before any marked changes were noted. It is likely that several weeks are required before adequate adaptive changes occur after small intestinal resection in man.

B. Human Studies

An elemental diet was first used successfully in the nutritional management of a patient with massive small intestinal resection by Thompson and colleagues[24] in 1969. The diet, similar to Flexical®, was administered slowly through a gastrostomy tube and evidence of adequate absorption was demonstrated. The patient was maintained in a satisfactory nutritional state for 101 days after 4 cm of the jejunum was anastomosed to the midtransverse colon after thrombosis of the superior mesenteric artery had occurred. The patient eventually died of acute bacterial endocarditis and at post-mortem examination dilatation of the stomach, duodenum, and colon was detected together with hypertrophy of the duodenum.

The first successful use of Vivonex® in the management of massive small intestinal resection was reported by Belin in 1971.[25] Voitk et al.[26] reported the use of the elemental diet Flexical® in the short gut syndrome in eight patients in 1973. A positive nitrogen balance was achieved in all patients and good weight gain reported. Adaptation sufficient to tolerate normal food was achieved in four patients. In this study, the elemental diet followed i.v. nutrition which was required as nutritional support in the early stages after surgery. Supplemental i.v. feeding may be required in such patients even after adaptive changes have occurred.[27]

The satisfactory use of a chemically defined diet in the management of the short bowel syndrome in children has also been reported.[28] In this study two infants were successfully taken off i.v. nutrition by continuous intragastric infusion of a chemically defined diet through a gastrostomy tube. The elemental diet provided adequate calories for growth and maintained positive fluid and electrolyte balance (see Chapter 16). Other similar successful uses of a chemically defined diet in the adaptive stage of short gut syndrome have been reported.

C. Conclusions

After massive small intestinal resections, nutritional support with i.v. feeding is generally initially required. At an early stage, however, it is desirable to introduce luminal nutrition so as to speed adaptive changes in the remaining gut. Although there is no evidence suggesting that chemically defined diets are better than ordinary food or other forms of enteral nutrition in inducing or speeding up adaptive changes in the remaining intestine, they may be helpful in providing adequate nutritional support in the period immediately following i.v. nutrition, and are also effective in inducing adaptation.

Elemental diets require little or no digestion and adequate absorption may be achieved more effectively than with other forms of enteral nutrition in the bowel remaining after massive intestinal resection. Elemental diets may thus be of value in the short bowel syndrome by virtue of three properties:

- Nutritional support (possibly following on from i.v. feeding)
- Adequate absorption in a short area of intestine with minimal digestion requirements
- Induction of intestinal adaptation, although they are probably no better than other forms of enteral nutrition in this respect

By virtue of their easy assimilation, such diets may thus be of value in the management of patients in the adaptive stage following massive resections. Further studies are required of the value of newer forms of enteral nutritional support such as whole protein liquid diets.

IV. COELIAC DISEASE AND OTHER MALABSORPTION STATES

Most patients with adult coeliac disease show a satisfactory clinical response shortly after starting therapy with a gluten-free diet. In some patients, however, the response is slow and some do not initially respond satisfactorily to the exclusion of gluten from the diet. Most patients exhibiting a good clinical response also show in time an improvement in the histological abnormalities present in the jejunal mucosa, although a return to complete histological normality may not be obtained, especially in adults. Indeed, clinical and histological improvement after gluten withdrawal from the diet is essential in confirming a diagnosis of coeliac disease. Patients with untreated adult coeliac disease have been shown to have a net secretion of water and electrolytes in the jejunum, demonstrated by the technique of small intestinal perfusion.[29,30] This abnormality of water and electrolyte transport across the jejunal mucosa may be slow to respond to the exclusion of gluten from the diet and may remain for many months after starting treatment.[29] Some patients with coeliac disease develop severe nutritional insufficiency due to longstanding malabsorption and are thus in a poor nutritional state by the time the diagnosis is made. Additional nutritional support may be required in some of these patients while the gluten-free diet is started as essential therapy. Coeliac disease is considered to be due to an allergy to gluten, which probably triggers an immunological response in the mucosa. The presence of gluten in the diet continues the mucosal damage. Many patients with coeliac disease also develop disaccharidase deficiency secondary to the mucosal damage induced by gluten.

It has been suggested that elemental diets may be of value in the initial management of patients with coeliac disease.[31,32] They may provide nutritional support to the patient with nutritional deficiency due to malabsorption and in view of their reported value in some patients with the short bowel syndrome in which adaptation may be induced by the presence of adequate luminal nutrition, it is theroretically possible that more rapid recovery of the jejunal mucosa toward normality may occur in the early stages of treatment by administering elemental diets. In addition the fact that the diets are hypoallergenic, gluten-free, and lactose-free may also serve to speed mucosal recovery.

A study has been reported to determine if the elemental diet Vivonex® in addition to a gluten-free diet could improve the secretory state of the jejunum and the histological abnormalities more rapidly than a gluten-free diet alone, when used for a period of 1 month in the initial management of patients with adult coeliac disease.[33] A jejunal biopsy was performed at the beginning and end of the 4-week period and the net absorption of water and electrolytes in the proximal jejunum determined at the same time by means of a triple lumen tube perfusion system. The mean absorption of water, sodium, and chloride before and after treatment in the patients treated with Vivonex® and gluten-free diet and gluten-free diet alone are shown in Table 1. The results showed that a 1 month course of treatment with the elemental diet together with a gluten-free diet resulted in no significant improvement in the absorption abnormality in the jejunum compared with the standard gluten-free diet alone. Histological examination of the jejunal biopsies at the beginning of the study revealed subtotal villous atrophy in seven of the eight patients and severe partial villous atrophy in one. After the test period repeat jejunal biopsies revealed only minor improvement in the histological appearances. It was noted, however, that in five of the patients (three of whom had received Vivonex®) some slight improvement of cellular infiltrate was noted in the jejunal biopsies with a reduction of plasma cell infiltrate being predominant. None of the patients were deemed to be markedly nutritionally deficient before the study and no changes in standard nutritional parameters were noted over the 1-month test period. The conclusions that can be drawn

Table 1
ABSORPTION OF WATER, SODIUM, AND CHLORIDE IN PATIENTS WITH ADULT COELIAC DISEASE BEFORE TREATMENT AND AFTER 1 MONTH OF THERAPY WITH GLUTEN FREE DIET (GFD) + VIVONEX (V) OR GLUTEN FREE DIET (GFD) ALONE

	Mean absorption (± SEM)		
	Water ($m\ell\ h^{-1}\ 30\ cm^{-1}$)	Sodium ($mmol\ h^{-1}\ 30\ cm^{-1}$)	Chloride ($mmol\ h^{-1}\ 30\ cm^{-1}$)
Before treatment	−61.3 ± 62.3	−8.9 ± 7.4	−12.9 ± 10.5
After 1 month GFD + V	−22.5 ± 14.6	−5.5 ± 3.0	−5.9 ± 2.6
Before treatment	−21.0 ± 8.2	−3.2 ± 1.3	−0.5 ± 1.1
After 1 month GFD alone	6.5 ± 9.1	−0.1 ± 0.7	−0.2 ± 0.4

from the study are that the elemental diet when used in conjunction with a gluten-free diet in the initial management of adult coeliac disease does not have an effect on the clinical features, jejunal absorption of water, and electrolytes and jejunal mucosal histology greater than that obtained by the use of a gluten-free diet alone. In view of these results there would appear to be no place for the use of an elemental diet in the initial treatment of patients with coeliac disease who do not have nutritional abnormality. It is possible that in patients who are more nutritionally deficient the use of an elemental diet may improve the nutritional status of the patients during the time that gluten-free diet exerts its beneficial effect on the mucosa. However, alternative enteral nutritional support may be of equal value in this respect. In those few patients with coeliac disease in whom gross nutritional deficiency is present at the time of diagnosis, i.v. nutrition may be required to restore nutritional status to normality.

There are many causes of small intestinal malabsorption and any one of these may lead to chronic nutritional deficiency requiring nutritional support. These causes include tropical sprue, drug-induced malabsorption, infiltrative diseases such as reticulosis, amyloidosis, and tuberculosis. Any one of these conditions may lead to nutritional deficiency over a period of time and nutritional support may be required. Chemically defined diets may be of value in providing such nutritional support in individual patients although there is no evidence that they are any better in this respect than other forms of supplementary feeding or other enteral nutritional regimes. The presence of small intestinal damage, if extensive, may also lead to some degree of malabsorption of the elemental diet itself, although this may also apply to other forms of enteral nutrition. There are no published data on the absorption of chemically defined diets and other forms of enteral nutrition in conditions associated with chronic malabsorption. In severe nutritional deficiency associated with any one of these malabsorption syndromes, i.v. nutritional support may be helpful and may be more specific in improving the nutritional status of the patient than any form of enteral nutrition, including elemental diets.

A. Conclusions

Patients with coeliac disease and other chronic malabsorptoin states may develop moderate or severe nutritional deficiency. When this is severe, i.v. nutrition may be required, but in less severe nutritional deficiency, enteral nutritional support is generally adequate. Although elemental diets may be effective in providing such support, there is no evidence that they are better in this respect than other forms of enteral nutritional support. The use of elemental diets as a source of improved luminal nutrition and their hypoallergenic nature does not appear to give them any advantage over a standard gluten-free diet in the initial management of coeliac disease. Intestinal structure and function do not improve more quickly when an elemental diet is used. Elemental diets therefore cannot be recommended in coeliac disease for other than moderate nutritional support if necessary.

V. BILE ACID-INDUCED DIARRHEA

Chemically defined diets have been shown to induce alterations of bile acid metabolism both in animals and man. This aspect has been discussed in Chapter 8. Both Vivonex® and Flexical® have been shown to reduce fecal bile acid excretion in animals, although the mechanism needs to be further investigated.

This observation suggested the potential use of elemental diets in the management of patients suffering from severe bile acid-induced diarrhea. This form of diarrhea, often known as cholerheic diarrhea, may follow severe disease of the terminal ileum (such as Crohn's disease) or ileal resection. The importance of the ileum for the absorpton of bile acids and the maintenance of their enterohepatic circulation has been well demonstrated both in dogs[34] and in man.[35,36] When the enterohepatic circulation has been broken due to interruption of bile acid absorption in the terminal ileum, there is a greatly increased load of bile acids entering the colon and severe, persistent diarrhea may result. This diarrhea is watery in nature and is characterized by urgency.[37] Its occurrence after ileal resection of less than 100 cm and its separation from the steatorrheic diarrhea of larger resections has been described.[38] The diarrhea is due to damage to the colonic mucosa, principally by dihydroxy bile acids, causing secretion of water and electrolytes.[39] The importance of the length of any associated colonic resection has been stressed in relation to the severity of diarrhea.[40] Treatment of this type of diarrhea with the bile acid sequestering agent cholestyramine may be successful,[41] but as bile acids are bound in both the small and large intestine, fat malabsorption over a period of time with worsening of steatorrhea, and supplementary fat-soluble vitamins are generally required.

On the basis of the reported alterations of bile acid metabolism with chemically defined diets and a reported reduction of fecal bile acid excretion in three healthy volunteers by Crowther et al.,[42] a study was performed to investigate the use of the elemental diet Vivonex® in the management of patients with bile acid-induced diarrhea. Fecal bile acid excretion before and during Vivonex® therapy was measured togehter with the severity of diarrhea, and the value of Vivonex® in the clincial management of the patients assessed.[43]

Six patients with cholerheic diarrhea after ileal resection were studied in this investigation. Four of the ileal resection had been performed for Crohn's disease, one for carcinoma of the cecum and one for mesenteric thrombosis. The length of ileum resected ranged from 10 to 100 cm. Two normal volunteers and four patients with noncholerheic diarrhea were also studied. Two 5-day stools were collected for each subject, the first being a control collection when the subjects were consuming a normal diet containing approximately 70 g fat per day and the second collection started 3 to 10 days after the normal diet had been replaced by Vivonex® administered alone. The effect of the elemental diet Vivonex® on fecal weight, fecal fat, stool frequency, and excretion of total fecal bile acids is shown in Table 2. Fecal wet weight was significantly reduced from 339 ± (Mean ± SEM) g/24 hr to 146 ± 13 g/24 hr for the six patients with cholerheic diarrhea during treatment with Vivonex® ($p<0.05$). Fecal dry weight was also significantly reduced, not only in the cholerheic diarrhea group but in all the subjects studied. Total fecal bile acids were significantly reduced in the patients with cholerheic diarrhea from a mean of 6.37 ± 1.64 (SEM) mmol/24 hr to 2.70 ± 1.12 mmol 1/24 hr after treatment with the elemental diet ($p<0.05$). Bile acid excretion was reduced in all six

Table 2
MEAN (± SEM) FECAL WET AND DRY WEIGHTS, AND BILE ACID EXCRETION IN PATIENTS WITH CHOLERHEIC DIARRHEA IN CONTROL PERIOD AND DURING VIVONEX THERAPY

	Before Vivonex®	During Vivonex®	
Fecal wet weight (g/24 hr)	339 ± 106	146 ± 13	$p < 0.05$
Fecal dry weight (g/24 hr)	46 ± 6	18 ± 4	$p < 0.05$
Total fecal bile acids (mmol/24 hr)	6.37 ± 1.64	2.70 ± 1.12	$p < 0.05$

patients and it was noteworthy that the largest reduction was observed in the patient with an intact ileo-cecal sphincter. Fecal fat excretion was also reduced using Vivonex® treatment. No marked change in fecal bile acid excretion was observed in patients with noncholerheic diarrhea and in normal subjects. The excretion of individual bile acids in the patients before elemental diet therapy and during treatment was also measured. In five of the patients with cholerheic diarrhea most of the excess fecal bile acids during the control period consisted of the primary bile acids cholic and chenodeoxycholic acids, as is usually found in patients after ideal resection. The relative proportions of the four bile acid peaks showed no real change during treatment with Vivonex®. During therapy with the elemental diet, all patients observed a reduction in the frequency of daily stools and it was noted that urgency was markedly reduced (Table 3). This study therefore suggests that the elemental diet Vivonex® may be valuable in the management with bile acid-induced diarrhea who may be resistant to treatment with cholestyramine. Although long-term treatment with an elemental diet by itself may not be feasible, short-term therapy may break the sequence of diarrhea in individual patients, while at the same time maintaining or improving the nutrition of the patient.

The patients in this investigation had severe cholerheic diarrhea following ileal resection. Another group of patients has also been reported in whom the fecal bile acid excretion was elevated due to severe ileal Crohn's disease without ileal resection.[44] These patients also benefited clinically from the use of the elemental diet Vivonex,® the number of bowel motions being greatly reduced, less watery in character, with less urgency being present.

In another recent study, ten patients with well-established ileostomies were studied with the elemental diet Vivonex® as sole nutritional source for a 10-day period.[45] The ileal fistula output fell markedly during treatment with the chemically defined diet (control period 578 ± 300 (± SEM) mℓ/day; Vivonex® 418 ± 190 mℓ/day; $p < 0.02$) There was also a significant reduction in the concentration of sodium, trypsin, and bile acids in the ileal output. The bile acid concentration fell from 0.911 ± 0.56 (SEM) mmol/mℓ to 0.662 ± 0.53mmol/mℓ ($p < 0.005$). It was concluded from this study that the use of the elemental diet Vivonex® causes changes in ileal fistula output which may be of benefit to patients with an enterocutaneous fistula Reasons for this benefit are the reduction of fluid output, the reduction of trypsin concentration, or of bile acids. This may also be helpful in the management of severe skin excoriation which may be related to excessive ileostomy fluid output. The use of the elemental diet in such patients over a short period as sole nutritional support not only maintains the patient in a good nutritional state but may also allow healing of the skin excoriations and thereby a return to subsequent normal oral food intake.[44]

Table 3
CLINICAL EFFECTS OF VIVONEX IN PATIENTS WITH BILE ACID-INDUCED DIARRHEA

	Before Vivonex®			During Vivonex®		
Patient	Number of Stools	Type	Urgency	Number of Stools	Type	Urgency
1	10—12	Watery	+	2—3	Semi-formed	0
2	4—6	Watery	+	3—4	Semi-formed	0
3	8—10	Watery	+	4—5	Watery	0
4	7—10	Watery	+	1—3	Formed	0
5	5—7	Semi-formed	+	1—3	Formed	0
6	3—4	Watery	+	1—3	Semi-formed	0

The cause of the reduced fecal bile acid excretion in patients with cholerheic diarrhea has not been entirely explained and it is to be noted that a reduction of fecal bile acid excretion aslo occurs to some extent in normal subjects. As elemental diets of such widely differing composition as Vivonex® and Flexical® appear to exert a similar effect, the low residue nature and fiber content may be the important common factor. These aspects are discussed in Chapter 8. Data are required on the effect of elemental diets on bile acid metabolism and fecal bile acid excretion, and also on the effect of specific enteral whole protein liquid feeds on bile acid metabolism.

A. Conclusions

There is much evidence from animal and human work that elemental diets alter bile acid metabolism. There are data to show that the elemental diet Vivonex® markedly reduces fecal bile acid excretion and may be of value in the chemical and clinical management of patients with bile acid induced diarrhea, following ileal resection or in patients with severe disease of the terminal ileum, as in Crohn's disease. Chemically defined diets may thus have a place in the short-term management of such conditions, providing a break in the diarrhea while at the same time maintaining or improving nutritional status. Further work is required on the effect of other elemental diets and other enteral preparations on bile acid metabolism and fecal bile acid excretion both in normal subjects and in patients with cholerheic diarrhea. Further work is also required on the mechanism of the alterations of bile acid metabolism which have been reported.

VI. OTHER DIARRHEAL STATES

Elemental diet therapy has been suggested as being of value in the management of some patients with irritable colon syndrome[46] and diverticular disease.[47,48] There is no convincing evidence of their value in either of these conditions and there seems to be no indication for their use in these diseases. It should be noted, however, that some patients with the irritable colon syndrome do have increased fecal bile acid excretion and this may be reduced in some patients by the use of an elemental diet. I have not found this form of treatment to be of value in the irritable colon syndrome or in diverticular disease.

In patients with postvagotomy diarrhea of continuous type, in which there may be an increased fecal bile acid excretion,[49] elemental diet therapy may be helpful in reducing fecal bile acid excretion and alleviating symptoms if therapy with cholestyramine is unhelpful, although this drug may be valuable in the treatment of many of these patients.[50] It is unlikely, however, that these patients have the concomitant nutritional problems which may be present in patients with Crohn's disease. It therefore is unlikely that elemental diets will prove to be of major practical value in the management of these patients.

An elemental diet has been reported to be of value in protracted infantile diarrhea.[51,52] In the study of Greene et al.[52] elemental and i.v. feeding together was compared with i.v. nutrition alone. Of eight children initially given the elemental diet, two were unable to tolerate the diet, and two others were given a whole protein, lactose-free enteral diet. The latter two had more diarrhea than those given the elemental diet. Duration of hospital stay was shorter in infants given oral nutritional support, but no difference was noted between those given elemental dets and those given whole protein liquid diets. Those given enteral nutrition were found to have a more rapid recovery of intestinal mucosal enzyme function, compared with those infants given i.v. nutrition.

REFERENCES

1. **Pincus, I. J., Citron, P. P., and Haverback, B. J.,** Nutritional support of gastrointestinal problems with Vivonex 100 in *Balanced Nutrition and Therapy,* Lang, K., Fekl, W., and Berg, G., Eds., Georg Theime Verlag, Stuttgart, 1971, 77.
2. **Stephens, R. V. and Randall, H. T.,** Use of a concentrated balanced liquid elemental diet for nutritional management of catabolic states, *Ann. Surg.,* 170, 642, 1969.
3. **Bury, K. D., Stephens, R. V., and Randall, T.,** Use of a chemically defined liquid elemental diet for nutritional management of fistulas of the alimentary tract, *Am. J. Surg.,* 121, 174, 1971.
4. **Voitk, A., Brown, R. A., Echave, V., McArdle, A. H., Gurd, F. N., and Thompson, A. G.,** Use of an elemental diet in the treatment of complicated pancreatitis, *Am. J. Surg.,* 125, 223, 1973.
5. **Kerstein, M. D. and Tonkens, R. M.,** Elemental diet in bile-induced pancreatitis, *Surg. Gynecol. Obstet.,* 143, 253, 1976.
6. **Blackburn, G. L., Williams, L. F., and Bistrian, B.,** New approaches to the management of severe acute pancreatitis, *Am. J. Surg.,* 131, 114, 1976.
7. **Paloyan, D. Siminovitz, D., and Bates, R. J.,** Guidelines in the management of patients with pancreatic abscess, *Am. J. Gastroenterol.,* 69, 97, 1978.
8. **Allan, J. D., Milner, J., and Moss, A. D.,** Therapeutic use of an artificial diet, *Lancet,* 1, 785, 1970.
9. **Allan, J. D., Mason, A., and Moss, A. D.,** Nutritional supplementation in treatment of cystic fibrosis of the pancreas, *Arch. Dis. Child.,* 126, 22, 1973.
10. **Berry, H. K., Kellogg, F. W., Hunt, M. M., Ingberg, R. L., Richter, L., and Gutjahr, J.,** Dietary supplements and nutrition in children with cystic fibrosis, *Arch. Dis. Child.,* 129, 165, 1975.
11. **Gupte, S.,** Treatment of cystic fibrosis, *Lancet,* 2, 521, 1974.
12. **Yassa, J. G., Prosser, R., and Dodge, J. A.,** Effects of an artificial diet on growth of patients with cystic fibrosis. *Arch. Dis. Child.,* 53, 777, 1978.
13. **Leonard, A. S., Levine, A. S., Wittner, R., Buchwald, H., and Varco, R. L.,** Massive small bowel resections, *Arch. Surg.,* 95, 429, 1967.
14. **Anderson, C. M.,** Long term survival with six inches of small intestine, *Br. Med., J.,* 1, 419, 1965.
15. **Kinney, J. M., Goldwin, R. M., Barr, J. S., and Moore, F. D.,** Loss of the entire jejunum and ileum, and ascending colon — management of a patient, *JAMA,* 179, 529, 1962.
16. **Wright, H. K. and Tolson, M. D.,** The short gut syndrome, Pathophysiology and treatment, *Current Problems in Surgery,* Chicago Year Book Medical Publishers, 1971.
17. **Weser, E.,** Intestinal adaption to small bowel resection, *Am. J. Clin. Nutr.,* 24, 133, 1971.
18. **Wilmore, D. W., Dudrick, S. J., Daly, J. M., and Vars, H. N.,** The role of nutrition in the adaptation of the small intestine after massive resectin, *Surg. Gynecol. Obstet.,* 132, 673, 1971.

19. **Voitk, A. J. and Crispin, J. S.,** The ability of an elemental diet to support nutrition and adaptation in the short gut syndrome, *Ann. Surg.,* 181, 220, 1975.
20. **Fenyo, G. and Hallberg, D.,** The influence of a chemical diet on the intestinal mucosa after jejunal ileal bypass in the rat, *Acta Chir. Scand.,* 142, 270, 1976.
21. **Touloukian, R. J., Metruka, B., and Hoil, C.,** Growth and nutrition of enterotomised rats fed an elemental liquid diet, *Surgery,* 69, 637, 1971.
22. **Dowling, R. H. and Gleeson, M. H.,** Cell turnover following small bowel resection and bypass, *Digestion,* 8, 176, 1973.
23. **Spiller, G. and Beigler, M. A.,** Time-dependent gastrointestinal adaptation of human subjects and non-human primates to liquid defined formula diets, *Z. Ernaehpungswiss. Suppl.,* 20, 48, 1977.
24. **Thompson, W. R., Stephens, R. V., Randall, H. T., and Bowen, J. R.,** Use of the "space diet" in the management of a patient with extreme short bowel syndrome, *Am. J., Surg.,* 117, 449, 1969.
25. **Belin, P.,** Use of Vivonex 100 in paediatric surgery in *Balanced Nutrition and Therapy,* Lang, K., Fekl, W., and Berg, G., Eds., Georg Thieme Verlag, Stuttgart, 1971, 95.
26. **Voitk, A. J., Echave, V., Brown, R. A., and Gurd, F. N.,** Use of elemental diet during the adaptive stage of short gut syndrome, *Gastroenterology,* 65, 419, 1973.
27. **Heizer, W. D. and Orringer, E. P.,** Parenteral nutrition at home for 5 years via arterial venous fistulae: Supplementary intravenous feedings for a patient with severe short bowel syndrome, *Gastroenterology,* 72, 527, 1977.
28. **Christie, D. L. and Ament, M. E.,** Dilute elemental diet and continuous infusion technique for management of short bowel syndrome, *J. Pediatrics,* 87, 705, 1975.
29. **Russell, M. I., Allan, J. G., Gerskowitch, V. P., and Robertson, J. W. K.,** A study by perfusion technique of the absorption abnormalities in the jejunum in adult coeliac disease, *Clin. Sci.,* 42, 735, 1972.
30. **Schmid, W. C., Phillips, S. F. and Summerskill, W. H. J.,** Jejunal secretion of electrolytes and water in non tropical sprue, *J. Lab. Clin. Med.,* 73, 772, 1969.
31. **Russell, R. I.,** Elemental diets, *Gut,* 16, 68, 1975.
32. **Jarnum, S. and Axelsson, C.,** Synthetic diet in internal medicine, *Z. Ernahrungswiss. Suppl.,* 20, 8, 1977.
33. **Russell, R. I., Atherton, S. T., Nelson, L. M., Robertson, E., and Lee, F. D.,** The effects of an elemental diet (Vivonex) on the absorption abnormalities and histological appearances of the jejunum in untreated adult coeliac disease, *Digestion,* 190, 335, 1979.
34. **Playoust, M. R., Lack, L., and Weiner, I. M.,** Effect of intestinal resection and bile salt absorption in dogs, *Am. J. Physiol.,* 208, 363, 1965.
35. **Austad, W. I., Lack, L., and Tyor, M. P.,** Importance of bile acids and an intact distal small intestine for fat absorption, *Gastroenterology,* 52, 638, 1967.
36. **Meihoff, W. E. and Kern, F.,** Bile salt malabsorption in regional ileitis, ileal resection and mannitol-induced diarrhoea, *J. Clin. Inv.,* 47, 261, 1968.
37. **Hofmann, A. F.,** The syndrome of ileal disease and the broken enterohepatic circulation: cholerheic enteropathy, *Gastroenterology,* 52, 752, 1967.
38. **Hofmann, A. F.,** Bile acid malabsorption caused by ileal resection, *Arch. Intern. Med.,* 130, 597, 1972.
39. **Mekhjian, H. S., Phillips, S. F., and Hofmann, A. F.,** Colonic secretions of water and electrolytes induced by bile acids: perfusion studies in man, *J. Clin. Inv.,* 50, 1569, 1971.
40. **Cummings, J. H., James, W. P. T., and Wiggins, H. S.,** Role of the colon in ileal resection diarrhoea, *Lancet,* 1, 344, 1973.
41. **Hofmann, A. F. and Poley, J. R.,** Cholestyramine treatment of diarrhoea associated with ileal resection, *N. Engl. J. Med.,* 281, 397, 1969.
42. **Crowther, J. S., Drasar, B. S., Goddard, P., Hill, M. J., and Johnston, K.,** The effect of chemically defined diets on the faecal flora and faecal steroid concentration, *Gut,* 14, 790, 1973.
43. **Nelson, L. M., Carmichael, H. A., Russell, R. I., and Atherton, S. T.,** Use of an elemnetal diet (Vivonex) in the management of bile acid induced diarrhoea, *Gut,* 18, 792, 1977.
44. **Russell, R. I. and Hall, M. J.,** Elemental diet therapy in the management of complicated Crohn's disease, *Scott. Med., J.,* 24, 291, 1979.
45. **Hill, G. L., Mair, W. S. J., Edwards, J. P., and Goligher, J. C.,** Decreased trypsin and bile acids in ileal fistula drainage during administration of a chemcially defined liquid elemental diet, *Br. J. Surg.,* 63, 133, 1976.
46. **Glotzer, D. J.,** Space diets: comment, *Gastroenterology* 61, 405, 1971.
47. **Moss, G.,** Physiological colostomy, *Arch. Surg.,* 106, 741, 1973.
48. **Rocchio, M. A., Mo Cha C. J., Haas, K. F., and Randall, H. T.,** Use of chemically-defined diets in the management of patients with acute inflammatory bowel disease, *Am. J. Surg.,* 127, 469, 1974.
49. **Allan, J. G., Gerskowitch, V. P., and Russell, R. I.,** The role of bile acids in the pathogeneiss of post-vagotomy diarrhoea, *Br. J. Surg.,* 61, 516, 1974.

50. **Allan, J. G. and Russell, R. I.,** Cholestyramine in the treatment of postvagotomy diarrhoea — a double blind controlled trial, *Br. Med., J.*, 1, 674, 1977.
51. **Sherman, J. O., Hamly, C., and Khachadurian, A. K.,** Use of an oral elemental diet in infants with severe intractable diarrhoea, *J. Paediatr.*, 86, 518, 1975.
52. **Greene, H. L., McCabe, D. R., and Merenstein, G. B.,** Protracted diarrhoea and malnutrition in infancy, changes in intestinal morphology and disaccharidase activities during treatment with total intravenous nutrition or oral elemental diets, *J. Paediatr.*, 87, 695, 1975.

Chapter 13

INFLAMMATORY BOWEL DISEASE

R. I. Russell

TABLE OF CONTENTS

I. INTRODUCTION

Elemental diets have been suggested as being of value in the management of some patients with Crohn's disease and ulcerative colitis. These inflammatory bowel diseases are, however, of different nature and etiology, and their natural history is different. In Crohn's disease exacerbations may occur and the disease generally runs a chronic relapsing course in which local complications such as fistulas and anorectal lesions may be troublesome over a long period, and malabsorption and nutritional deficiency frequently develop. Surgery is not an effective cure as in ulcerative colitis, and recurrences and complications frequently develop following surgical intervention. Patients with ulcerative colitis are also subject to intermittent acute exacerbations which are satisfactorily controlled in the most part by the use of corticosteroid therapy, and long-term sulfasalazine reduces the incidence of exacerbations of the disease. If the disease is difficult to remit or if serious complications develop, proctocolectomy is a complete cure.

Crohn's disease is thus more frequently associated with chronic ill health than ulcerative colitis and can be less easily and less effectively dealt with by surgery. It is thus more likely that nutritional support such as elemental diets would be of value in patients with Crohn's disease than in ulcerative colitis. This treatment, however, has been used in both types of inflammatory bowel disease.

There are several reasons why chemically defined diets may be helpful in patients with inflammatory bowel disease. They may provide nutritional support in patients who are, by virtue of longstanding disease, nutritionally deficient. They may also be of value in the management of local complications of inflammatory bowel disease because of their low residue nature and specific composition. A third potential use of elemental diets in inlammatory bowel disease is as "primary therapy" for the disease, in that they may induce a remission of the disease process. It is the purpose of this chapter to consider the value of elemental diets in each of these ways in the management of patients with Crohn's disease and ulcerative colitis.

II. CROHN'S DISEASE

Patients with Crohn's disease are frequently malnourished and may develop malnutrition associated with severe absorption problems in the small intestine.[1,2] They are also liable to develop severe anal and rectal problems such as chronic fistulas, local ulcerations, infections and fissures.[3,4] Diarrhea is also a problem in many patients and frequently prevents adequate healing of perianal, anal, and rectal lesions. The diarrhea itself may be due to extensive mucosal damage in the jejunum, ileum, or colon with consequent malabsorption of fat, water, electrolytes, or bile acids.[2,5,6] Jejunal Crohn's disease may cause malabsorption of fat with the development of steatorrhea, and water and electrolyte malabsorption or secretion may also occur. There is evidence that damage to jejunal absorption mechanisms may be more widespread than is frequently apparent from radiological or histological investigations.[7] Severe terminal ileal Crohn's disease may lead to malabsorption of conjugated bile acids with subsequent increased faecal excretion of bile acids resulting in cholerheic diarrhea. In some patients ileal resection may have been performed which may also result in bile acid-induced diarrhea. The combination of severe malabsorption, chronic fistulas, fissures, anal and perianal infections, and ulceration (often associated with the development of perirectal abscesses) leads to nutritional deterioration in many patients with the development of nutritional deficiency.

Nutritional insufficiency in any patient with Crohn's disease is liable to have multiple etiology and be associated with chronic and recurrent local complications. Patients with Crohn's disease are liable to develop acute on subacute intestinal obstruction, often in the ileum, which may necessitate surgery; this may become necessary in an unfavorable situation when the patient has severe nutritional deficiency. Growth retardation may occur in children with Crohn's disease and in one study was found in 17% of the children studied.[8] Improvement of the nutritional status of such children may lead to an improvement in linear growth.

Elemental diets may be theoretically valuable in Crohn's disease for a number of different reasons and frequently several indications are present in any individual patient. The assessment of any particular form of therapy in a disease such as Crohn's disease which is characterized by remissions and exacerbations, is extremely difficult, and these difficulties have been highlighted in the use of drugs such as corticosteroids, sulfasalazine, and azathioprine. Very few satisfactory controlled studies of these drugs in Crohn's disease have been performed. The assessment of a form of treatment such as elemental diets in Crohn's disease is equally difficult, particularly in view of several possible beneficial effects which they may have. No controlled data is available in which elemental diets have been compared with other forms of enteral nutrition or intravenous feeding in comparable groups of patients. Such data clearly requires to be obtained, although much of the published information on the clinical value of elemental diets in Crohn's disease is of interest and value.

Bowel rest and nutritional support are both important in the management of Crohn's disease. The use of chemically defined diets combines both forms of therapy and may be of value in many patients with Crohn's disease.

A. Elemental Diets in the Nutritional Management of Crohn's Disease

As previously described, many patients with longstanding Crohn's disease have severe nutritional insufficiency which is of multiple etiology. Negative nitrogen balance is common in these patients and a number of surgical failures in Crohn's disease are related directly to the poor nutritional state of the patient. Many patients with Crohn's disease require intravenous nutrition, and there are numerous reports of the successful use of this therapy in the management of Crohn's disease.[9-12] Patients with severe nutritional deficiency should be considered immediately for intravenous feeding rather than any form of enteral or elemental nutritional support. The potential hazards of intravenous feeding are worth risking because of the benefits which can be gained in severe nutritional deficiency by this form of therapy in Crohn's disease.[13]

The value of elemental diets in providing nutritional support in Crohn's disease with less severe nutritional insufficiency has been well-substantiated. In patients with Crohn's disease with some degree of nutritional deficiency, elemental diets may be helpful in improving the nutritional state, and in those with a relatively normal nutritional state, nutritional normality can be maintained with chemically defined diets. At the same time their low residue nature and specific formulations may provide other benefits to these patients. The value of elemental diets in providing adequate nutritional support in patients with Crohn's disease over a short-term period was shown by Stephens and Randall[14] in 1969, and confirmation provided by Bury et al.[15] and Voitk and colleagues.[16] In the latter study, using Flexical, 13 patients were treated 17 times for an average of 22 days with the elemental diet. All gained weight and demonstrated positive nitrogen balance. In general the elemental diet was able to provide nutrition while allowing bowel rest, and was considered to have satisfactorily improved the nutritional state in a number of these patients prior to surgery. The maintenance of nutrition with the elemental diet Vivonex® in patients with inflammatory bowel disease and fistulas was reported successfully by Rocchio et al.[17] in 1974. More prolonged use of this elemental diet in patients with inflammatory bowel disease, providing 2000 to 5000 calories a day without significant complication allowed the maintenance of a positive nitrogen balance and resulted in clinical improvement.[18] Short-term use of the elemental diet Flexical® was also found to provide effective nutrition in catabolic states associated with Crohn's disease, often accompanied by the healing of local intestinal lesions.[19] Although the relationship between improved nutrition and successful surgery in Crohn's disease is undoubted, there is debate as to the relationship of improvement of the nutritional state of patients with Crohn's disease and clinical improvement of the disease itself. This has recently been highlighted by Earnest and Hammerman[20] who reported that the clinical improvement in patients with Crohn's disease on an elemental diet is likely to be related to factors other than improved nutrition as clinical improvement occurred in many of their patients even when a positive nitrogen balance was not achieved.

The value of the elemental diet Vivonex® in long-term nutritional support in Crohn's disease has also been reported.[21] Eight patients were studied who had lost on average 30% (18 to 37%) of their normal weight. Three preoperative patients who had been unable to maintain their weight on a normal diet were able to restore 10% per month of the lean tissue mass which had been lost, and in five patients who had undergone bowel resection for Crohn's disease the postoperative rate of improvement of lean tissue mass was 18.5% per month on the elemental diet. In these patients the elemental diet was used for up to 360 days and the study confirmed that such a diet is capable of arresting and reversing chronic weight loss in patients who are capable of full cooperation in the treatment regime.

Nutritional deficits associated with Crohn's disease in children may lead to growth retardation.[22] An indication of the effectiveness of nutritional support in these children is the reversal of growth retardation. Most of these patients require intravenous feeding, and this has been shown to be effective in reversing growth retardation in this group.[23] In one recent case report, reversal of growth retardation was achieved by the use of the elemental diet Vivonex® in a young boy with Crohn's disease[24] and similar results have recently been reported using a continuous intragastric infusion of Vivonex® for 6 weeks in four children with Crohn's disease.[25] After cessation of elemental diet therapy, three of the four children continued to grow; over a period of 4.5 months from the beginning of treatment, they gained an average of 5.0 $\pm$ 1.6 kg weight and grew 3.5 $\pm$ 0.3 cm. Reversal of growth retardation in seven children with Crohn's disease was also demonstrated in another recent study, using planned oral nutritional treatment with supplements of either Vivonex® or a complete oral liquid diet, Ensure®.[48]

Thus it would appear that the principal elemental diets Vivonex® and Flexical® may be of value in maintaining nutritional status in patients with Crohn's disease with normal nutritional status or with some degree of nutritional deficiency. It is possible, however, that similar benefit can be obtained in such patients using other forms of enteral support. The use of an elemental diet may not be necessarily essential in such enteral nutritional support. Controlled data are required to compare the value of elemental diets and other enteral preparations in this group of patients, such as complete oral liquid diets.

B. The Use of Elemental Diets in The Management of Symptoms and Local Complications of Crohn's Disease

1. Acute Symptoms of Crohn's Disease.

When chemically defined diets first started being used in patients with Crohn's disease, initially for such as fistulas, there were reports of improvements of symptomatolgy of the Crohn's disease in many of these patients. Since that time, many such reports have appeared. Voitk et al.[16] in a prospective study of seven patients with Crohn's disease treated with Flexical® reported improvement in diarrhea together with weight gain and positive nitrogen balance in all patients. Three of the patients had been referred for nutritional management because of deterioration following surgery and all had active disease in the remaining gut. The elemental diet reversed the downward course and none of the patients required further surgery. Rocchio[18] also reported improvement in patients with acute Crohn's disease using the elemental diet Vivonex®. Bounous et al.[19] reported relief of symptoms in nine patients with Crohn's disease using Flexical® and commented on the difficulty in planning adequate controlled trials of nutritional therapy or of any specific therapy in a disease such as Crohn's disease which has a remitting natural history. They also discussed the possibility that the use of the elemental diet may not necessarily be better than other forms of enteral nutrition in improving the symptoms of the disease. These studies were uncontrolled and relate to small numbers of patients.

Further favorable reports of the management of acute symptoms of Crohn's disease by elemental diets were provided by Jarnum,[25] Berg,[26] Base et al.[27] and Pichler[28] each using Vivonex®. In each of these studies clinical improvement occurred with the use of the chemically defined diet. At the same time nutritional improvement occurred, but no controlled information was available on the specific effect of the elemental diet on the disease process.

Segal et al[29] treated eight patients who had active Crohn's disease with the elemental diet Vivonex® prior to treatment with Levamisole; the patients were on no other specific therapy. The elemental diet was administered for 14 days before treatment with Levamisole was started and it was found that symptoms settled during this period. In an extension of the same study, these authors have recently reported improvement in the acute symptoms in 29 of 32 acute exacerbations within a 4 week period of starting treatment with Vivonex®.[50]

A further study reporting the management of 11 patients with acute Crohn's disease with Vivonex® was reported by Axelsson and Jarnum.[30] The duration of dietary therapy was decided from the clinical course, the average being 26 days (range 11 to 55 days). Symptomatic improvement was obtained in two of the 11 patients with severe disease and five with moderate disease activity. Two patients with severe disease activity showed no improvement during treatment. Assessment of the effect of the elemental diet by itself was not performed and most of the patients had oral prednisolone during treatment. Eight patients with Crohn's disease were followed up and four remained unoperated and free of symptoms 22 to 35 months after the study. No real assessment can be made of the effect of the elemental diet on disease activity or in inducing remission in Crohn's disease from this report. The same authors attempted to assess the effect of Vivonex® on the activity of Crohn's disease by studying intestinal protein exudation using ^{131}I albumin.[31] Four patients with Crohn's disease were studied for 1 to 7 weeks. Steroid therapy was also used during the acute treatment period.^{131} I albumin studies showed no significant change of albumin degradation and thus, by inference, of intestinal protein loss in these patients, although clinical improvement occurred in three of the four patients studied. The authors concluded that measurement of intestinal protein leakage is of no predictive value as regards the effect of treatment of Crohn's disease with the elemental diet, and considered that diminishing protein exudation is likely to be a late phenomenon during a course of clinical remission. An alternative explanation is that the symptomatic improvement occurring with Vivonex therapy may not infer remission of the disease process. Another study of small bowel Crohn's disease treated with Vivonex did, however, show some reduction of gastrointestinal (GI) protein loss.[32] Vivonex® was administered for 4 to 8 weeks to seven patients with hypoalbuminemia from jejuno-ileal Crohn's disease. Protein loss, assessed by intravenous^{51} $CrCl_3$, was reduced from the equivalent of a mean of 190 mℓ plasma cleared per day (range 118 to 274 mℓ/day) before treatment to a mean of 99.5 mℓ/day (range 42 to 21 mℓ/day)after therapy. ($p<0.05$). Clinical and nutritional improvement also occurred. This 47.5% reduction of GI protein loss may be indicative of a direct improvement due to Vivonex therapy, but the numbers in the study were small and the ranges of protein loss figures large. Further controlled data in larger numbers of patients is required.

Another recent study on 23 consecutive adult patients with an acute exacerbation of Crohn's disease who were treated either with the elemental diet Vivonex® or intravenous nutrition followed by the introduction of a low residue diet. The symptoms responded favorably to treatment in most patients, postoperative fistulas closed in some patients and enterocutanous fistulas settled in all five patients with this condition.[33]

Most of the reports of the successful use of elemental diets in inducing remission of symptoms in patients with Crohn's disease are anecdotal and not well controlled. It is possible however, that some improvement of symptomatology may occur in some patients with the use of an elemental diet. Improvement may be mediated by the low residue nature, nutritional improvement, hypoallerginicity, or alteration of bowel flora. It does seem, however, that good results have been attained with both Vivonex® and Flexical® in individual patients and as these elemental diets are of widely different composition, it seems possible that the common factor of low residue nature and nutritional improvement may be more important than their specific composition. Controlled studies are required to investigate the use of elemental diets and other forms of enteral nutrition in the management of acute symptomatology in Crohn's disease. It is important in such studies that other treatment such as prednisolone, azathioprine or sulfasalazine should not also be used. Complete oral liquid diets also provide nutritional support with minimal residue and may in theory be as effective as elemental diets in the management of acute symptoms in Crohn's disease.

2. Local Complications of Crohn's Disease

There is convincing evidence on the use of elemental diets in the management of some of the local complications of Crohn's disease. Following the report of the successful use of the elemental diet in healing of fistulas and reduction of intestinal fistula output by Wolfe et al.,[34] a number of studies reported benefit and healing of fistulas in Crohn's disease by the use of elemental diets.[17-19] The low residue nature of elemental diets providing bowel rest may allow healing to occur in these patients with fistulas associated with Crohn's disease. At the same time the nutritional status of the patient is likely to be maintained or improved, thus increasing the likelihood of healing. Other low residue enteral feeds may be equally effective in this respect and some of these patients may require intravenous nutrition because of severe nutritional insufficiency. Intravenous feeding also provides bowel rest and may also encourage healing of these lesions.

The use of elemental diets in healing fissures and anorectal lesions in Crohn's disease has also been reported by a number of authors, generally as case reports,[35] and their use to settle acute inflammatory lesions prior to surgery has also been favorably reported. These two indications in the management of local complications of Crohn's disease were also reported by Russell and Hall, [36] who reviewed the use of the elemental diet Vivonex® in the management of complicated Crohn's disease. Patients found to benefit included those with severe local perianal and anal problems, subacute ileal obstruction and ileostomy problems associated with the skin excoriation following proctocolectomy for extensive colonic Crohn's disease. This latter use of an elemental diet, leading to a reduction in ileostomy output has also been reported by Hill et al.[37]

C. Elemental Diets as 'Primary Therapy' in Crohn's Disease

An early study of the use of an elemental diet in Crohn's disease raised the possibility that this form of therapy, providing nutritional support and bowel rest, may be "primary therapy".[16] This suggestion was encouraged by the observation that symptoms improved when the treatment was used. As we have seen, a nunber of susequent studies have reported symptomatic improvement with elemntal diet therapy.[18,19,25-33] Although there are indications for elemental diets or other forms of nutritional support in some patients with Crohn's disease, and advantages in providing bowel rest in others, the term "primary therapy" infers a different and more specific effect on the disease process itself. The same problem applies to the use of intravenous nutrition in Crohn's disease, which also provides nutritional support together with bowel rest. Intravenous nutrition as "primary therapy" has been suggested by a number of authors.[38-41] The term "primary therapy" requires to be defined more specifically so that controlled trials of intravenous nutrition or various forms of enteral support can be performed.[42] Specific parameters of disease activity require to be indentified and defined. This is difficult in a disease such as Crohn's which is charaterized by repeated natural exacerbations and remissions. Such specific clinical, laboratory, and histological parameters of Crohn's disease activity have not as yet been satisfactorily defined. There is no convincing evidence at present that nutritional therapy combined with bowel rest (either intravenous nutrition or elemental diets) acts as primary therapy in Crohn's disease. Some preliminary diets may have an additional and more "specific" effect than might be expected from nutritional support and bowel rest alone,[32,43] but much stronger and better controlled data are required before any definitive statement can be made on the value of elemental diets as "primary therapy" in Crohn's disease.

III. ULCERATIVE COLITIS

In many of the reports of the use of elemental diets in Crohn's disease, there have been patients reported with acute ulcerative colitis in which this treatment has been given. This has been recorded by a number of authors.[16,18,25-30,44,47] The use of the term "inflammatory bowel disease" has included both ulcerative colitis and Crohn's disease, and in many reports no differentiation of these conditions has been attempted.

Although improvement in diarrhea was noted in most of the patients reported, no controlled information is available and the patients at the same time were being treated with standard therapy for acute ulcerative colitis, notably with corticosteroid therapy. It is unlikely that elemental diets by themselves are of value in the management of acute ulcerative colitis. Standard therapy with corticosteroids is effective in ulcerative colitis much more so than in Crohn's disease and nutritional insufficiency in ulcerative colitis is less likely to occur than in Crohn's disease. It seems unlikely, therefore, that there is much place for the use of elemental diets in the management of acute ulcerative colitis, and there is no evidence of a "primary" effect of elemental diets in the treatment of ulcerative colitis.

IV. CONCLUSIONS

Elemental diets may be helpful in the short- and long-term management of nutritional insufficiency in patients with Crohn's disease, but in any individual patient with severe nutritional deficiency intravenous nutrition is likely to be necessary. Elemental diets may sometimes lead to some improvement of acute symptoms of Crohn's disease, although good controlled data on this is required. Chemically defined diets, by providing bowel rest, may be helpful in the management of local complications of Crohn's disease such as anorectal and perianal lesions — fissures, fistulas, — in allowing subacute small intestinal obstruction to settle before surgery, or in allowing healing of skin excoriations near an ileostomy by reducing ileostomy fluid output. The value of elemental diets as "primary therapy" in Crohn's disease is as yet unproven. There remains however, a possibility that this form of therapy, by improving nutritional status and providing bowel rest, may have a specific "primary" effect on the activity of the disease. Controlled studies of this aspect of elemental diet therapy are required. The comparison of nutritional, acute symptomatic local, and "primary therapy" effect of elemental diets with that provided by other forms of enteral nutrition and intravenous nutrition also require to be studied under proper controlled conditions.

There is no convincing evidence of a specific effect of elemental diets in improving either symptomatology of ulcerative colitis or as primary therapy in this condition. In some individuals symptomatology may be improved by the use of elemental diets although the use of standard medical therapy, notably with corticosteroids, is much more successful and more specific in this condition. In some individuals with ulcerative colitis nutritional support may be necessary and in some of these patients elemental diets or other other forms of enteral nutrition may be of some value. In severe cases intravenous nutrition may be required.

REFERENCES

1. **Creamer, B. and Lockhart-Mummery, H. F.,** Crohn's disease — clinical aspects in *The Small Intestine,* Creamer, B., Ed., Heinemann, London, 1974, 161.
2. **Smith, A. N. and Balfour, T. W.,** Malabsorption in Crohn's disease, in *Crohn's Disease — Clinics in Gastroenterology,* Brooke, B. N., Ed., W. B. Saunders, London, 1972, 433.
3. **Lockhart-Mummery, H. F.,** Anal lesions of Crohn's disease, in *Crohn's Disease — Clinics in Gastroenterology,* Brooke, B. N., Ed., W. B. Saunders, London, 1972, 377.
4. **Steinberg, D. M., Cooke, W. T., and Alexander-Williams, J.,** Abscess and fistula in Crohn's disease, *Gut,* 14, 865, 1973.
5. **Creamer, B. and Lochart-Mummery, H. F.,** Crohn's disease — clinical aspects, in *The Small Intestine* Creamer, B., Ed., Heinemann, London, 1974, 161.
6. **Sleisenger, M. H. and Brandborg, I. L.,** Crohn's disease (transmural enteritis) in *Malabsorption,* W. B. Saunders, London, 1977, 185.
7. **Allan, R. N., Steinberg, D. M., Dixon, G. K., Cooke, W. T.,** Changes in the bidirectional sodium flux across the intestinal mucosa in Crohn's disease, *Gut,* 16, 201, 1975.
8. **McCaffrey, T., Nasr, K., Lawrence, A. M., and Kirsner, J. B.,** Severe growth retardation in children with inflammatory bowel disease, *Paediatrics,* 45, 386, 1970.
9. **Dudrick, S. J. and Ruberg, R. L.,** Principles and practice of parenteral nutrition, *Gastroenterology,* 61, 901, 1971.
10. **Mullen, J. L., Hargove, W. C., Dudrick, S. J., Fitts, W. T., and Rosato, C. F.,** Ten years experience with intravenous hyperalimentation and inflammatory bowel disease, *Ann. Surg.,* 187, 523, 1978.
11. **Vogel, C. M., Corwin, T. R., and Bane, A. E.,** Intravenous hyperalimentation in the treatment of inflammatory diseases of the bowel, *Arch. Surg.,* 108, 460, 1974.
12. **Driscoll, R. H., Jr. and Rosenberg, R. I.,** Total parenteral nutrition in inflammatory bowel disease, *Med. Clin. North Am.,* 62, 185, 1978.
13. **Russell, R. I.,** Intravenous nutrition and elemental diets in gastrointestinal disease, in *Scientific Foundations of Gastroenterology,* Sircus W. and Smith, A. N., Eds., Heinemann, London, 1980, 130.
14. **Stephens, R. V. and Randall, H. T.,** Use of a concentrated balanced liquid elemental diet for nutritional management of catabolic states, *Ann. Surg.,* 170, 642, 1969.
15. **Bury, K. D., Turnier, E., and Randall, H. T.,** Nutritional management of granulomatous colitis with perianal ulceration, *Can. J. Surg.,* 15, 108, 1972.
16. **Voitk, A. J., Echave, V., Feller, J. H., Rowan, R. A., and Gurd, F. N.,** Experience with elemental diet in the treatment of inflammatory bowel disease, *Arch. Surg.,* 107, 329, 1973.
17. **Rocchio, M. A., Mo Cha, C., Haas, K. F., and Randall, H. T.,** Use of chemically defined diets in the management of patients with high output gastrointestinal cutaneous fistulas, *Am. J. Surg.,* 127, 148, 1974.
18. **Rocchio, M. A., Mo Cha, C., Haas, K. F., and Randall, H. T.,** Use of chemically defined diets in the management of patients with acute inflammatory bowel disease, *Am. J. Surg.,* 127, 469, 1974.
19. **Bounous, G., Devroede, G., Haddad, H., Beaudry, R., Perey, B. J., and Lejeune, L. P.,** Use of an elemental diet for intestinal disorders and for the critically ill, *Dis. Colon Rectum,* 17, 157, 1974.

20. **Earnest, D. and Hammerman, K.,** Nitrogen balance during elemental diet treatment of patients with inflammatory bowel disease and steatorrhoea, *Gastroenterology,* 74, 1121, 1978.
21. **Goode, A., Hawkins, T., Feggetter, J. G. W., and Johnson, I. D. A.,** Use of an elemental diet for long-term nutritional support in Crohn's disease, *Lancet,* 1, 122, 1976.
22. **McCaffrey, T., Nasr, K., Lawrence, A. M., and Kirsner, J. B.,** Severe growth retardation in children with inflammatory bowel disease, *Paediatrics,* 45, 386, 1970.
23. **Layden, T., Rosenberg, J., Nemchausky, B., Elson, C., and Rosenberg, I. H.,** Reversal of growth arrest in adolescents with Crohn's disease after parenteral alimentation, *Gastroenterology,* 70, 1017, 1976.
24. **Younoszai, M. K.,** Growth in a teenage boy with ganulomatous enteritis fed elemental diets *Am. J. Dis. Child.,* 131, 235, 1977.
25. **Jarnum, S.,** Treatment with alimentary diet in gastrointestinal disease, *Infusionstherapie,* 3, 27, 1975.
26. **Berg, G.,** Langfristige Ernahrung mit chemisch definierder Diät, *Infusionstherapie,* 3, 4, 1975.
27. **Base, W., Ferenci, P., Pesendorfer, F. X., Aigner, O., and Wewalka, F.,** Ernahrunspropleme bei Dunn-Und Dickdarmerkrankungen, *Infusionstherapie,* 3, 6, 1976.
28. **Pichler, B.,** Geschmackliche Verbesserung der bilanzierten synthetischen Diat, *Infusionstherapie,* 4, 52, 1977.
29. **Segal, A. W., Levi, A. J., and Loewi, G.,** Levamisole in the treatment of Crohn's disease, *Lancet,* 2, 382, 1977.
30. **Axelsson, C. and Jarnum, S.,** Assessment of the therapeutic value of an elemental diet in chronic inflammatory bowel disease, *Scand. J. Gastroenterol.,* 12, 89, 1977.
31. **Axelsson, C. and Jarnum, S.,** Influence of an elemental diet on protein exudation in chronic inflammatory bowel disease, *Digestion,* 16, 77, 1977.
32. **Logan, R. F. A., Gillan, J., Farrington, C., and Ferguson, A.,** Treatment of small bowel Crohn's disease with an elemental diet (Vivonex), *Gut,* 20, A905, 1979.
33. **Fromm, H., Gebal, M., Schroeter, U., Canzler, H., and Schmidt, F. W.,** Treatment of Crohn's disease in the acute stage. Results of diet therapy, *Dtsch. Med. Wocheschr.,* 103, 377, 1978.
34. **Wolfe, B. M., Keltner, R. M., and Willman, V. L.,** Intestinal fistula output in regular elemental and intravenous alimentation, *Am. J. Surg.,* 124, 803, 1972.
35. **Giorgini, G. L., Stephens, R. V., and Thayer, W. R.,** The use of "medical bypass" in the therapy of Crohn's disease: report of a case, *Digestive Dis.,* 18, 153, 1973.
36. **Russell, R. I. and Hall, M. J.,** Elemental diet therapy in the management of complicated Crohn's disease, *Scott. Med. J.,* 24, 291, 1979.
37. **Hill, G. L., Mair, W. S. J., Edwards, J. P., Morgan, D. B., and Goligher, J. C.,** Effect of a chemically defined liquid elemental diet on the composition and volume of ileal fistula drainage, *Gastroenterology,* 68, 676, 1975.
38. **Fischer, J. E., Foster, G. S., and Abel, R. M.,** Hyperalimentation as primary therapy for inflammatory bowel disease, *Am. J. Surg.,* 125, 165, 1973.
39. **Reilly, J., Ryan, J. A., Strole, W., and Fischer, J. E.,** Hyperalimentation in inflammatory bowel disease, *Am. J. Surg.,* 131, 192, 1976.
40. **Fleming, C. P., McGill, D. B., and Berkner, S.,** Home parenteral nutrition as primary therapy in patients with extensive Crohn's disease of the small bowel and malnutrition, *Gastroenterology,* 73, 1077, 1977.
41. **Strobel, C. T., Byrne, W. J., and Ament, M. E.,** Home parenteral nutrition in children with Crohn's disease: an effective management alternative, *Gasteroenterology,* 77, 272, 1979.
42. **Rosenberg, I. H.,** Nutritional support in inflammatory bowel disease, *Gastroenterology,* 77, 393, 1979.
43. **O'Morain, C.,** Elemental diets in the treatment of Crohn's disease, *Proc. Nutr. Soc.,* 38, 403, 1979.
44. **Wall, A. J. and Kirsner, J. B.,** The management of ulcerative colitis and granulomatous colitis, *Mod. Treat.,* 8, 944, 1971.
45. **Zetzel, L.,** Ulcerative colitis, in *Current Therapy,* Conn, H. F., Ed., W. B. Saunders, London, 1973, 356.
46. **Shoemaker, W. C., Bryan-Browne, C. W., and Elvyn, D. H.,** Therapy of nutritional failure, *Semin. Drug Treat.,* 3, 301, 1973.
47. **Smith, D. W. and Lee, R. M.,** Nutritional management in duodenal fistula, *Surg. Gynecol. Obstet.,* 103, 666, 1956.
48. **Morin, C. L., Roulet, M., Roy, C. C., Weber, A.,** Continuous elemental enteral alimentation in children with Crohn's disease and growth failure, *Gastroenterology,* 79, 1205, 1980.
49. **Kirschner, B. S., Klich, J. R., Kalman, S. S., de Favaro, M. V., Rosenberg, I. H.,** Reversal of growth retardation in Crohn's disease with therapy emphasizing oral nutritional restitution, *Gastroenterology,* 80, 10, 1981.
50. **O'Morain, C., Segal, A. W., and Levi, A. J.,** Elemental diets in treatment of acute Crohn's disease, *Br. Med. J.,* 281, 1173, 1980.

Chapter 14

ELEMENTAL DIETS AND CANCER

J. M. Trotter and K. C. Calman

TABLE OF CONTENTS

I. INTRODUCTION

The nutritional and metabolic consequences of malignant disease are numerous and incompletely understood. Most patients with advanced malignancy have demonstrable abnormalities in carbohydrate, fat, and protein metabolism together with evidence of vitamin and mineral deficiencies. The combination of these metabolic abnormalities contributes to the causation of cancer cachexia. This syndrome accounts for a significant proportion of the deaths from malignant disease and, in contradistinction to uncomplicated starvation, is characterized by a hypercatabolic state in association with anorexia which results in malnutrition, weight loss and, wasting of lean body mass.

The problems of cancer cachexia are frequently compounded by the primary therapeutic modalities employed in the management of cancer: surgery, radiotherapy, and cytotoxic chemotherapy. It can be appreciated, therefore, that the nutritional problems and requirements of the patient with malignant disease can occur more frequently and be more diverse than those associated with nonmalignant illness.

Protein-calorie malnutrition adds significantly to the problem of cancer cachexia as a result of reduced oral food intake. In many patients this is the result of anorexia which can be so intense that patients lose all incentive to eat. Appropriate nutritional support can reverse at least in part the protein-calorie malnutrition of malignant disease but is probably unable to reverse some of the other metabolic abnormalities induced by the underlying neoplasm such as an elevated metabolic rate and insulin resistance. Eradication of the neoplasm therefore remains of prime therapeutic importance. Nutritional support can, however, improve appetite and well-being and this can not only be a major psychological boost but may also improve the quality of life.

Because untreated malignancy is almost invariably progressive, the application of nutritional support has more recently concentrated on its use as an adjunct to cancer therapy. There is no doubt that malnutrition contributes to weakness and debility, delayed wound healing, predisposition to bed sores, impaired immunity, and increased morbidity and mortality. The rationale for nutritional support in cancer has been to reduce these complications of protein-calorie malnutrition and, by so doing, improve the poor therapeutic response of the malnourished patient and reduce the morbidity from treatment.[2]

With this background, the use of elemental diets for nutritional support in malignant disease is considered with particular reference to the indications for their use, the problems encountered and the benefits of therapy. Experimental data and potential future research will be discussed where appropriate.

II. NUTRITION AND CANCER ETIOLOGY

Much has been written about the possible role of nutrients in the causation of cancer. It has been estimated that 80 to 90% of epithelial tumors in man are related to dietary factors.[3] There is, however, no objective evidence to date that dietary modification in man can reduce the incidence of malignant disease although there is substantial data which suggests this could be possible. Dietary modification in the rat can influence established tumor growth (see below) and Castleden[4] has recently suggested that an elemental diet can reduce the incidence of intestinal tumors in dimethylhydrazine-treated rats and that survival is prolonged. For this study male Wistar rats were treated with dimethlhydrazine (DMH) weekly. DMH is known to have high specificity for the production of intestinal tumors in rats. The animals were divided into groups, one group receiving an elemental diet every 12 hours. This group lost weight for the first 10 to 14 days and thereafter the rate of gain in weight was similar to control groups. By Week

23 all rats treated with higher doses of DMH had died of drug toxicity, except for rats treated with an elemental diet, all of which remained alive. Bowel tumor incidence was determined by autopsy, the rats fed an elemental diet being killed at Week 23 for this purpose. The reduction of tumors in the "elemental diet" group was significant at the $P < 0.001$ level. At a lower dose of DMH no rats died of toxicity in any group but bowel tumor incidence in the elemental diet group was again significantly reduced ($p < 0.001$). The rats on elemental diets were, however, eating sawdust from their litters and the author suggested that it was possible this additional dietary fiber content contributed to the altered tumor incidence. It is of interest that Rogers and Newherne[5] found, in the same tumor model, reduced survival and increased incidence of colonic tumors with increased dietary fat and reduced choline and methionine. The tumor inhibitory properties of induced methionine deficiency is mentioned further below.

III. HISTORICAL PERSPECTIVES

The early development of liquid elemental diets in the laboratory animal involved the original work of the effects of such diets on tumors. This early work is discussed elsewhere (see Chapter 6), but mention will be made of the work in relation to tumors. Sugimura et al.[6] compared the nitrogen balance of normal and tumor-bearing albino male rats of the Sprague-Dawley (N.I.H.) strain fed with a "chemically defined diet." Rats were fed the experimental diet for 10 to 14 days before starting the study at which time half the rats were implanted with Walker 256 carcinosarcoma. The diets were force fed four times daily and differences in average weights, carcass weights, and nitrogen balance compared. Tumor-bearing rats gained an average of 41 g in weight compared with controls of 9.5 g. Nearly all the weight gain was tumor since carcass weights were very little different between the groups. In addition, nitrogen balance results suggested there was fluid retention in tumor-bearing animals rather than an increase in lean body mass, and that the tumor was acting as a "nitrogen trap". The nitrogen balance remained positive in tumor bearing rats for the duration of the experiment and it was concluded that the tumor bearing rats may have been using the dietary nitrogen more effectively.

Sugimura et al.[7] also looked at the effect of amino acid modification of chemically defined diets on tumor growth. Using the same tumor model discussed above, slowing of tumor growth was found with a diet deficient in the amino acids leucine, methionine, and valine. Similar results have been obtained by other workers using different tumor models.[8,9] Applications of diets deficient in amino acids to the treatment of human tumors has not been widely investigated primarily because of the low palatability of such diets and their low therapeutic index. Most recent work in amino acid deprivation has been associated with the use of amino acid analogs and enzyme inhibitors such as asparaginase and methioninase. Induction of methionine deficiency has potential therapeutic potential because of the known inhibitory effect of a deficiency of the amino acid in a number of experimental tumor models.[10]

IV. SPECIAL PROBLEMS IN ADMINISTRATION OF ELEMENTAL DIETS AND MONITORING OF NUTRITIONAL STATUS IN CANCER PATIENTS

One of the biggest problems facing the cancer nutritionist is not so much what type and amount of nutritional supplement to give but how to get the anorectic cancer patient to swallow any at all. The anorexia of malignant disease and its causes have been extensively reviewed.[11] (Table 1). Anorexia can even be the cause of malnutrition in patients with a small tumor volume. To compound the problem, cancer patients often

Table 1
CAUSES OF ANOREXIA IN MALIGNANT DISEASE

A. Caused by the malignancy
- 1. Metabolic
  - Malignant cachexia
  - Taste abnormalities
  - "Anorectic peptides" } Postulated
  - Amino acid abnormalities } Postulated
  - Hormone abnormalities } Postulated
- 2. Mechanical
  - Gastric stasis, delayed gastric emptying
  - Bowel obstruction

B. Caused by therapy
- 1. Antineoplastic chemotherapy
- 2. Radiation therapy
- 3. Surgery — head and neck; thoracic; abdominal
- 4. Other drugs — antibiotics; analgesics; tranquillizers; allopurinol

C. Psychogenic — anxiety; depression; pain

have abnormalities of taste which further reduces their appreciation of food. In particular, low taste thresholds to urea are not infrequent and are thought to be a cause of the aversion to meat which is a common feature of malignant disease.[12] These factors mean that palatability of food is a crucial factor in the ability of the cancer patient to consume an adequate diet. In this respect, elemental diets rate poorly because of their low fat content and free amino acids. Oral supplementary feeding of the cancer patient with elemental diets is possible in some patients but in most there is low acceptance of these products. This has certainly been our experience and others have reported a similar problem.[13] In the latter report, patients were randomized to receive either a normal diet or a normal diet plus elemental diet supplements while receiving abdominal irradiation. The object of the study was to determine whether radiation damage to the gut could be reduced by dietary supplementation with an elemental diet. The "limiting factor", however, was "poor patient compliance" due to the poor palatability of the elmental diet. Attempts to improve the acceptance by patients of the product by using various flavors, ice slush, or even alcoholic beverages were not successful. The low palatability of elemental diets has also been documented by De Wys and Herbst[14] who found that an elemental supplement when compared in a panel of predominantly milk-based whole protein oral products was given low preference scores by both cancer patients and normal controls. In another panel of products, this time predominantly defined formula diets (elemental and hydrolyzed) the only one to obtain a positive mean preference score was a nonsynthetic milk-based supplement.

Although it is sometimes possible to persuade out-patients at an oncology clinic to persevere with these oral supplements, nearly all patients admitted to hospital for nutritional support with cancer cachexia will require tube feeding to ensure that sufficient calories and protein are provided. Nasogastric tubes are generally satisfactory for the purpose and with the use of the recently introduced fine-bore tubes, well-tolerated. Easy satiety, abdominal fullness, gastric retention, and persistant nausea and vomiting can usually be overcome by lowering infusion rates and reducing the concentrations of supplement for a day or two (Table 2). If these problems persist, naso-duodenal or naso-jejunal feeding may be necessary. Energetic nutritional supplementation in the cancer patient will usually achieve a positive nitrogen balance and associated weight gain.[15] There is usually a delay of about a week before significant increments in weight gain are seen. However, most patients who achieve adequate protein and calorie ingestion not only feel better, but have an improved appetite. The reasons for the improvement in appetite are unknown.

The enteral route for nutritional support is to be preferred where possible and even subacute bowel obstruction, malabsorption, esophageal strictures, and fistulas can often be managed by enteral feeding.

The methods of assessing and monitoring nutritional status are discussed in detail in Chapter 4. Sufficient numbers of these tests should be employed in the nutritionally supplemented cancer patient to ensure that adequate essential nutrients are being provided. The hypercatabolism that frequently attends malignant disease means that high energy and protein diets are usually necessary to maintain anabolism. Basic requirements for tube feeding are 130 to 150 KJ (30 to 35 kcal) of energy per kg body weight per day. The nitrogen:calorie ratio should be between 150:1 and 200:1. Careful attention to vitamins and minerals is necessary because patients with malignant disease frequently have evidence of multiple vitamin and mineral deficiencies.[16] It may be necessary to supply additional supplements of vitamins and minerals to cancer patients on tube feeding, particularly if nutritional screening reveals deficits and no normal food is being taken orally. Zinc for example is important in maintaining normal taste, probably has an important role in appetite control, and is essential for normal tissue healing. Urinary excretion of zinc, however, may be as high as three times normal values in some malignancies.[17] Care should be exercised when using diets with fixed formulation which may be hazardous in certain situations. They may for example, provide excessive sodium, potassium, and protein loads in patients with hepatic and renal disease or compound hypercalcemia by providing additional dietary calcium. In addition, many cancer patients demonstrate abnormal glucose tolerance when subjected to glucose loading[18] and this can be accentuated by the use of corticosteroids which are used as part of treatment in some combination chemotherapy protocols, for the management of raised intracranial pressure, nerve root compression, and hypercalcemia. It may be beneficial, or occasionally necessary to add insulin to the nutritional regime, the dose being titrated to the individual patient. This approach to treatment is not altogether without potential theroretical value in malignant disease and it has recently been suggested to be of possible practical application.[19] There is a need for this use of insulin to be carefully studied to determine its role as a potent anabolic agent in stimulating protein synthesis.

V. THERAPEUTIC USES OF ELEMENTAL DIETS IN THE CANCER PATIENT

Nutritional support in the cachectic cancer patient with protein-calorie malnutrition is a valuable adjunct to therapy. Wherever possible nutritional support should be by the enteral route. The problems of palatability of elemental diets often makes tube feeding necessary. It should be clearly stated, however, that elemental diets are not necessarily better in providing nutritional support than are the large number of whole protein liquid diets available for oral and tube feeding. Many of these whole protein preparations are more palatable than elemental diets because of the type of nitrogen source and their

Table 2
SUGGESTED REGIMES FOR THE INTRODUCTION OF DEFINED FORMULA DIETS IN CANCER PATIENTS

	Vivonex standard		Flexical	
	Dry weight (g)	Reconstituted volume (mℓ)	Dry weight (g)	Reconstituted volume (mℓ)
Day 1	160	1200	125	1000
Day 2	240	1800	125	1000
Day 3	320	1800	250	2000
Day 4	400	1800	350	2000
Day 5 (maximum concentration)	480	1800	450	2000

higher fat content. There is divergent opinion at present as to whether elemental diets are absorbed better from the small intestine than partially hydrolyzed protein and whether these in turn are better absorbed than whole protein diets. When the gut is intact and digestive secretions are normal, whole protein feeds are as effective as elemental diets, are cheaper and, in our experience, better tolerated. Silk[20] and others have suggested that dipeptides and tripeptides are better absorbed than free amino acids. However, in situations where "luminal hydrolysis is likely to limit absorption", Silk suggests than an "oligopeptide nitrogen source . . . might be indiciated". Even the occurrence of an intestinal fistula of malignant origin is not necessarily an indication for a low residue diet. Celestin[21] considers that malnutrition is the main reason for persistance of fistulas and that there is no evidence that "lack of residue or complete absorption" are necessary for fistulas to heal. The use of elemental diets may therefore, particularly in respect to malignant disease, be used less in the future for general nutritional support and more for specific indications such as severe exocrine pancreatic insufficiency, the "short bowel" syndrome, and for surgical bowel preparation.

Bearing these points in mind, elemental diets have been used extensively for nutritional support in malignant disease with good effect.[22-27] (Table 3). Elemental diets have been shown to be useful in healing intestinal fistulas[28-30] Prior to the use of adequate nutritional support patients with gastrointestinal (GI) fistulas had a poor prognosis, malnutrition being the greatest cause of death. Starved patients with fistulas have a mortality of about 60%.[31] In patients with malignant disease, the gravity of the situation is no better. In fact, although a significant proportion of malignant fistulas heal with appropriate nutritional support, in the absence of control of tumor growth, about one third of such patients die despite energetic nutritional support.[31]

Fine bore tube feeding can be continued for long periods and is therefore valuable for the patient with a high grade esophageal stricture in whom surgical techniques have failed or are not contemplated. This form of feeding can be readily continued on an outpatient basis once a regime has been established. As with all forms of nutritional support, monitoring the nutritional status is necessary (Chapter 4) so that supplementary calories, minerals, or vitamins can be provided as necessary.

A. Surgery, Cancer, and Elemental Diets

The use of elemental diets in surgery is discussed in Chapter 11, and the principles discussed therein are relevant to the patient with malignant disease. The more advanced the cancer, the more likely is nutritional depletion, and the more reason for perioperative nutritional support. The use of elemental diets to reverse catabolism prior to surgery in

Table 3
USES OF ELEMENTAL DIETS IN CANCER PATIENTS

Related to the Cancer	Protein-calorie malnutrition
	Cancer cachexia
	Anorexia
	Difficulty with mastication and swallowing
	Fistulas/Sinuses
	Bowel obstruction (sub acute)
	Malabsorption
	Esophageal strictures
	Protein losing enteropathy
	Exocrine pancreatic insufficiency
	Bed sores
Surgery	Short bowel syndrome
	Blind loops
	Preoperative
	Bowel preparation
	Fistulas
	Postoperative anorexia
Radiotherapy	Anorexia/Taste abnormalities
	Nausea/Vomiting
	Mucositis, oral ulceration
	Esophagitis
	Radiation enteritis — acute and chronic
Chemotherapy	Anorexia/taste abnormalities
	Nausea/vomiting
	Weight loss
	Malabsorption
	Protection of toxicity — gut
	— hematological

11 malnourished patients has been reported, three of whom had esophageal strictures secondary to esophapeal carcinoma.[32] Mitty et al.[33] discuss the use of elemental diets in surgery and propose in part the following indications for their use: hypoalbuminemia, preoperative preparation, postoperative anorexia, severe sepsis, enterostomy feeding, esophageal carcinoma, abdominal carcinomatosis, GI fistula, and radiation enteritis. All these problems are potential complications of malignant disease.

Two cases of paracolostomy abscess as a result of traumatic perforation of a colostomy have been reported to heal without the intervention of surgery by a combination of elemental diet and intravenous hyperalimentation. Both patients had had colostomies performed for malignant disease.[34]

B. Radiotherapy and Elemental Diets

The nutritional consequences of radiation therapy have been recently reviewed.[13] Radiation therapy to the brain can cause nausea and vomiting. Oral mucositis, xerostomia, pharyngitis, anorexia, and dental caries and abscesses are complications of radiation to the head and neck. Taste abnormalities induced by radiotherapy may persist for up to four months. Esophagitis can be severe following thoracic irradiation and esophageal stenosis and perforation are late sequelae. Radiation to the large and small bowel is often accompanied by nausea, vomiting, and diarrhea, and frequently accompanied by malabsorption of carbohydrates, fats, and proteins. These problems are the features of acute radiation enteritis which can progress to a chronic form. Acute radiation enteritis is associated with a reduction in intraluminal enzymes such as disaccaridase. In addition, protein losing enteropathy is well recorded.[35] Chronic enteritis is associated with fibrosis and episodic bowel obstruction, mucosal ulceration and perforation. Diarrhea and blood loss add to the malnutrition. The problems of enteritis increase as radiation dose is escalated. Whole abdominal pelvic irradiation can produce significant weight loss. Fifty-nine of 67 patients (88%) being treated with whole abdominal irradiation for non-Hodgkin's lymphoma lost an average of 3.5 Kg in weight over the 6 weeks of treatment.[13]

Elemental diets have been used to provide nutritional support during radiotherapy and have been suggested to protect against radiation-induced enteropathy.[36] Weight and serum protein levels were maintained in patients on this diet and controls had a higher incidence of diarrhea. Long term enteral nutrition with an elemental diet taken by mouth has been described in a patient with chronic radiation enteritis.[37] For a period of six months this patient, with an adenocarcinoma of the ovary, was maintained in good nutrition and fecal analysis after five months of enteral nutrition revealed no evidence of fat or nitrogen malabsorption. A randomized trial was commenced at Stanford University Medical Center in an attempt to determine the extent, if any, of protection against radiation-induced enteritis by a defined formula diet in patients having radiotherapy to a "uniform portion of the small bowel."[13] Patients were randomized to receive either an elemental (defined formula) diet as dietary supplement three times per day or no such supplement. At 6 months there was no difference between the groups in any of the study parameters (which included small bowel X-rays and small bowel biopsies and various laboratory indices) but the numbers studied at the time of the report were small. It is possible that insufficient elemental diet was ingested by these patients because of unpalatability to determine whether a protective role on the gut does, or does not exist. In the experimental animal, it has been reported that intestinal lesions produced by radiation in the mouse can be reduced by an elemental diet taken orally.[38] It was postulated that the beneficial effects may have been due to reduced pancreatic secretion (see Chapter 8).

All these observations need to be continued and extended to look at the value of dietary support for other nutritional sequelae of radiation therapy.

C. Elemental Diets and Antineoplastic Chemotherapy

Cytotoxic treatment of cancer produces a spectrum of nutritional disorders which range from minor and inconsequential to life-threatening and even fatal. Nearly all cytotoxic drugs produce a degree of nausea, vomiting, and anorexia. Taste abnormalities caused by cytotoxics are common. Mucositis, pharyngitis, esophagitis, diarrhea, constipation, malabsorption, and hepatic toxicity also occur, the incidence dependent upon the drug being used. Some of these drugs are also prone to increasing or exacerbating a latent radiation esophagitis or skin reaction. Reactivation of a latent radiation reaction is known as a "recall phenomenon". Many of the currently used combination chemotherapy protocols, where three, four, or sometines more drugs are used together, result in increased host toxicity with frequent nutritional problems. Weight loss of 4 Kg or more per course of chemotherapy is common in the absence of nutritional suoport. These nutritional deficits can be corrected in most instances with energetic enteral hyperalimentation without the need for parenteral nutrition.[39,40]

Most of the work with elemental diets and chemotherapy has been concerned with the gut-induced toxicity of the antineoplastic drug, 5-fluorouracil. This drug commonly causes a degree of GI toxicity at therapeutic doses, manifested by nausea, vomiting, and diarrhea. The intestinal lesion involves the epithelial cells which become vacuolated, flattened and necrotic. 5-FU also reduces ileal dipeptidase activity thereby interferring with the normal terminal (final) digestion and absorption of proteins. Free amimo acids do not require any digestion prior to absorption and therefore may be more readily absorbed than whole protein and oligopeptide diets in the situation where dipeptidase concentration is reduced. A 40% reduction in the absorption rates of glucose and water and dipeptide activity at 3 and 5 days after 5-FU administration has been reported in rats.[41] Bounous, et al.[42] pioneered work on this subject and reported protection from the toxic effects of 5-FU with the use of an elemental diet. In a later study[43] rats fed a diet containing casein hydrolysate (10% wt/wt) when compared with those on a whole casein diet were found to have increased tolerance to the toxic effects of 5-FU as measured by changes in serum albumin and weight. Concentration of two brush border enzymes were significantly lower in the 5-FU treated rats than in the control rats. Unfortunately, brush border enzymes were not determined for the rats fed the elemental diet. It was postulated that diets with free amino acid content could be better absorbed in these circumstances than mixtures of oligopeptides. Miller et al.[44] reported weight gain of 20 g in rats given a single intraperitoneal dose of 5-FU plus an elemental diet compared with 40 g weight loss in control rats given a normal diet and the same dose of 5-FU. There were fewer deaths in the elemental diet groups. These results support the view that elemental diets have a protective effect against 5-FU induced gut toxicity. Stanford et al.[45] reported the opposite. In this short paper five groups of rats were given different diets. The control group received a standard diet and the other groups received one of four defined formula diets. In each group 20 animals received diet alone and 50 animals received the same diet plus 5-FU subcutaneously for 6 days. The toxicity of 5-FU as measured by mortality, number of positive blood cultures, fall in serum albumin, and colonic goblet cell counts was proportional to the degree of protein hydrolysis in the diet and therefore highest for those diets with total hydrolysis. In the latter groups blood cultures were almost 100% positive.

Gardner and Heading[46] examined the effects of elemental diets on enzymatic and absorptive activities in rat small intestine and the effects of these diets on 5-FU toxicity. It was found that changes in intestinal peptide hydrolases depended on the nitrogen source. Levels of cytoplasmic dipeptidases in gut epithelial cells were the same at 10 days with both elemental diet treated rats and those rats on normal diet. It was concluded that the effects on the enzymes were probably due to overall composition of diet rather than the degree of protein hydrolysis.

Clearly, therefore, the situation in the experimental animal is far from resolved. More careful controlled experiments are needed comparing hydrolysates with free amino acids, and using comparable drug doses, schedules and routes of administration. The establishment of a standard reference diet in the experimental animal is needed to improve reproducibility between laboratories and for this purpose one of the readily available commercial defined formula diets has been suggested.[46]

Beneficial effects of elemental diets in protecting the human gut from the toxic effects of 5-FU have been reported.[47] Twenty-four patients were investigated, all with advanced metastatic carcinoma, and were given either normal hospital food or a protein hydrolysate diet. All patients received 12 mg/kg body weight of 5-FU for six to nine consecutive days by intravenous infusion. Patients on the "elemental" diet lost no weight although in the control group there was a statistically significant weight loss. Rectal biopsies demonstrated fewer rectal lesions in the patients on the "elemental" diet than in those patients eating a normal diet. Elemental diets may reduce pancreatic secretions but normal diets increase these secretions (see Chapter 8) and this is one postulated mechanism to explain how elemental diets might reduce 5-FU toxicity. In man, elemental diets need to be compared with other nutritional supplements to determine whether adequate provision from any food source can provide the same protection. The results of further studies are awaited with interest. In addition, the role of nutritional support including elemental diets, has yet to be investigated with respect to cytotoxic drugs other than 5-FU which cause GI toxicity. Methotrexate, for example, also causes epithelial damage in the rat intestine.[48]

D. Pediatric Oncology

The role of elemental diets in pediatric oncology has been largely unexplored. A recent review of nutrition in children with cancer scarcely mentions enteral nutrition as a method of nutritional support.[49] The same article does, however, suggest that the incidence of malnutrition in children with cancer is high and of the order of 37.5%.

Children with partial to complete small bowel obstruction may be therapeutically benefited by a gluten-free, milk free, low fat, low residue diet.[50] In this study, children with small bowel fibrosis following radiotherapy plus chemotherapy all responded to dietary therapy as the only form of treatment. At the same center subsequent use of such a diet in children undergoing abdominal radiotherapy has resulted in "no cases of severe, acute, or delayed enteritis."

Therapeutic success in childhood neoplastic diseases has improved dramatically in recent years. As in adult oncological practice, there is reason to believe that adequate nutritional support will reduce morbidity and may improve response rates and survival. Clearly, there is considerable scope for exploring aspects of nutritional support in children, and in particular, the role of supplementary nutrition during chemotherapy.

VI. CONCLUSIONS

The value of enteral nutritional support in patients with malignant disease has been presented with particular emphasis on its use as a valuable adjunct to the major treatment modalities of surgery, radiotherapy, and chemotherapy. The benefit of nutritional supplementation for all degrees of nutritional depletion has been emphasized. The role of elemental diets and defined formula diets in these situations has been presented together with experimental data where appropriate. While few nutritionists would doubt the potential value of nutritional supplementation, most would have to agree that there is as yet little data on the relative merits of different oral diets (e.g., whole protein vs. defined formula) for different situations. There is clearly a large potential for further clinical trials and research in this area.

REFERENCES

1. **Calman, K. C.,** Nutritional support in malignant disease, *Proc. Nutr. Soc.*, 37, 87, 1978.
2. **Copeland, E. M., III,** Intravenous hyperalimentation as an adjunct to cancer patient management, *Ca.*, 28, (6), 322, 1978.
3. **Doll, R.,** Strategy for detection of cancer hazards in man, *Nature*, 265, 589, 1977.
4. **Castleden, W. M.,** Prolonged survival and decrease in intestinal tumours in dimethelhydrazine-treated rats fed a chemically defined diet, *Br. J. Cancer*, 35, 491 1977.
5. **Rogers, A. E. and Newberne, P. M.,** Dietary enhancement of intestinal carcinogenesis by DMH in rats, *Nature (London)*, 246, 49, 1973.
6. **Sugimura, F., Birnbaum, S. M., Winitz, M., and Greenstein, J. P.,** Quantitative nutritional studies with soluble chemically defined diets. VII. Nitrogen balance in normal and tumour bearing rats following forced feeding, *Arch. Biochem. Biophys.*, 81, 439 1959.
7. **Sugimura, F., Birnbaum, S. M., Winitz, M., and Greenstein, J. P.,** Quantitative nutritional studies with water-soluble chemically defined diets each lacking in one essential amino acid, *Arch. Biochem. Biophys.*, 81, 448, 1959.
8. **Theurer, R. C.,** Effect of essential amino acid restriction on the growth of female C57 BL mice and their implanted BW10232 adenocarcinomas, *J. Nutr.*, 101, 223, 1971.
9. **Skipper, H. E. and Thomson, J. R.,** A preliminary study of the influence of amino acid deficiencies on experimental cancer chemotherapy, in *Amino Acids and Peptides with Antimetabolite Activity*, Wolstenholme, G. E. W. and O'Connor, C. M., Eds., CIBA Foundation Symp., Churchill, London, 1958, 33.

10. **Tisdale, M. J.,** Methionine dependence of tumour cells, *Br. J. Cancer,* 40, 303, 1979.
11. **De Wys, W.,** Anorexia in cancer patients, *Cancer Res.,* 37, 2354, 1977.
12. **De Wys, W.,** Abnormalities of taste sensations in cancer patients, *Cancer,* 36, 1888, 1975.
13. **Donaldson, S. S. and Lenon, R. A.,** Alterations of nutritional status: impact of chemotherapy and radiation therapy, *Cancer,* 43, 2036, 1979.
14. **De Wys, W. D. and Herbst, S. H.,** Oral feeding in the nutritional management of the cancer patient, *Cancer Res.,* 37, 2429, 1977.
15. **Copeland, E. M., Daly, J. M., Ota, D. M., and Dudrick, S. J.,** Nutrition, cancer and intravenous hyperalimentation, *Cancer,* 43, 2108, 1979.
16. **Soukop, M., and Calman, K. C.,** Nutritional support in patients with malignant disease, *J. Human Nutr.,* 33, 197, 1979.
17. **Schwartz, M. K.,** Role of trace elements in cancer, *Cancer Res.,* 35, 3481, 1975.
18. **Holroyde, C. P., Gabuzda, T. G., Putnam, R. C., Paul, P., and Reichard, G. A.,** Altered glucose metabolism in metastatic carcinoma, *Cancer Res.,* 35, 3710, 1975.
19. **Schein, P. S., Kisner, D., Haller, D., Blecher, M., and Hamosh, M.,** Cachexia of malignancy: potential role of insulin in nutritional management, *Cancer,* 43, 2070, 1979.
20. **Silk, D. B. A.,** Physiology of protein absorption, *Res. Clin. Forums,* 1, 29, 1979.
21. **Celestin, L. R.,** Residue — sense and nonsense, *Res. Clin. Forums,* 1, 91, 1979.
22. **Kaminski, M. V., Jr.,** Enteral hyperalimentation, *Surgery Gynecol. Obstet.,* 143, 12 1976.
23. **Valassi, K.,** Nutritional management of cancer patients in a variety of therapeutic regimens, *Arch. Phys. Med. Rehabil.,* 58, 393, 1977.
24. **Calman, K. C.,** Elemental diets in cancer management, in *The Role of Elemental Nutrition, Proc. Symp., Selby Fork Hotel, 1975,* Johnston, I. D. A., Ed., Medical Congresses and Symposia Consultants, England, for Eaton Laboratories, 1976, 30.
25. **Bounous, G., Devroede, G., Haddad, H., Beaudry, R., Perey, B. J., and Le Jeune, L. P.,** Use of an elemental diet for intestinal disorders and for the critically ill, *Dis. Colon Rectum,* 17, 157, 1974.
26. **Hoover, C. J., Maini, H. S., Bistrian, B. R., Schlamm, H. T., Wade, J. F., and Blackburn, G. L.,** Use of a defined formula diet to prevent malnutrition in advanced cancer patients. Abstracts of papers presented 1st Ann. Congress Am. Soc. Parenteral and Enteral Nutrition, Chicago, 1977, *J. Parenteral Enteral Nutr.,* 1, 14A, 1977.
27. **Valdivieso, M.,** Commentary: A defined formula diet as exclusive source of nutrition in patients with cancer, in *Conference on Defined Formula Diets for Medical Purposes, 1975,* Shils, M. E., Ed., American Medical Association, Chicago, 1977, 80.
28. **Bury, K. D., Stephens, R. V., and Randall, H. T.,** Use of a chemically defined, liquid elemental diet for nutritional management of fistulas of the alimentary tract, *Am. J. Surg.,* 121, 1974, 1971.
29. **Voitk, A. J., Echave, V., Brown, R. A., McArdle, A. H., and Gurd, F. N.,** Elemental diet in the treatment of fistulas of the alimentary tract, *Surg. Gynecol. Obstet.,* 137, 68, 1973.
30. **Grundy, D. J.,** Small bowel fistula treated with low-residue diet, *Br. Med. J.,* 2, 531, 1971.
31. **Rocchio, M. A., Cha., C. J. M., Haas, K. F., and Randall, H. T.,** Use of chemically defined diets in the management of patients with high output gastrointestinal cutaneous fistulas, *Am. J. Surg.,* 127, 148, 1974.
32. **Nealon, T. F., Jr.,** Enteral hyperalimentation, *Surg. Gynecol. Obstet.,* 143, 12, 1976.
33. **Mitty, W. F., Jr., Nealon, T. F., Jr., and Grossi, C.,** Use of elemental diets in surgical cases, *Am. J. Gastroenterol.,* 65, 297, 1976.
34. **Reynolds, H. M., Jr., Frazier, T. G., and Copeland, E. M.,** Treatment of para-colostomy abscesses without proximal diverting colostomy: report of two cases, *Dis. Colon Rectum,* 19, 458, 1976.
35. **Vatistas, S. and Hornsey, S.,** Radiation induced protein loss into the gastrointestinal tract, *Br. J. Radiol.,* 39, 547, 1966.
36. **Bounous, G., La Bel, E., Shuster, J., Gold, P., Tahan, W. T., and Bastin, E.,** Dietary protection during radiation therapy, *Strahlentherapie,* 149, 476, 1975.
37. **Haddad, H., Bounous, G., Tahan, W. T., Devroede, G., Beaudry, R., and Lafond, R.,** Long term nutrition with an elemental diet following intensive abdominal irradiation: report of a Case, *Dis. Colon Rectum,* 17, 373, 1974.
38. **Hugon, J. S. and Bounous, G.,** Elemental diet in the management of the intestinal lesions produced by radiation in the mouse, *Can. J. Surg.,* 15, 18, 1972.
39. **Ching, N., Mills, C., Grossi, C., Hughes, J., Zurawinsky, H., Jham, G., and Nealon, T. F.,** The maintenance of optimal nutritional status in chemotherapy treatment, *Proc. Am. Soc. Clin. Oncol.,* 19, 319, 1978.
40. **Nixon, D. W., Bethel, R. A., and Heymsfield, S. B.,** Nasogastric hyperalimentation through a polyethylene catheter:an alternative to central venous hyperalimentation in cancer patients, *Proc. Am. Soc. Clin. Oncol.,* 19, 209, 1978.
41. **Gardner, M. L. G., Samson, R. R., and Heading, R. C.,** Changes in absorption and enzymatic activities and on 5-fluorouracil toxicity in rat small intestine, *Clin. Sci. Mol. Med.,* 54, 411, 1978.

42. **Bounous, G., Hugon, J. S., and Gentile, J. M.,** Elemental diet in the management of the intestinal lesion produced by 5-F.U. in the rat, *Can. J. Surg.,* 14, 298, 1971.
43. **Bounous, G. and Maestracci, D.,** Use of an elemental diet in animals during treatment with 5-F.U., *Cancer Treat. Rep.,* 60, 17, 1976.
44. **Miller, J. M., Valbuena, R. M., and Remigo, M. R.,** Protection by an elemental diet against the toxic intestinal changes of 5-fluorouracil in rats, *Abdom. Surg.,* 19, 25, 1977.
45. **Stanford, J. R., Carey, L. C., King, D. R., and Anderson, G. W.,** Adverse effects of elemental diets on tolerance for fluorouracil (5-F.U.) toxicity in rats, *Surg. Forum,* 27, 42, 1976.
46. **Gardner, M. L. G. and Heading, R. C.,** Effects of "elemental" diets on absorption and enzymatic activities and on 5-fluorouracil toxicity in rat small intestine, *Clin. Sci. Mol. Med.,* 56, 243, 1979.
47. **Bounous, G., Gentile, J. M., and Hugon, J.,** Elemental diet in the management of the intestinal lesion produced by 5-fluorouracil in man, *Can. J. Surg.,* 14, 312, 1971.
48. **Robinson, J. W. L., Antonioli, J. A., and Vannotti, A.,** The effect of methotrexate on the rat intestine, *Gastroenterologie,* 105, 129, 1966.
49. **Van Eys, J.,** Malnutrition in children with cancer: incidence and consequence, *Cancer,* 43, 2030, 1979.
50. **Donaldson, S. S., Jund, T. S., Ricour, C., Sarrazin, D., Lemerle, J., and Schweisguth, O.,** Radiation enteritis in children: a retrospective review, clinicopathologic correlation and dietary management, *Cancer,* 35, 1168, 1975.

Chapter 15

ELEMENTAL DIETS AS NUTRITION IN BURNED PATIENTS

Joseph A. Moylan

TABLE OF CONTENTS

I. INTRODUCTION

One of the major factors following initial stabilization of a significant thermal injury is nutritional support of the burn patient. Attention to this important aspect of burn care has not only improved survival but has minimized the morbidity associated with this postinjury problem. There are two components of the postburn nutritional dilemma, one related to increased nutritional requirements and the other impaired intake secondary to chronicity of the healing process and long-term pain. Increased evaporative water loss, greater radiated heat losses and increased metabolic rate make a daily dietary demands frequently three to five times greater than normal. This acute and chronically ill patient has great difficulty in ingesting sufficient quantities of food to meet these needs. If the metabolic demands are not met by an adequate level of intake, body stores must be used, especially a preferential use of protein primarily from skeletal muscle.[1] The consequence of a caloric deficit is a decrease in muscle tissue mass that is reflected by a weight loss at 1 kg/3500 to 4500 calories that are expended. Weight change is the most consistent and reliable clinical indicator of long-term caloric balance.

Both the extent and duration of the exaggerated metabolic demands are determined by the severity of the injury reflected as burn size. These profound requirements extend even into the period following complete healing of the burn wound itself (Figure 1). The initial increase in body weight which is a consequence of fluid resuscitation is followed by a sustained period of weight loss which may at times exceed 1% of the preburn weight per day.[2] The use of special dietary programs is the only effective way to prevent this significant and disastrous weight loss. In fact, if weight loss is permitted to continue indefinitely it may be itself lethal depending upon the patient's preinjury state of nutrition. Other significant consequences of inadequate nutrition include unhealthy granulation tissue, poor skin graft take, delayed epithelization of partial thickness burns. In the absence of greatly enhanced caloric intake, the derangement of cellular metabolism especially the alteration of intracellular electrolytes has been observed.[3] There is both increase systemic and pulmonary sepsis which is due in part to impaired cellular and humoral immune mechanisms. The economic impact of prolonged convalescence, exacerbated by inadequate nutrition is also a very important consequence which can be reversed by attention to nutritional support.

II. INDIVIDUAL REQUIREMENTS

A. Water

Besides specific nutritional requirements during the early phase of his postburn period, the thermal injury patient has an increased need for water primarily because of exaggerated evaporative water losses. These can be estimated at between 0.5 and 1.5 mℓ per percent burn per kilogram body weight per day. In the initial few days following the injury, this requirement may be partially met by mobilization of the greatly expanded extracellular fluid volume which resulted from the shock resuscitation. However, following return of the body weight to its preburn state, this evaporative water loss must be met totally by exogenous replacement. Monitoring the daily urine output and routine serum chemistries, especially sodium and blood urea nitrogen, can be used to assess the state of hydration. Ordinarily, these needs are not difficult to meet and affords the physician an opportunity to administer the large volumes of fluids necessary for adequate caloric replacement, even in patients with marginal cardiopulmonary reserve.

B. Calories

Caloric requirements following burn injuries are profoundly increased. This large caloric need is a function of both body weight and severity of injury (Figure 2). It has

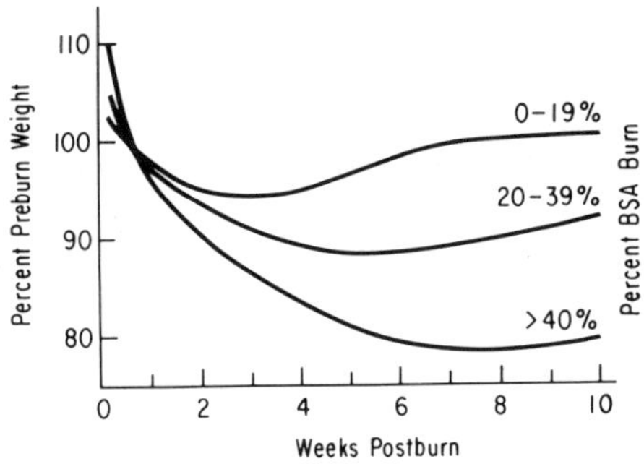

FIGURE 1. Expected weight loss of burn patients in absence of special nutritional program.

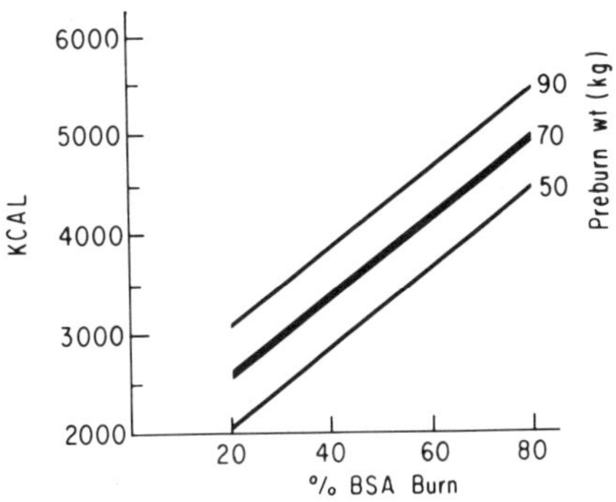

FIGURE 2. Daily calorie requirement for major burn victims.

been shown that severe burn injuries in adult patients may require as much as 6000 to 8000 cal/day.[4] This increased demand may last many weeks until the wound is completely epithelized or skin grafting performed. Additional complications such as the effects of emotional stress, infection, or multiple operations may significantly increase the caloric requirement above daily levels imposed by the burn injury itself. Since during the initial phase of the resuscitation and immediately before and after operative procedures, the patient usually receives no caloric replacement, the physician should actually provide considerably higher than estimated daily needs to offset these losses. While optimally approximately 20% of the the daily calories should come from fats, diets which are extremely high in carbohydrate calories have been effective in reversing this negative caloric balance.

C. Protein

Increased protein needs following thermal injury are a result of the hypermetabolic state as well as the healing requirements. In addition, nitrogen loss may have resulted from the direct tissue injury itself and from the significant wounds exudate. The patients with moderate size burn injuries up to 30% of the body surface can lose 25 g of protein a day from the wound exudate. The patients with larger burn injuries may lose up to 60 g of protein per day until the wound is completely healed. Protein requirements of 200 to 300 g a day are not uncommon in major burns in adult patients.

For proper utilization of administered protein, a proper calorie and nitrogen ratio is necessary. Approximately 150 total calories are required per gram of dietary nitrogen for adequate protein metabolism. Protein ingested in excess of this ratio will be used as an energy source rather than for protein synthesis. The corollary to this statement is that protein intake needed to obtain positive nitrogen balance is influenced by the total caloric consumption. Increased protein requirements are highest during the initial month following a major burn injury and then decrease slowly. The severely burned patients with 250 g of protein requirement during the initial severe catabolic phase would characteristically achieve positive nitrogen balance with 100 to 150 g after approximately 30 days and this will gradually reduce to 75 to 100 g/day in the convalescence phase presuming that there were no other significant complications such as sepsis and that wound coverage is achieved.[5] (Figure 3).

III. TOTAL ENTERAL SUPPORT

Total enteral support of severely burned patients has been demonstrated to be possible without the use of intravenous hyperalimentation. Important details in managing these patients include accurately defining the daily caloric and nitrogen requirements for each patient to assure adequate replacement to meet the increased metabolic demands. Soroff et al.[6] calculated nitrogen requirements of 20 to 25 $g/m^2/day$ which is approximately 3 g protein per kg per day. Curreri[4] recently derived an empirical formula which is valuable in estimating the caloric needs based on both body size and magnitude of burn injury. Caloric needs = [25 × preburn weight] + [40 × % TBS Burn]. Daily calorie counts, frequent measurements of body weights to assess the effectiveness of the replacement program and cooperation between the nursing and dietary personnel are required to assure that the patient achieves his caloric quota each day. While intravenous hyperalimentation offers an alternate method to achieve caloric intake in seriously burned patients, there is especially high infection risk in this group secondary to sepsis from intravenous catheters. Many studies have shown significant sepsis complication rates using hyperalimentation with high mortality in spite of supernormal caloric replacement.[7] In addition, serious metabolic complications may develop in the severely critical patients with this type of alimentary support.

The standard hospital diet is often not effective in nutritional replacement because of a decreased appetite secondary to pain, depression, and multiple surgical procedures. Elemental diet affords the burn care team an effective means either for supplement to the standard hospital diet or total support. Commercially available elemental diets containing a calorie per cc are usually high in carbohydrate and protein and low in fat. Because of the high evaporative water losses and fluid volume that are necessary to replace this, great quantiites of calories and protein in a calorie per cc solution can be administered without compromising cardiopulmonary reserve. It is not unusual to administer 7 to 8 liters of fluid per day. The goal of the program is to keep weight loss at less than 10% of the preinjury weight. Body mass loss greater than 10% are associated with significant morbidity and mortality.

Nutritional monitoring is an important aspect of the patient's care to ensure optimal recovery. Even with the most appetizing menus, the patient with a significant thermal injury may not take full adequate amounts of protein and calorie from the hospital tray. When an adequate intake cannot be achieved and a deficit of more than 200 calories is noted on two consecutive days, enteral feeding via feeding tube should be used.[8] Another part of the monitoring program should include serum electrolyte and glucose determinations, at least daily during the initial phase to prevent hyperglycemia, hypernatremia, dehydration, and hypokalemia. Frequent checks of urine glucose are vital when any

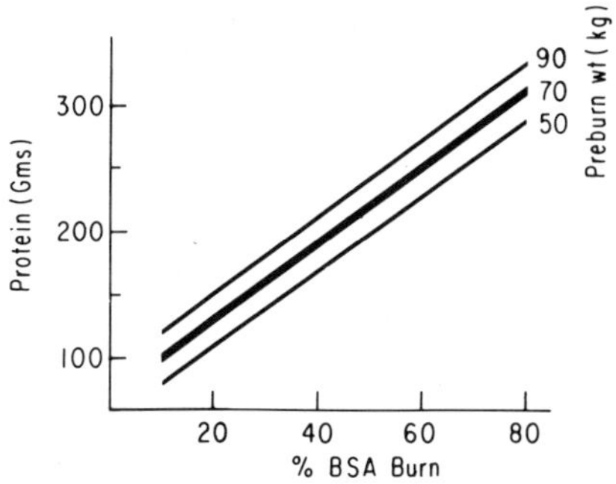

FIGURE 3. Daily protein requirement for major burn victims.

supernormal dietary regimen is followed. Glycosuria produces an osmotic diuresis and can result in hyperosmolar, hyperglycemic, nonketotic dehydration which may be fatal in the burn patient. Glycosuria greater than 2% requires treatment either by temporarily decreasing the number of calories until pancreatic insulin response is appropriate or by administering exogenous insulin.

As stated above, elemental nutrients can be used either as a nutritional supplement or total support system. Once the caloric program has been defined, the elemental diet liquid can be used between meals and provide as much as 50 to 60% of the caloric and nitrogen replacement. In addition, limitations of non- or low-caloric fluids such as water or soda should be maintained during this period since even the most motivated patients have difficulty in achieving total replacement. If, however, evaporative water losses are excessive, more free water can be allowed to meet these external losses once the optimal caloric replacement has been achieved.

Nasogastric or enteral feeding should be reserved for patients unable to ingest sufficient oral nutrition to fulfill their nitrogen and caloric requirements as documented by weight loss and failure to achieve a prescribed caloric quota each day. As a rule, a deficit of 200 or more calories below the designated 24-hr calorie requirement on two consecutive days is an indication for enteral feeding. With a nasogastric tube in place, the elemental diet, easily administered even through small feeding tubes, should be continuously administered. An additional benefit of 24-hr feeding is the minimization of stress and gastrointestinal (GI) bleeding secondary to Curling's ulcers which are common complication of patients with major burn injuries. It appears that the continuous neutralization of gastric acid is the best way of achieving such protection.

Since burn patients may be more prone to esophageal stricture and tracheoesophageal fistulas due to long-term tube placement, the use of a small soft silastic #8 French tube is recommended. This tube can be passed transnasally into the stomach with a weighted end and be left in for long periods of time without any morbidity. Care should be taken to make sure that gastric emptying is adequate prior to placement of one of these tubes as aspiration through this small tube to detect gastric ileus is limited.

Morbidity from elemental diets may consist of diarrhea which increases fluid losses in a patient population already at risk. In addition, electrolyte imbalance could develop. This can be easily controlled by antimotility agents in the majority of patients but must be appreciated early. Palatability of the solutions is another problem with oral supplementation and may require use of a nasogastric tube in these patients.

An elemental diet is easily absorbed, and requires little predigestion. This is extremely important since the burn patient's GI tract initially behaves as if a functional "short gut syndrome" is present as evidenced by some degree of malabsorption. The actual mechanism of this temporary GI dysfunction is unclear but may be due to catabolism of the small bowel villi as a protein source for glyconeogenesis or decreased regeneration of the absorptive surface of the small bowel. Selection of an elemental diet low in fat may be important if poor fat absorption is documented by fat in the stools and diarrhea.

Careful attention to electrolyte balance must be made in these patients. After the initial phase of fluid resuscitation, sodium replacement is usually not necessary because of the great expanded extracellular volume. However, later on in the patient's intermediate phase of care, addition of sodium to the elemental diet may be necessary. Also, supplemental potassium in the range of 80 to 250 meqs/day is often indicated especially when a high caloric intake is achieved.

Supplemental vitamin therapy should be utilized with an elemental diet. Usual supplements recommended include ascorbic acid (2 g) riboflavin (50 mg), thiamin (50 mg), nicotinamide (500 mg), folic acid (1.5 mg), vitamin B_{12} (4 μ). These can be administered orally in capsules or added as a liquid into the elemental diet. Since most elemental diets are low in fats, caution should be observed with prolonged use of this technique. Fatty acid deficiency may develop as has been demonstrated in patients on total intravenous hyperalimentation. Fats should be added to the dietary program as soon as tolerated.

IV. CONCLUSIONS

The burn injury results in significant increases in metabolic requirements. These are reflected by a two- to three-fold increase in calorie and protein replacement required to achieve positive nitrogen balance. These supernormal dietary requirements can be achieved utilizing an elemental diet either has a supplement or as a total parenteral replacement. Complications appear minimal, with careful attention to adequate fluid, vitamin, and electrolyte replacement. The elemental diet affords the burn team an effective method of assuring adequate caloric and nitrogen replacement.

REFERENCES

1. **Border, J. R.,** Metabolic response to short-term starvation, sepsis, and trauma, in *Surgery Annual,* Cooper, P., and Nyhus, L., Eds., Appleton-Century-Crofts, New York, 1970.
2. **Newsome, T. W., Mason, A. D., Jr., and Pruitt, B. A., Jr.,** Weight loss following thermal injury, *Ann. Surg.,* 178, 215, 1973.
3. **Curreri, P. W.,** Metabolic and nutritional aspects of thermal injury, *Burns,* 2, 16, 1976.
4. **Curreri, P. W., Richmond, D., and Marvin, J., Baxter, C. R.,** Dietary requirements of patients with major burns, *J. Am. Diet Assoc.,* 65, 415, 1974.
5. **Sutherland, A. B.,** Nitrogen balance and nutritional requirement in the burn patient, A reappraisal, *Burns,* 2, 238, 1976.
6. **Soroff, H. S., Pearson, E., and Artz, C. P.,** An estimation of the nitrogen requirements for equilibrium in burned patients, *Surg. Gynecol. Obstet.,* 112, 159, 1961.
7. **Wilmore, D. W., Curreri, P. W., and Spitzer, K. W., Spitzer, M. E.,** Supranormal dietary intake in thermally injured hypermetabolic patients, *Surg. Gynecol. Obstet.,* 132, 881, 1971.
8. **Larkin, J. M., and Moylan, J. A.,** Complete enteral support of thermally iniured patients, *Am. J. Surg.,* 131, 722, 1976.

Chapter 16

THE USE OF ELEMENTAL DIETS IN PEDIATRICS

D. L. Christie

TABLE OF CONTENTS

I. INTRODUCTION

This chapter will discuss the use of elemental diets and specialized formulas in the pediatric patient. Emphasis has been placed upon the special nutritional requirements needed for pediatric patients as well as the importance of nutritional assessment in evaluating infants who will receive specialized nutritional support. There is a considerable discussion regarding the use of elemental formulas in protein-sensitive enteropathies, as this is a common and clinically relevant problem in early infancy. The chapter will not discuss the use of elemental diets in pediatric patients with cancer, Crohn's disease, or thermal injuries as these topics have been discussed thoroughly in previous chapters.

II. NUTRITIONAL ASSESSMENT

When significant malnutrition is suspected, the physical examination should include anthropometric measurements. It is important to accurately assess the degree of malnutrition before considering the use of elemental diets in infants and children. Routine measurements of body weight, height, or length, if less than 3 years of age, are the minimum measurements required. Head circumference should be obtained, as it is an index of brain growth and may correlate with brain cell number. Further measurements that are useful in pediatric patients are triceps skinfold thickness, midupper arm circumference, arm muscle circumference, and arm muscle area. Measurement of the triceps skinfold is an indirect estimate of body fat or caloric stores. Arm muscle circumference is an indicator of body protein reserves. It is derived from measurements of midarm circumference and triceps skinfold in centimeters. The arm muscle area is also a measure of body protein reserves and is particularly useful in children. This can be calculated by knowing the midupper arm circumference and the triceps fatfold in centimeters.[1-3](Table 1).

Evaluation of visceral protein status should also be ascertained prior to starting specialized nutritional support. Total protein, albumin, and transferrin are all useful measurements of visceral protein status. Transferrin appears to be a more sensitive indicator of protein-calorie malnutritinn than serum albumin. Serum albumin is still a reliable indicator of protein status as there is a significant correlation between serum albumin levels and arm muscle circumference.[1]

Immune status can be assessed by total lymphocyte count as well as skin tests in children older than 1 year of age. These would include Candida, mumps, and SKSD.

Kanawati and McLaren[4] proposed an "index of thriving" consisting of weight, height, head circumference, and midarm circumference measurements in relation to international standards (Figures 1 and 2). Infants with mid-arm circumference/head circumference ratios of less than 0.250 are classified as having severe protein-calorie malnutrition.

Accurate and thorough nutritional assessment can help one identify the children with severe malnutrition who require intensive nutritional support. Pediatric patients in need of specialized nutrition are those

1. Whose weight or height is greater than two standard deviations below normal or 80% of standard.
2. Whose arm muscle area is less than the fifth percentile (Table 2).
3. Whose serum albumin is less than 3 g/100 mℓ.
4. Whose transferrin concentration is less than 150 μg/100 mℓ.
5. Whose lymphocyte count is less than 1500 m^2.
6. Whose midarm circumference to head circumference ratio falls below 0.310.

Table 1
CALCULATION OF ARM MUSCLE AREA

M	=	$[(Ca - \pi s)^2]/4\pi$
M	=	Arm muscle area in square centimeters
Ca	=	Midupper arm circumference in centimeters
S	=	Triceps fatfold in centimeters
π	=	3.14

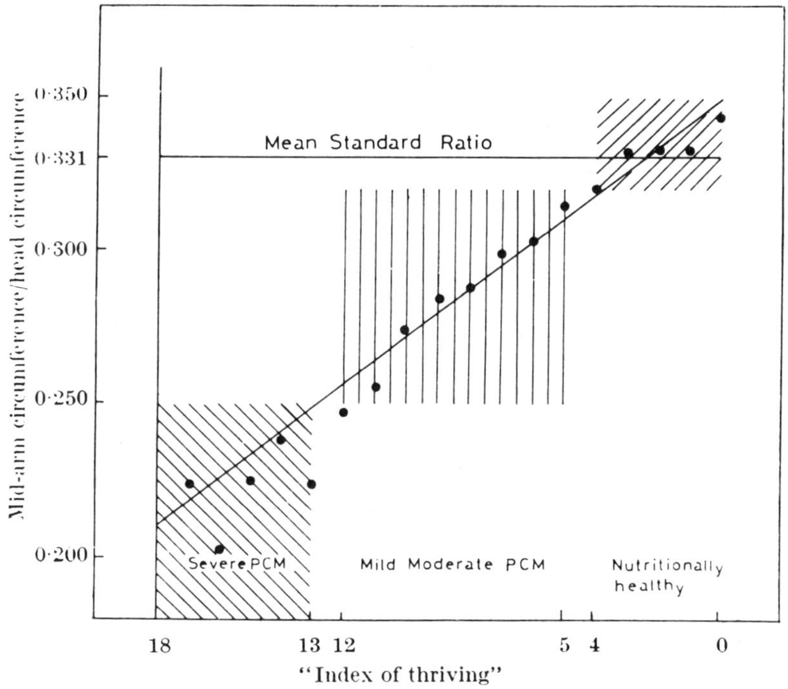

FIGURE 1. Midarm circumference/head circumference ratio and the "index of thriving" for 1,276 children, 45 with acute marasmus. (From Kanawati, A. A. and McLaren, D. S., *Nature,* 228, 574, 1970. With permission).

III. NUTRITIONAL NEEDS OF INFANTS AND CHILDREN

The recommended daily caloric requirements and dietary allowances for infants and children are found in Tables 3-6. The premature or low birth-weight infant has a total caloric requirement on a per kilogram basis of 120 cal/day. Most low birth-weight infants will achieve satisfactory growth with calorie intakes averaging 110 to 150 cal/kg/day. Formulas that are fed to infants should provide approximately 67 cal/dℓ (20 cal/oz).[5] On occasion, high caloric densities can result in faster rates of growth. However, sufficient water must be given to provide for normal renal excretion in low birth-weight infants. Infants with infection, diarrhea, or other stresses that alter water balance should be given formulas of low renal solute load. They should not be fed formulas of caloric densities greater than 81 cal/dℓ (24 cal/oz).

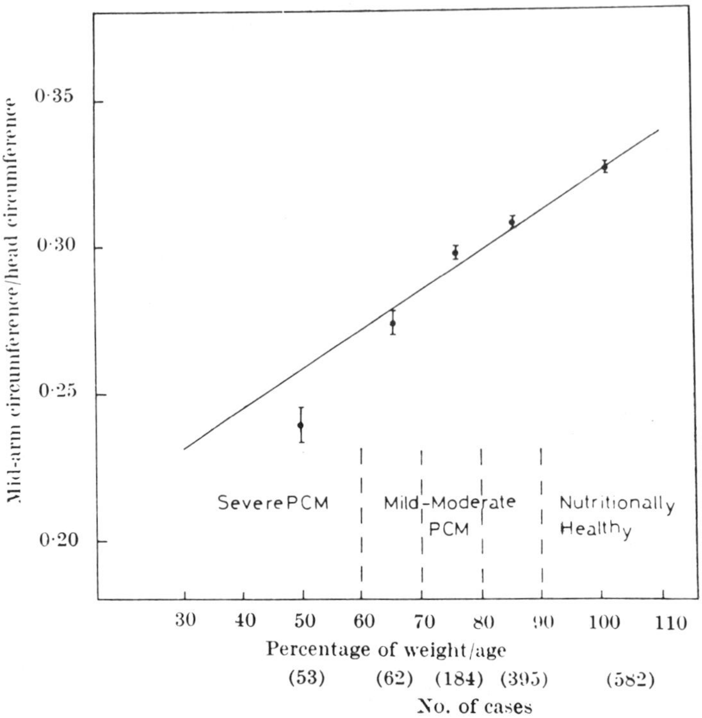

FIGURE 2. Relationship between the midarm circumference/head circumference ratio and the percentage weight/age. (From Kanawati, A. A. and McLaren, D. S., *Nature*, 228, 574, 1970. With permission).

Optimal protein intake for low birth-weight infants is between 2.25 and 5 g/kg/day when fed a cow's milk formula. The amino acid composition of formulas or diets fed to premature infants is important. Snyderman[6] demonstrated that the removal of cystine or tyrosine from the diet resulted in decreased growth and nitrogen retention. Premature infants requiring cystine also failed to show an increase in plasma cystine after a methionine load. This means an absence of the enzyme, cystathionase, in the liver of premature infants.[7] High levels of cystathionine in plasma of premature infants fed high protein formulas means that the conversion of methionine to cystine is not present.[8] Formulas deficient in cystine may need the addition of this amino acid if fed to premature infants. A commercial preparation is now available for intravenous use (L-cysteine 50 mg/mℓ — Abbott Laboratories).

Low birth-weight infants absorb fat, especially saturated fats such as butter fat, rather poorly. Vegetable oils are much better absorbed so that formulas now contain vegetable oils or mixtures of vegetable oils and animal fats. Infant feedings should supply a minimum of 3% of the total calories in the form of linoleic acid or 300 mg of linoleic acid should be fed per 100 kcal given to the infant. This will meet the infant's requirement for essential fatty acids. Formulas or elemental diets containing less than the required linoleic acid concentration should be supplemented on a daily basis.[5]

Intestinal disaccharidases are developed early in fetal life. Maltase and sucrase reach mature levels by the sixth to eighth month of gestation. Lactase does not reach mature levels until term. The low birth-weight infant generally is able to adequately digest disaccharidases. There is some evidence, however, that the addition of sucrose to cow's milk formula instead of lactose will result in a decreased incidence of diarrhea and

Table 2
ARM MUSCLE AREA PERCENTILES (SQUARE CENTIMETERS)

Age	Male 5th	Female 5th
0—5 mo	5.2	5.9
6—17mo	7.9	7.5
1½—2½ yr	9.7	8.8
2½—3½ yr	10.2	9.2
3½—4½ yr	11.0	10.4
4½—5½ yr	11.7	11.1
5½—6½ yr	12.7	11.6
6½—7½ yr	13.4	12.1
7½—8½ yr	15.0	13.2
8½—9½ yr	15.2	14.7
9½—10½ yr	16.0	15.2
10½—11½ yr	18.0	15.5
11½—12½ yr	18.7	17.8
12½—13½ yr	20.1	19.0
13½—14½ yr	22.3	21.8
14½—15½ yr	23.7	21.2
15½—16½ yr	27.4	23.1
16½—17½ yr	33.7	23.1

Table 3
MEAN HEIGHTS AND WEIGHTS

Category	Age (yrs)	Weight (kg)	Height (cm)	Energy Needs (with range) (kcal)	
Infants	0.0—0.5	6	60	kg × 115	(95—145)
	0.5—1.0	9	71	kg × 105	(80—135)
Children	1—3	13	90	1300	(900—1800)
	4—6	20	112	1700	(1300—2300)
	7—10	28	132	2400	(1650—3300)
Males	11—14	45	157	2700	(2000—3700)
	15—18	66	176	2800	(2100—3900)
Females	11—14	46	157	2200	(1500—3000)
	15—18	55	163	2100	(1200—3000)

metabolic acidosis in low birth-weight infants.[9] The delay in maturation of lactase in some low birth-weight infants may be of clinical significance.

IV. THE USE OF ELEMENTAL DIETS IN INTRACTABLE DIARRHEA OF INFANCY

The intractable diarrhea syndrome of infancy is defined as an unremitting, severe diarrheal state not responding to conventional therapy and associated with large losses of fluid, electrolytes, and proteins.[10] Caloric insufficiency is present and leads to protein-calorie malnutrition. The protein-calorie malnutrition leads to an abnormal utilization

Table 4
RECOMMENDED DAILY DIETARY ALLOWANCES

		Fat-soluble vitamins		
Category	**Age (yrs)**	**Vitamin A (μg/RE)[a]**	**Vitamin D (μg)[b]**	**Vitamin E (mg $\alpha-$ TE)[c]**
Infants	0.0—0.5	420	10	3
	0.5—1.0	400	10	4
Children	1—3	400	10	5
	4—6	500	10	6
	7—10	700	10	7
Males	11—14	1000	10	8
	15—18	1000	10	10
Females	11—14	800	10	8
	15—18	800	10	8

[a] Retinol equivalents. 1 retinol equivalent = 1 μg retinol or 6 μg β carotene.
[b] As cholecalciferol. 10 μg cholecalciferol = 400 IU of vitamin D.
[c] $\alpha-$tocopherol equivalents. 1 mg d-α tocopherol = 1 $\alpha-$TE.

Reproduced from "Recommended Dietary Allowances" 9th ed., 1980 with the permission of the National Academy Sciences, Washington, D.C.

Table 5
RECOMMENDED DAILY DIETARY ALLOWANCES

		Water-soluble Vitamins						
Category	**Age (yrs)**	**C (mg)**	**Thiamin (mg)**	**Riboflavin (mg)**	**Niacin (mg NE)**	**B-6 (mg)**	**Folacin (μg)**	**B-12 (μg)**
Infants	0.0—0.5	35	0.3	0.4	6	0.3	30	0.5
	0.5—1.0	35	0.5	0.6	8	0.6	45	1.5
Children	1—3	45	0.7	0.8	9	0.9	100	2.0
	4—6	45	0.9	1.0	11	1.3	200	2.5
	7—10	45	1.2	1.4	16	1.6	300	3.0
Males	11—14	50	1.4	1.6	18	1.8	400	3.0
	15—18	60	1.4	1.7	18	2.0	400	3.0
Females	11—14	50	1.1	1.3	15	1.8	400	3.0
	15—18	60	1.1	1.3	14	2.0	400	3.0

Reproduced from "Recommended Dietary Allowances" 9th ed., 1980 with the permission of the National Academy Sciences, Washington, D.C.

Table 6
RECOMMENDED DAILY DIETARY ALLOWANCES

		Minerals					
Category	**Age (yrs)**	**Calcium (mg)**	**Phosphorus (mg)**	**Magnesium (mg)**	**Iron (mg)**	**Zinc (mg)**	**Iodine (μg)**
Infants	0.0—0.5	360	240	50	10	3	40
	0.5—1.0	540	360	70	15	5	50
Children	1—3	800	800	150	15	10	70
	4—6	800	800	200	10	10	90
	7—10	800	800	250	10	10	120
Males	11—14	1200	1200	350	18	15	150
	15—18	1200	1200	400	18	15	150
Females	11—14	1200	1200	300	18	15	150
	15—18	1200	1200	300	18	15	150

Reproduced from "Recommended Dietary Allowances" 9th ed., 1980 with the permission of the National Academy Sciences, Washington, D.C.

of proteins and sugar because of reduced pancreatic enzyme secretions and severe damage of the small bowel mucosa. This results in reduced disaccharidase and dipeptidase activities in the brush border of the small bowel mucosa. The protracted diarrhea also involves impaired reabsorption of the endogenous nitrogen as well as altered duodenal and jejunal bacterial flora. There is a net secretion of fluid into the lumen of the jejunum with continued impaired synthesis of small bowel intestinal mucosa. This sequence of events leads to a further decrease in digestion and absorption of all nutrients and further exacerbates the protein-calorie malnutrition.

Diets containing free amino acids and little fat have potential benefit in patients with intractable diarrhea. Free amino acids will not require digestion from pancreatic proteases or the dipeptidases present in the brush border of the small bowel. Also, free amino acid diets will eliminate the risk of abnormal peptide transfer. This abnormal peptide transfer of intact protein molecules across the damaged mucosa can cause an increased risk of inducing protein sensitivity. Diets free of excess fat will eliminate the problems related to bacterial overgrowth and deconjugation of bile salts as well as pancreatic insufficiency with decreased lipase activity.

Many diseases have been found to cause intractable diarrhea of early infancy. These include inflammatory disorders of the gastrointestinal (GI) tract, such as infectious diarrhea and allergic gastroenteropathy; enzymatic or biochemical disorders of the GI tract, such as pancreatic insufficiency and monosaccharide or disaccharide malabsorption; anatomical disorders of the GI tract, such as Hirschsprung's disease or massive intestinal resection; hormonal disorders, such as neural crest tumors; and recently bile acid malabsorption secondary to ileal dysfunction.[11]

However, in a significant percent of infants, no diagnosis can be made in spite of extensive evaluation. Because these infants with no specific diagnosis often have significant small bowel mucosal disease and pancreatic insufficiency, elemental diets have been tried as a therapeutic modality on an empiric basis. Greene et al.[12] studied 16 infants with protracted diarrhea and malnutrition. All of these patients had diarrhea for at least 40 days and had a weight more than two standard deviations below that expected for age. All were unable to respond to conservative treatment which consisted of short-term fasting and intravenous fluids. The serum protein:albumin concentration in all 16 patients was 4.5:2.0 g/dℓ. Greene compared eight infants on total parenteral nutrition alone to eight infants on a regimen of partial total parenteral nutrition plus a continuous infusion of an elemental diet. Multiple small bowel biopsies were performed prior to beginning treatment, several days after treatment was begun, and after treatment had finished. Initial biopsies in the infants with intractable diarrhea showed a severe small bowel mucosal disease. All of the patients had deficient disaccharidase activities (Figure 3) and deficient levels of trypsin activity in duodenal fluid. Greene's study showed that trypsin activity in the duodenal secretions was significantly higher in the biopsies of patients treated with the elemental diet as compared to those treated by total parenteral nutrition alone. Also, sucrase and maltase activities were significantly higher earlier in the elemental diet-treated group as compared to the patients treated with total parenteral nutrition. The study suggests that a more complete recovery was achieved earlier in the group treated with an elemental diet.

Sherman et al.[13] used an elemental diet in intractable diarrhea in 27 infants under a year of age. They used both a high nitrogen and standard nitrogen formula. These investigators demonstrated positive nitrogen balance in both groups of infants and a mean weight gain of 4.6 $\pm$ 3.9g/kg/day in the standard elemental diet formula compared to 9.2 $\pm$ 4.5 g/kg/day in the high nitrogen fed group (Table 7). Feeding of the high nitrogen formula resulted in acceptable nitrogen retention and weight gain which was significantly better than the standard formula diet. However, significant elevations of

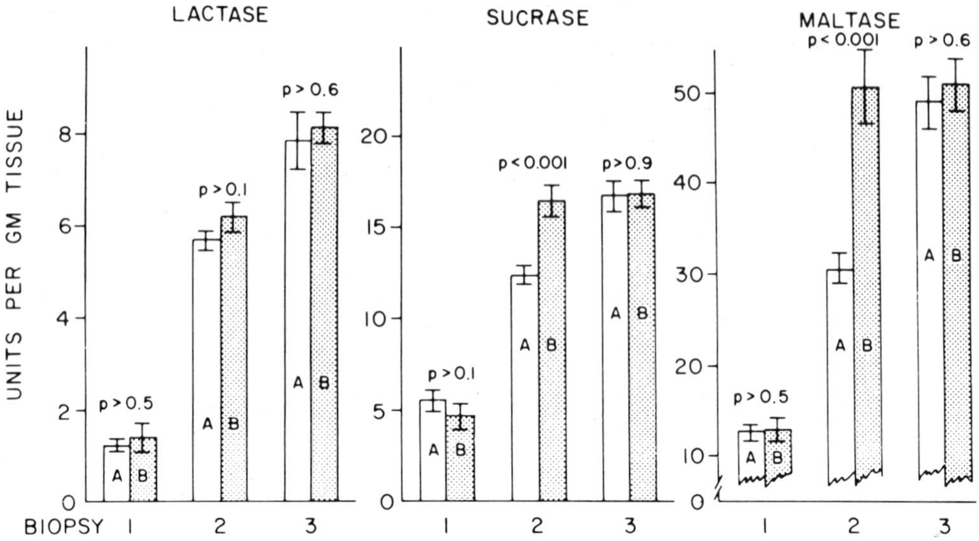

FIGURE 3. Comparison of intestinal disaccharidase activities. Activities expressed as moles of substrate metabolized per minute per gram wet weight of tissue. Group A treated with total parenteral nutrition by central vein, Group B treated with dilute parenteral feedings plus enteral elemental diet. (From Greene, H. L., McCabe, D. R., and Merenstein, G. B., *J. Pediatr.*, 87, 695, 1975. With permission).

Table 7
COMPARISON OF AMINO ACID INTAKE, NITROGEN BALANCE, AND WEIGHT GAIN[13]

Diet (18% wlv)	Amino Acid intake (g/kg/day)	Nitrogen balance (mg/kg/day)	Mean weight gain (g/kg/day)	Length of treatment (days)
Vivonex® standard	2.25	+163 ± 75	4.6 ± 3.9	66
Vivonex® high-nitrogen	4.58	+332 ± 82	9.2 ± 4.5	78

several amino acids occurred while on the high nitrogen diet. Cystine, which was not found in the elemental diet, remained low in both treatment groups. Two patients also had an elevation of SGPT while on the high nitrogen formula. Sherman's study demonstrated that an elemental diet would give positive nitrogen balance and growth but that abnormalities in plasma and amino acids were present during constant infusion of this formula (Figures 4 and 5).

Lindblad et al.[14] compared the amino acid composition to an elemental diet and breast milk (Fiqure 6) and measured plasma free amino acid levels in patients with protracted diarrhea and protein-calorie malnutrition. They were able to demonstrate a gain in weight in 11 infants with protracted diarrhea. They found high levels of proline and phenylalanine in the plasma aminogram of these infants prior to treatment with the elemental formula. After the initial treatment, the plasma aminogram showed very low branch-chained amino acids and cystine levels (Figure 7). Their investigation supported the previous assumptions that cystine was an essential amino acid in malnourished infants. They also noted that the elemental diet in use (Vivonex®) had sodium and chloride concentrations that were too high while vitamin D, iron, and zinc concentrations were lower than that required for most infants.

In summary, elemental diets are useful in patients with intractable diarrhea syndrome. Because infants may have multiple vitamin and trace mineral deficiencies as part of their

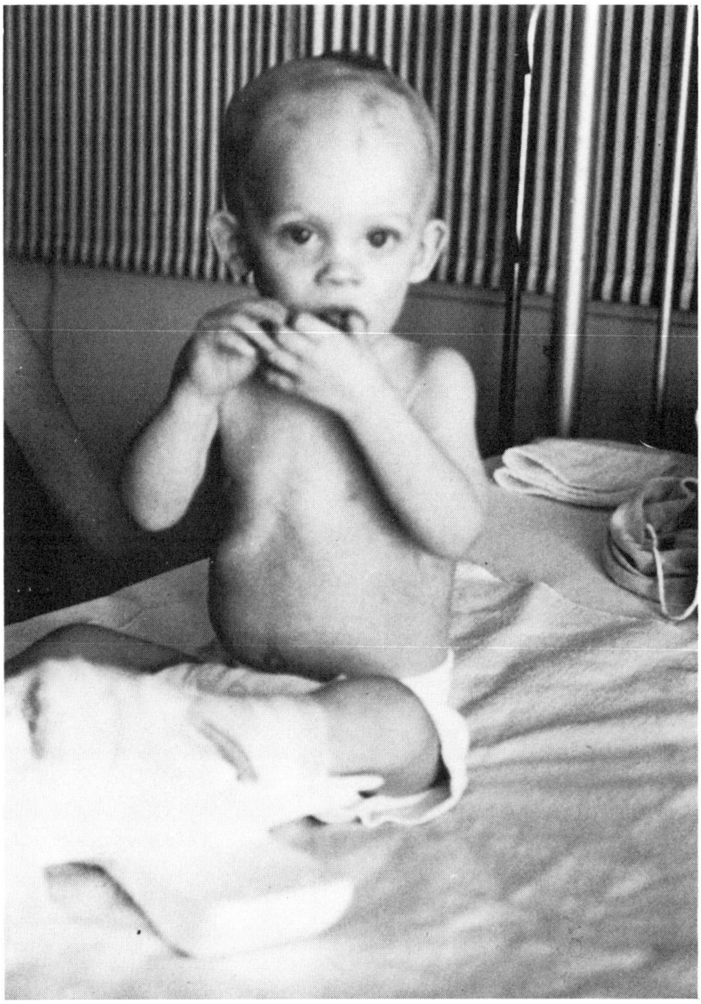

A

FIGURE 4. (A) Infant with intractable diarrhea syndrome on admission to hospital. (B) Evaluation demonstrated severe small bowel mucosal abnormality with absent villi. Treatment was total parenteral nutrition and continuous enteral infusion of an elemental diet. No etiology was ascertained. Infant eventually tolerated a regular diet.

intractable diarrhea syndrome, it is important to be aware of the recommended daily allowances of these vitamins and minerals and to supplement them where the diet appears to be inadequate. If a clinical syndrome compatible with deficiency of any of these vitamins or minerals develops, immediate supplementation is indicated.

V. THE USE OF ELEMENTAL DIETS IN SHORT BOWEL SYNDROME

The use of specialized diets or elemental formulas in infants with short bowel has many theoretical advantages. Minimal small bowel mucosal length is required for intraluminal digestion and mininal mucosal surface for digestion and absorption when

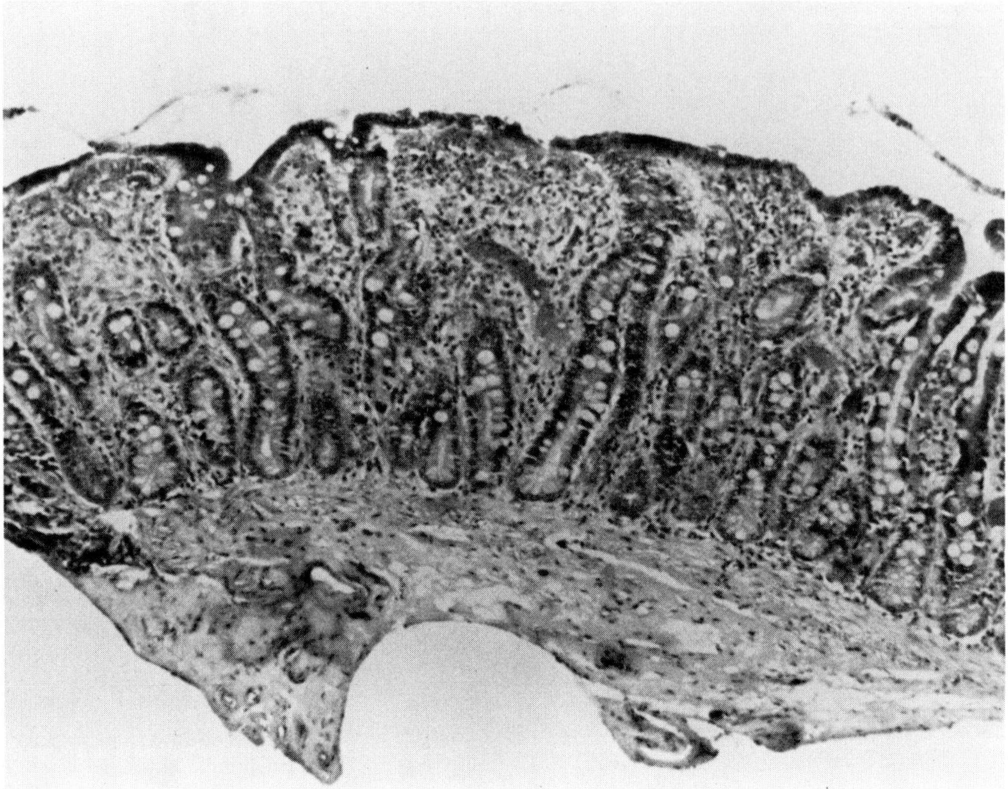

4-B

elemental formulas are used. When relative disaccharidase deficiency is present because of decreased small bowel surface area, the glucose in elemental diets will still be actively transported across the intestine into the capilaries. The amino acids in elemental diets do not require pancreatic proteases for intraluminal hydrolysis or oligopeptidases in the brush border of the small intestinal mucosa for further digestion The need for bile acids and pancreatic lipase is minimal because specialized formulas do not contain fat in any significant quantity; or if present, fat is usually in the form of median-chain triglycerides.

Previous studies have demonstrated that infants with short bowel syndrome have significant steatorrhea, decreased bile acid concentration in duodenal secretions, and abnormal intestinal vitamin B_{12} absorption (Figure 8).[15] Infants with distal resection of the small intestine have more significant steatorrhea and vitamin B_{12} malabsorption because of the loss of the normal sites for absorption of bile acids and vitamin B_{12} (Figure 8). With time, some adaptation occurs as steatorrhea decreases regardless of what portion of the small bowel is resected. However, infants with a distal resection may have a continued decrease in the critical micellar concentration of bile salts in the lumen of the small intestine and also vitamin B_{12} malabsorption. A compelling reason to use oral nutrition in infants with significant small intestinal resection is animal evidence indicating that an increase in height of the small intestinal villi and an increase in the number of enterocytes occurs when nutrients are delivered to the GI tract orally rather than by intravenous methods.[16]

The main problem in using elemental diets in infants with short bowel is the "dumping syndrome" which occurs because of the osmolality of the formulas. Most investigators

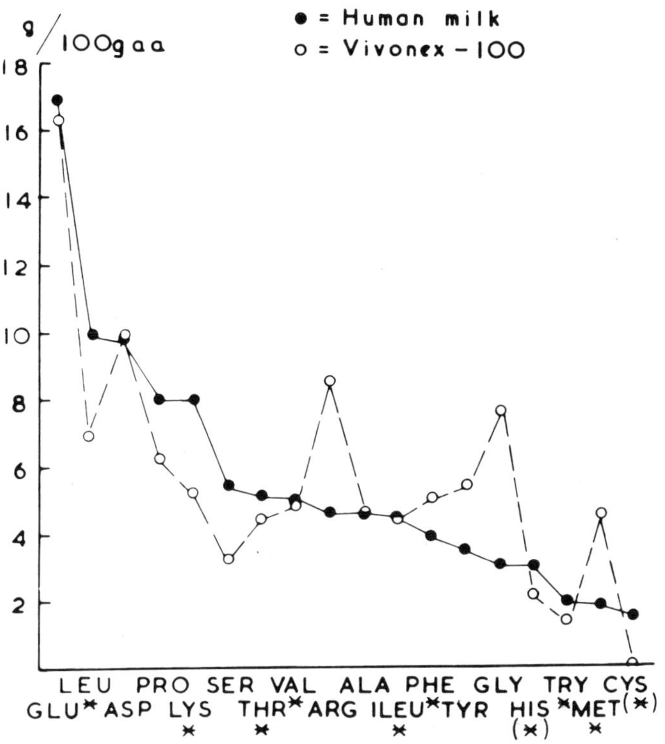

FIGURE 5. The amino acid composition of Vivonex® as compared to that of human milk. Essential amino acids are indicated by an asterisk. (From Lindblad, B. S., Rahimtoola, R. J., Hafiz-ur-Rehman, Ahmad, S. S., Fancy, K., Singha, L., and Hussain, S. S., *Acta Paediatr. Scand.*, 67, 335, 1978. With permission).

recommend using a dilute diet of approximately 166 mOsm/ℓ with a caloric concentration of 0.3 kcal/mℓ.[17] These formulas are usually infused via a gastrostomy tube continuously over a 24-hr period. The initial rate of infusion in infants with short bowel syndrome is usually 50 cc/kg/day. The volume infused is gradually increased to provide adequate calories for growth. Some infants may require infusion rates of 160 to 300 cc/kg/day.[17-18] After adequate infusion at the dilute one third strength, the diets are usually advanced to one half and finally to two thirds concentration. The strength of the formula is generally not increased unless the infant gains weight steadily and reducing substances are absent from the stool. The concentration of the formula and the amount of diet infused are never increased at the same time.

Constant rate enteral nutrition has the advantage of enabling the patient to be gradually switched from total parenteral nutrition to oral nutrition when bolus feedings cause excessive fecal volume.[19] During the switch from complete total parenteral nutrition to complete oral nutrition, it is important not to exceed the maximum absorption rates of the remaining small intestine. One investigator recommends that the maximum rate of water infusion should not exceed 0.06 mℓ/min/cm, that the lipid rate should not exceed 1.71 ± 0.11 mg/min/cm, and the carbohydrate rate should not exceed 3 mg/min/cm.[18] The combined use of total parenteral nutrition and oral alimentation requires attention to fluid and electrolyte balance. Daily input and output should be carefully recorded. Table 8 demonstrates one method of recording daily changes in nutritional and metabolic status.

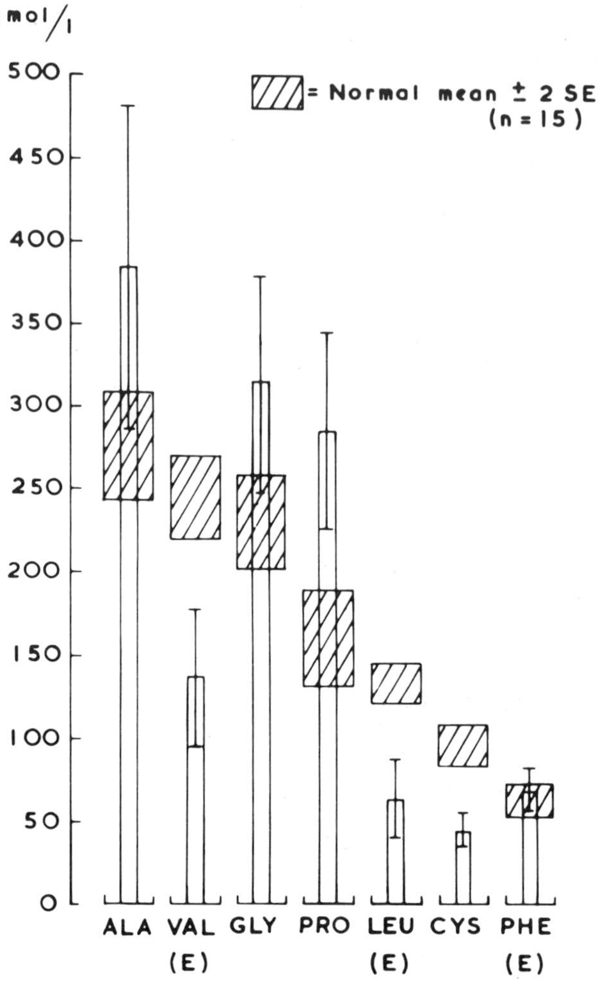

FIGURE 6. The free amino acid levels of plasma after introduction of Vivonex®. Mean ± 2 S.E. are given for those amino acids whose plasma levels change characteristically in malnutrition. (From Lindblad, B. S., Rahimtoola, R. J., Hafiz-ur-Rehman, Ahmad, S. S., Fancy, K., Singha, L., and Hussain, S. S., *Acta Paediatr. Scand.*, 67, 335, 1978. With permission).

VI. THE USE OF ELEMENTAL DIETS IN PROTEIN-SENSITIVE ENTEROPATHIES

Numerous authors have documented the presence of small bowel mucosal disease in infants secondary to cow milk protein and soy milk protein.[20-21] These infants usually present in early infancy with diarrhea, vomiting, abdominal distention, weight loss, and malnutrition. Lactose intolerance occurs secondary to loss of lactase enzyme. Small bowel mucosal abnormalities have been documented and can range from a mild villus abnormality to a severe mucosal defect. The infants clinically improve when the offending protein is removed from the diet. When rechallenged, the jejunal mucosa becomes abnormal again. A xylose tolerance test will demonstrate a drop between pre- and post-challenge levels. Histological relapse occurs even without clinical symptoms in some patients. Occasionally these infants can be sensitive to multiple proteins, with cow's and

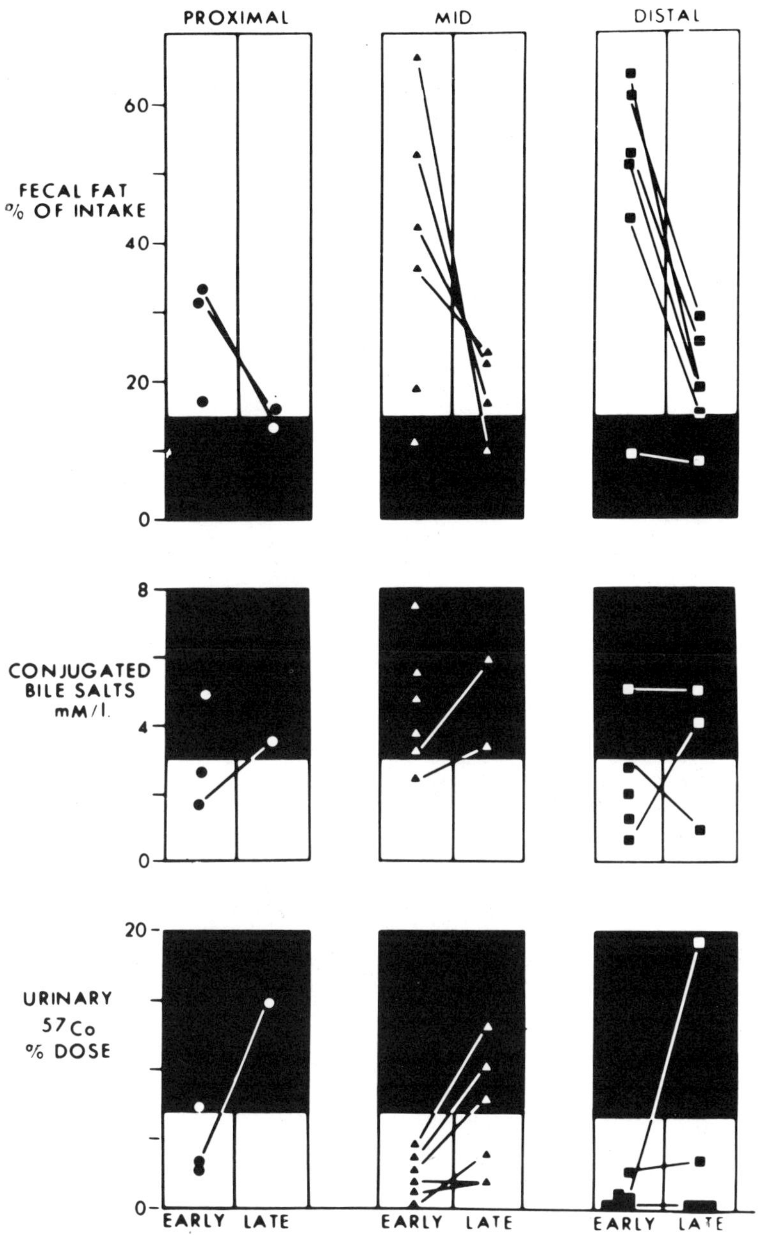

FIGURE 7. Comparison of initial with later values of fecal fat, conjugated bile salts, and results of Schilling test in infants with absence or resection of proximal, mid, or distal small intestine. Shaded areas indicate normal range. (From Bohane, T.D., Haka-Ikse, K., Baggar, W. D., Hamilton, J. R., and Gall, D. G., *J. Pediat.*, 94, 552, 1979. With permission).

soy milk protein combined as the two common offending antigens. However, rarely the hypoallergenic formulas containing casein hydrolysate peptides also cannot be tolerated (Figures 9 and 10).

An elemental diet has theoretical usefulness in patients with protein-sensitive enteropathies because of the low antigenecity in free amino acid preparations. Galant et al.[22] could demonstrate no evidence of immunogenicity in animals fed elemental diets by

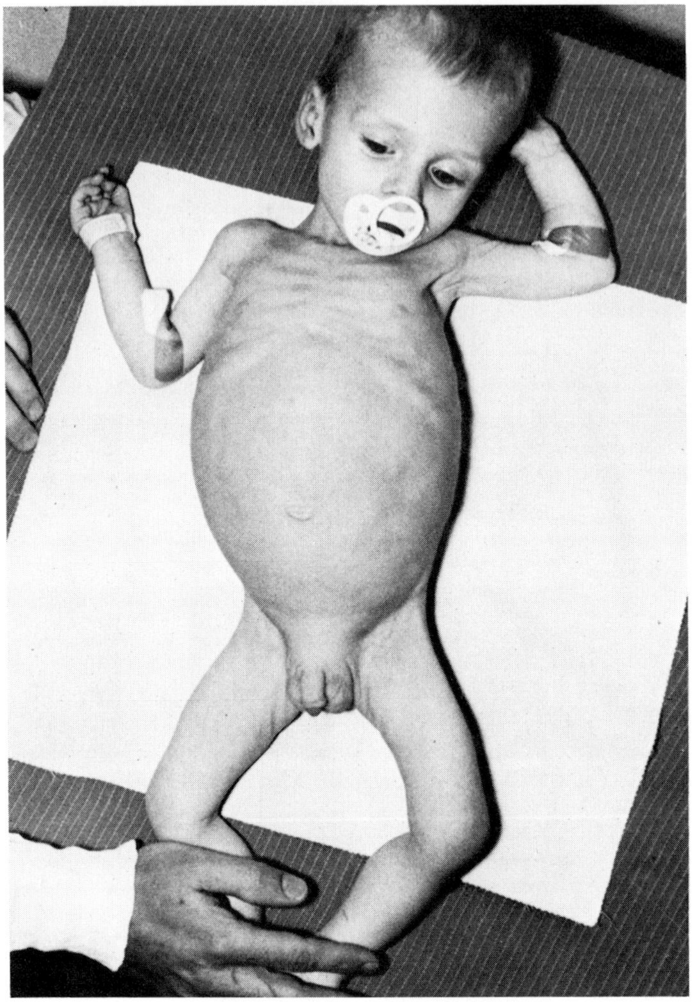

FIGURE 8. Ten-month-old infant who was admitted to the hosptial with a history of intractable diarrhea of early infancy which presented with dehydration and severe metabolic acidosis on a cow's milk protein formula. Rotaviral infection was documented at two weeks of age. The infant demonstrated a continued failure to thrive on multiple formulas including soy-based, casein hydrolysate-based, and meat-based protein. Small bowel biopsy demonstrated a moderately abnormal villus architecture.

either precipitant or the passive cutaneous anaphylaxis method. These investigators also could demonstrate no cross-reactivity between elemental diets and milk or egg antigens. This is not the case with the commonly fed formulas. Walker et al.[23] studied 25 infants fed casein hydrolysate, milk protein, or soy protein formulas to determine the degree of antigenicity. They demonstrated that infants fed the casein hydrolysate formula for the first 3 months of life had lower hemagglutinin antibody titers to subsequent challenge with milk or soy protein formulas than infants who were given the soy or milk protein formula since birth. Iyngkaran et al.[24] showed that cow's milk protein damaged the small bowel mucosa in young infants who were recovering from acute infectious enteritis. Disaccharidase enzymes — lactase, sucrase, and isomaltase — were all decreased in these infants so that the majority had a clinical carbohydrate intolerance secondary to

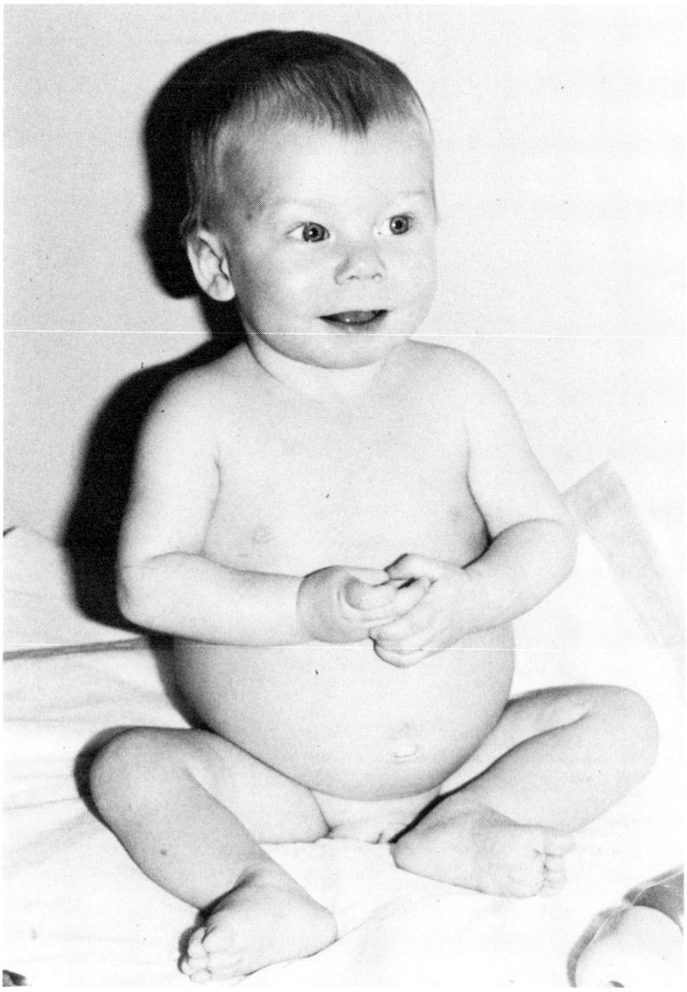

FIGURE 9. The infant in Figure 8, 4 months later, after treatment with an elemental diet containing glucose, oligosaccharides, free amino acids, and minimal fat. Infant continues to do well on the elemental formula with added trace elements and vitamins. Repeat small bowel biopsy was normal.

damage from the cow's milk protein. These authors believe that cow's milk protein and lactose should be excluded from the diet of infants with acute infectious gastroenteritis. Most authors advocate that the diagnosis of protein-sensitive enteropathy be based upon clinical symptoms — usually, diarrhea and vomiting — while receiving the offending protein with improvement while on a diet free of the offending protein. The biopsy of the jejunal mucosa will be abnormal at the time the infant originally presents with the illness but should show a normal or minimally abnormal biopsy after being off the protein for 8 weeks. Histological relapse then should be documented after reexposure to the offending antigen. Some investigators have demonstrated abnormal xylose tolerance tests and changes in immunoglobulin and complement levels pre- and postchallenge with either soy or cow's milk protein. Other investigators have recently found increased IgE antibodies in the mucosa of the small bowel.[25]

The usefulness of an elemental diet in infants with multiple protein sensitivities is not only in treatment but also in diagnosing which type of protein is causing the clinical

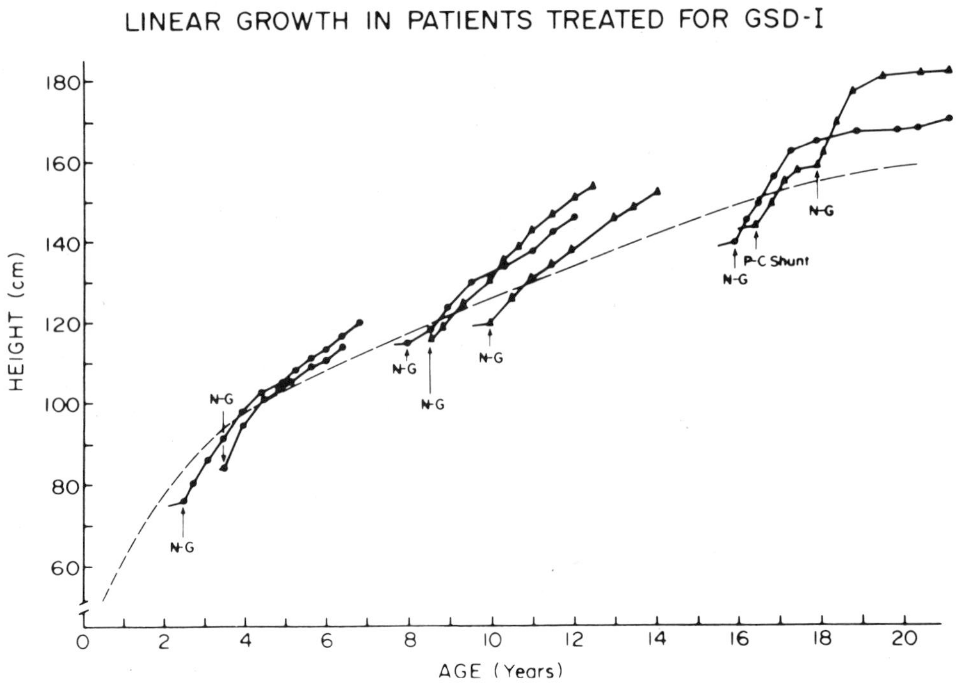

FIGURE 10. Growth of seven patients during treatment with nocturnal feedings. (From Greene, H. L., Slonim, A. E., Burr, I. M., and Moran, J. R., *J. Pediatr.*, 96, 590, 1980. With permission).

syndrome. The occasional infant who demonstrates significant small bowel mucosal disease because of intolerance to multiple proteins will be benefitted by an elemental diet, as this is generally the only formula tolerated. The infant can regain his weight and his small bowel mucosa will return to normal. Challenge can then be instituted with the offending protein to determine if small bowel mucosal damage will ensue.

Recently, an adult patient with refractory celiac sprue was found to recover after removal of nongluten dietary proteins — namely, egg, chicken, and tuna.[26] By using an elemental diet between each food challenge, the investigators were able to determine what offending proteins were causing the severe small bowel mucosal disease. The use of the elemental diet enables the physician to introduce selected proteins over a period of time to determine whether symptoms follow the introduction of these specific antigens. By using the elemental formula between each challenge, one can be reasonably sure that the offending protein causing the disease will be identified by this method.

VII. THE USE OF ELEMENTAL DIETS IN GLYCOGEN STORAGE DISEASE

In 1974, Greene and coworkers[27] reported the use of intragastric glucose feedings in patients with glucose 6-phosphatase deficiency. They postulated that blood/glucose levels below approximately 70 mg/dℓ would cause a release of glucagon and catechols which would stimulate glycogen degradation to glucose 6-phosphate. The absence of glucose 6-phosphatase would impair release of glucose to correct the falling blood/glucose concentration. This results in augumented glycogenolysis which causes excess formation of lactate, triglycerides, and uric acid. They hypothesized that treatment with exogenous glucose to maintain blood/glucose levels above 70 mg/dℓ would inhibit release of catechols and glucagon.

These investigators have now reported a study on seven patients over a 5-year period.[28] The children were given continuous intragastric infusions of Vivonex® high nitrogen at night during the 5-year period. During the day, the patients were allowed to eat a normal caloric diet, except for allowing approximately 70% of the calories as carbohydrate, 10% to 15% as protein, and the remainder as fat. Diets were given at a 3-hour interval during the day. The investigators found that continuous intragastric infusions of Vivonex® caused a significant decrease in SGOT, lactate, urate, and bleeding time, as well as triglycerides, and an increase in blood glucose levels. As impressive was the rate of accelerated growth. All patients were less than the third percentile for age in height. After 5 years of therapy, all patients studied were greater than the third percentile (Figure 11).[28] Some of the patients grew 1 cm/month during the first year of treatment. Thus, the use of continuous infusion of an elemental diet enabled the metabolic abnormalities of glycogen storage disease Type I to be significantly improved.

VIII. THE USE OF ELEMENTAL DIETS IN CYSTIC FIBROSIS

Infants and children with cystic fibrosis have significant problems with malabsorption of nutrients and have increased needs for protein and essential fatty acids. A recent review discussed the aspects of malnutrition in cystic fibrosis.[29] The use of elemental diets has not been firmly established for use in patients with cystic fibrosis (see Chapter 12). Allan and co-workers[30] originally claimed that artificial diets can improve growth in patients with cystic fibrosis. However, Dodge and colleagues[31] recently showed that only 36% of patients with cystic fibrosis had a clinically significant improvement in height or weight when fed an elemental diet for 12 months. They recommended using an elemental formula only on a short-term basis in patients with failure to thrive. Other workers have recently claimed that elemental diets when given nocturnally would also speed growth in patients with cystic fibrosis. This report has yet to be further substantiated.[32]

IX. THE USE OF SPECIAL DIETS FOR INFANTS WITH INBORN ERRORS OF AMINO ACID METABOLISM

Complete discussion of the various specialized diets for use in patients with hereditary amino acid disorders is beyond the scope of this chapter. Numerous references are available regarding these types of diets.[33] These diets generally contain an adequate amount of the harmful amino acid to provide the metabolic requirements for the body, including the requirement for growth, without causing excess accumulation of amino acid or its derivatives. Lofenalac® is a commercial product that is low in phenylalanine. The casein hydrolysate is processed to remove most of the phenylalanine for these infants. Carbohydrate in Lofenalac is from corn syrup solids and tapioca starch and the fat is from corn oil. Phenylalanine-free products are advantageous for older children because they enable the child to choose some foods containing phenylalanine in order to meet the daily requirements of this essential amino acid. Two products are available for these children, PKU-aid® and Phenyl-free®.

Patients with maple syrup urine disease require a restriction of the branched-chain amino acids — leucine, valine, and isoleucine. Two products are available for use in these infants, MSUD-aid and MSUD Diet Powder. MSUD Diet Powder contains crystalline amino acids, except for the branch chain amino acids and appropriate amounts of the fats, carbohydrates, vitamins, and minerals. Product 3200-AB is a hydrolysate formula that is low in phenylalanine and tyrosine and is used in patients with hereditary tyrosinemia. Three products are available for homocystinuria where restriction in methionine and supplementation of cystine is indicated. These products are Methionaid. Product 3200-K, and Low Methionine Isomil.

X. THE USE OF MODULAR FORMULAS IN INFANTS AND CHILDREN

Recently, physicians have realized the importance of being able to modify the amount and type of carbohydrate, protein, and fat in oral feeding mixtures to tailor the formula to the type of malabsorption syndrome present in a particular infant. Two problems that have been instrumental in development of specialized modular formulas for treatment in pediatric patients has been a realization of the importance of osmolality, and the evidence that carbohydrate modification is indicated in patients with severe small bowel mucosal disease. High osmolality formulas are commonly responsible for nausea, vomiting, and gastric retention in infants. There is evidence that the osmolality of the formula is responsible for the dumping syndrome with water secretion increased at the intestinal level. Also, the possibility of necrotizing enterocolitis in premature infants related to high osmolality feedings has been raised.[34]

Glucose oligosaccharides from corn syrup solids are now being added to formulas to decrease osmolality and improve the transport of carbohydrate across the small bowel mucosa. Corn syrup solids are digested by maltase and isomaltase before transport across the small bowel intestine. Because maltase levels are much higher than lactase and sucrase levels in infants recovering from GI illness, corn syrup solids are advantageous in diseases where small intestinal damage is present.[35] Fat can be added in varying concentrations from the minimal 3% of linoleic acid needed to prevent essential fatty acid deficiency to diets containing 40% to 60% mediun-chain triglycerides.

Klish and colleagues[36] advocated the use of a modular formula for use in patients with chronic diarrhea. This formula contains calcium sodium caseinate and electrolytes with no added sugar or fat. The formula is usually used in a concentration of 3 g powder per dℓ H_20 which provides 2.2 g of protein. Any carbohydrate can be added including glucose, sucrose, or fructose to provide a final concentration of approximately 5 to 7 g/dℓ. Vitamins must be added to this formula since none are present. Fat can be added at any time during the therapy. These authors reported favorable use of the modular formula in patients with acquired glucose intolerance, chronic intractable diarrhea of infancy, short bowel syndrome, or when weaning an infant from total parenteral nutrition to a regular diet. Another modification of this formula (Table 8) provides 6% of the calories as fat in the form of linoleic acid with a glucose polymer as the carbohydrate. The formula has an osmolality of only 237 because of the use of the glucose oligosaccharide. Trace elements, minerals, and vitamins are added in order to meet recommended daily allowances. The formula is particularly promising for use in short bowel syndrome where fat malabsorption is generally the major abnormality present.

Pregestimil was introduced in 1971 to be used with infants who had severe malabsorption of protein, long-chain fatty acids, and disaccharides. It contained free amino acids and oligopeptides as well as medium-chain triglycerides and dextrose. The formula proved useful in a variety of GI problems in infants. However, the original osmolality of the Pregestimil® was 627 mOsm/kg of water. Because of the potential problems related to high osmolality, Pregestimil® formula has been changed by replacing the dextrose and some of the modified tapioca starch with corn syrup solids which contains approximately 75% of the carbohydrates as tetrasaccharides.[37] The content of the casein hydrolysate was reduced slightly and cystine, tryosine, and tryptophan were increased in the diet. The medium-chain triglyceride was decreased and corn oil was increased so that the longchain triglyceride now provides 60% of the fat calories. The resulting

Table 8
SPECIALIZED FORMULAS FOR USE IN PEDIATRIC PATIENTS

	Protein source	% kcal	CHO source	% kcal	Fat source	% kcal
Pregestimil®	Casein hydrolysate	11	85% corn syrup solids, 15% modified tapioca starch	54	40% MCT, 60% corn oil and soy lecithin	35
Modular Formula	Sodium caseinate	10	Glucose polymer	84	Safflower oil	6
Product 3232-A	Casein hydrolysate	13	Needs CHO added, 59 g/qt	50	88% MCT, 12% corn oil	37
Chicken-based protein	Strained chicken 200 g	16	Glucose polymer 72 g	45	23% LCT from chicken fat, 14% safflower oil	37

osmolality change was to 338 mOsm/kg of water. This formula has only recently been introduced but should be useful because of the lowered osmolality and the presentation of the carbohydrate in a form that should be easily transported across the small intestinal villus.

Larcher and co-workers[38] have advocated the use of a formula containing comminuted chicken plus long-chain triglyceride from chicken fat and a glucose polymer, with added electrolytes and trace elements and minerals for use in infants with intractable diarrhea. Table 9 shows the constituents of this formula when used for treatment in early infancy. The authors recommend using this diet in early infancy with intractable diarrhea for 2 to 3 months before reintroducing disaccharides and cow's milk protein. Thorn et al.[39] recently evaluated this diet with a mineral and trace metal supplement and demonstrated a positive balance of trace elements while on this particular formula. No other studies are available on the use of a comminuted chicken formula in pediatric patients. The formula is promising because of its ease of manufacture and its low cost.

Product 3232-A is the original Pregestimil® formula without added carbohydrate in either disaccharide or monsaccharide form. The product does contain modified tapioca starch which is used as a stablizer. The nitrogen source is still casein hydrolysate and 60% of the fat source is medium-chain triglycerides and corn oil. To prepare a formula which would provide 20 kcal/fl oz. 59 g of a carbohydrate must be added to one quart with water and 83.5 g of the Pregestimil® powder. This formula has little advantage over other products presently on the market as the new Pregestimil® formulation provides a decreased osmolality and other formulas are available which will give as high or higher concentration of medium-chain triglycerides in the diet.

XI. HOW TO USE ELEMENTAL DIETS AND SPECIALIZED FORMULAS IN PEDIATRIC PATIENTS

The majority of infants should be given continuous infusion of the elemental diet over a 24-hr period for several days to weeks before contemplating feeding these formulas by bolus or nipple. Gastrostomy or infant feeding tubes should be used. The feeding tubes should usually be size 5 to 9 French and are generally either made of silicone or polyurethane compounds. Several brands are available for use in pediatric patients and include Keofeed (Headco, Inc., California) and Dobbhoff (Biosearch Medical Products, Inc., New Jersey). These tubes can be generally introduced into the stomach through the nasogastric passage without difficulty. It is important to check patency and positon by X-ray prior to starting the infusion of the formula. At times, a wire guide may be needed for proper placement of the tube in the stomach. The Cook-Blaslabel wire guide can be used for placement of tubes.

Formula is usually begun at one third concentration at a rate of 50 mℓ/kg/day. The rate can be gradually increased as tolerated to 165 cc/kg/day by approximately 96 hr. The patient must be observed for glucosuria or diarrhea when the diet is first begun. In the absence of diarrhea and glucosuria, the rate can be increased on a 24-hr basis until adequate rate and strength are achieved. The rate of infusion and the concentration of the formula should never be increased at the same time. Continuous-drip formulas are best administered by an infusion pump to avoid excess infusion into the stomach and to provide adequate drip rates. During the period of transition from a dilute concentration to the concentration which will provide adequate calories, stool frequency, and weight should be recorded daily. The majority of stools should be tested for reducing substances with a Clinitest® tablet and for pH with a Nitrazine Paper. The recognition of reducing substances greater than 1% to 2% is an indication that the diet is being advanced too rapidly.

There are many potential complications that can occur with continuous infusion of specialized formulas. Proper placement of the tube is essential to decrease the possibility of aspiration. Infants and small children should have the head of their bed elevated during the time of infusion. Any symptoms that are compatible with aspiration should necessitate stopping the infusion and removing the tube immediately. Diarrhea is the most common side effect of continuous enteral nutrition. Dumping syndrome secondary to high osmolality can be elminated or decreased by starting out at a very dilute concentration at a rate less than the daily fluid requirement. Metabolic and complications include hyperosmolar hyperglycemic nonketotic dehydration, fluid overload, and serum electrolyte abnormalities. In the beginning, electrolyte and glucose levels should be monitored frequently. If the infant is having a large amount of liquid stool during the infusion, electrolyte concentrations in the stools should be monitored; and additional fluids and electrolytes should be given intravenously during the period of adaptation. Antidiarrheal agents such as Lomotil® or Loperamide are to be discouraged because of the risk of causing ileus with abdominal distention and collection of fluid intraluminally. Basic monitoring must include strict intake and output plus daily weights and urine checks, as mentioned above, for glucose and reducing substances (Table 9). Besides the measurement of electrolytes and glucose, BUN on a twice-weekly basis is indicated during the early continuous infusion technique.

Table 9
ALIMENTATION FLOW SHEET

Case No.

Name

B-Date

F18-18 I-1 11-78

	FORMULA	DEXTROSE SOLUTIONS				AMINO ACID SOLUTIONS									INTRALIPID
	Full Strength Formula	D5W	D10W	D15W	D20W	4.25%	2.125%	2.125% D10W	2.125% D15W	2.125% D20W	2.125% D25W	4.25% D10W	4.25% D20W	4.25% D25W	10%
CAL/CC	0.66	0.17	0.35	0.52	0.69	0.11	0.05	0.40	0.58	0.75	0.90	0.45	0.80	0.98	1.10

INTAKE													OUTPUT			URINE TESTS			
DATE	WT.	TYPE OF FORMULA	DIET CC'S	PO CAL	IV CC'S	IV CAL	HA CC'S	HA CAL	IL CC'S	IL CAL	TOTAL CC KG	TOTAL CAL KG	URINE	STOOL	GAST DRG	RS	ACE	PRO	SG

REFERENCES

1. **Grant, A.,** *Nutritional Assessment Guidelines,* 2nd ed., Cutter Laboratories, Berkeley, 1979.
2. **Zerfas, A. J., Shorr, I. J., and Neumann, C. G.,** Office assessment of nutritional status, *Pediatr. Clin. North Am.,* 24, 253, 1977.
3. **Fomon, S. J.,** *Nutritional Disorders of Children,* U.S. Department of Health, Education, and Welfare (HSA) 76-5612, Rockville, Md., 1976.
4. **Kanawati, A. A. and McLaren, D. S.,** Assessment of marginal malnutrition, *Nature,* 228, 574, 1970.
5. American Academy of Pediatrics, Committee on Nutrition, Nutritional needs of low-birth-weight infants, *Pediatrics,* 60, 519, 1977.
6. **Snyderman, S. E.,** The protein and amino acid requirements of the premature infant, in *Metabolic Processes in the Foetus and Newborn Infant,* Jonxis, J. H. P., Vesser, H. R. A., and Troelstra, J. A., Eds., William and Wilkins, Baltimore, 1971.
7. **Sturman, J. A., Gaull, G., and Raiha, N. C. R.,** Absence of cystathionase in human fetal liver: Is cystine essential?, *Science,* 169, 74, 1970.
8. **Valman, H. B., Brown, R. J. K., Palmer, T.,** et al. Protein intake and plasma amino acids of infants of low birth weight, *Br. Med. J.,* 4, 789, 1971.
9. **Fosbrooke, A. S. and Wharton, B. A.,** "Added lactose" and "added sucrose" cow's milk formulae in nutrition of low birth-weight babies, *Arch. Dis. Child.,* 50, 409, 1975.
10. **Sunshine, P., Sinatra, F. R., and Mitchell, C. H.,** Intractable diarrhoea of infancy, *Clin. Gastroenterol.,* 6, 445, 1977.
11. **Balistreri, W. F., Partin, J. C., and Schubert, W. K.,** Bile acid malabsorption — A consequence of terminal ileal dysfunction in protracted diarrhea of infancy, *J. Pediatr.,* 89, 21, 1977.
12. **Greene, H. L., McCabe, D. R., and Merenstein G. B.,** Protracted diarrhea and malnutrition in infancy: Changes in intestinal morphology and disaccharidase activities during treatment with total intravenous nutrition or oral elemental diets, *J. Pediatr.,* 87, 695, 1975.
13. **Sherman, J. O., Hamly, C. -A., and Khachadurian, A. K.,** Use of an oral elemental diet in infants with severe intractable diarrhea, *J. Pediatr.,* 86, 518, 1975.
14. **Lindblad, B. S., Rahimtoola, R. J., Hafiz-ur-Rehman, Ahmad, S. S., Fancy, K., Singha, L., and Hussain, S. S.,** Plasma free amino acid levels during the initial rehabilitation of protein-energy malnutrition with protracted diarrhoea using a free amino acid-glucose diet, *Acta Paediatr. Scand.,* 67, 335, 1978.
15. **Bohane, T. D., Haka-Ilse, K., Biggar, W. D., Hamilton, J. R, and Gall, D. G.,** A clinical study of young infants after small intestinal resection, *J. Pediatr.,* 94, 552, 1979.
16. **Feldman, E. J., Dowling, R. H., McNaughton, J.,** et al., Effect of oral versus intravenous nutrition on intestinal adaptation of small bowel resection in the dog, *Gastroenterology,* 70, 712, 1976.
17. **Christie, D. L. and Ament, M. E.,** Dilute elemental diet and continuous infusion technique for managenent of short bowel syndrome, *J. Pediatr.,* 87, 705, 1975.

18. **Hartline, J. V.,** Continuous intragastric infusion of elemental diet: Experiences with ten infants having small-intestinal diseases, *Clin. Pediatr.*, 16, 1105, 1977.
19. **Ricour, C.,** Constant rate enteral nutrition, A transition from total parenteral nutrition to voluntary intake, in *Total Parenteral Nutrition. Premises and Promises*, Ghadimi, H., Ed., John Wiley & Sons, New York, 1975, 601.
20. **Whitington, P. F. and Gibson, R.,** Soy protein intolerance: Four patients with concomitant cow's milk intolerance, *Pediatrics*, 59, 730, 1977.
21. **Iyngkaran, N., Davis, K., Robinson, J. J., Boey, C. G., Sumithran, E., Yadav, M., Lam., S. K., and Puthucheary, S. D.,** Cow's milk protein-sensitive enteropathy, *Arch. Dis. Child.*, 54, 39, 1979.
22. **Galant, S. P., Franz, M. L., Walker, P., Wells, I. D., and Lundak, R. L.,** A potential diagnostic method for food allergy: clinical application and immunogenicity evaluation of an elemental diet, *Am. J. Clin. Nutr.*, 30, 512, 1977.
23. **Eastham, E. J., Lichauco, T., Grady, M. I., and Walker, W. A.,** Antigenicity of infant formulas: role of immature intestine on protein permeability, *J. Pediatr.*, 93, 561, 1978.
24. **Inygkaran, N., Abdin, Z., Davis, K., Boey, C. G., Prathap, K., Yadav, M., Lam., S. K., and Puthucheary, S. D.,** Acquired carbohydrate intolerance and cow milk protein-sensitive enteropathy in young infants, *J. Pediatr.*, 95, 373, 1979.
25. **Rosekrans, P. C. M., Meijer, C. J. L. M., Cornelisse, C. J., van der Wal, A. M., and Lindeman, J.,** Use of morphometry and immunohistochemistry of small intestinal biopsy specimens in the diagnosis of food allergy, *J. Clin. Pathol.*, 33, 125, 1980.
26. **Baker, A. L. and Rosenberg, I. H.,** Refractory sprue: Recovery after removal of nongluten dietary proteins, *Ann. Intern. Med.*, 89, 505, 1978.
27. **Burr, I. M., O'Neill, J. A., Karzon, D. T., Howard, L. J., and Greene, H. L.,** Comparison of the effects of total parenteral nutrition, continuous intragastric feeding, and protacaval shunt on a patient with type I glycogen storage disease, *J. Pediatr.*, 85, 792, 1974.
28. **Greene, H. L., Slonim, A. E., Burr, I. M., and Moran, J. R.,** Type I glycogen storage disease: Five years of management with nocturnal intragastric feeding, *J. Pediatr.*, 96, 590, 1980.
29. **Chase, H. P., Long, M. A., and Lavin, M. H.,** Cystic fibrosis and malnutrition, *J. Pediatr.*, 95, 337, 1979.
30. **Allan, J. D., Mason, A., and Moss, A. D.,** Nutritional supplementation in treatment of cystic fibrosis of the pancreas, *Am. J. Dis. Child.*, 126, 22, 1973.
31. **Yassa, J. G., Prosser, R., and Dodge, J. A.,** Effects of an artificial diet on growth of patients with cystic fibrosis, *Arch. Dis. Child.*, 53, 777, 1978.
32. **Bradley, J. A., Axon, A. T. R., and Hill, G. L.,** Nocturnal elemental diet for retarded growth in a patient with cystic fibrosis, *Br. Med. J.*, 1, 167, 1979.
33. American Academy of Pediatrics, Committee on Nutrition, Special diets for infants with inborn errors of amino acid metabolism, in *Pediatric Nutrition Handbook*, O'Brien, D. and Forbes, G. B., Eds., American Academy of Pediatrics, Evanston, Ill., 1979, 219.
34. Editorial, Hypertonic elemental feeding of very premature infants and necrotizing enterocolitis, *Nutr. Rev.*, 34, 135, 1976.
35. **Burke, V., Kerry, K. R., and Anderson, C. M.,** The relationship of dietary lactose to refractory diarrhoea in infancy, *Aust. Paediatr. J.*, 1, 147, 1965.
36. **Klish, W. J., Potts, E., Ferry, G. D., and Nichols, B. L.,** Modular Formula: An approach to management of infants with specific or complex food intolerance, *J. Pediatr.*, 88, 948, 1976.
37. **Graham, G. G., Klein, G. L., and Cordano, A.,** Nutritive value of elemental formula with reduced osmolality, *Am. J. Dis. Child.*, 133, 795, 1979.
38. **Larcher, V. F., Shepherd, R., Francis, D. E. M., and Harries, J., T.,** Protracted diarrhoea in infancy, *Arch. Dis. Child.*, 52, 597, 1977.
39. **Thorn, J. M., Aggett, P. J., Delves, H. T., and Clayton, B. E.,** Mineral and trace metal supplement for use with synthetic diets based on comminuted chicken, *Arch. Dis. Child.*, 53, 931, 1978.

Chapter 17

OTHER USES OF ELEMENTAL DIETS

R. I. Russell

TABLE OF CONTENTS

I. INTRODUCTION

In this chapter various other potential uses of elemental diets are considered. These include the following:

- Preparation of the colon for diagnostic procedures
- Allergies and immunological problems
- Phenylketonuria and mental deficiency
- Kwashiorkor
- Obesity
- Hepatic insufficiency and failure
- Renal disease

II. PREPARATION OF THE COLON FOR DIAGNOSTIC PROCEDURES

Elemental diets have minimal residue and this property may be utilized in the preparation of the colon for diagnostic procedures such as colonic radiology and colonoscopy. For these procedures it is essential that the colon is empty of feces for effective examination to be made.

Standard low residue diets given for up to 5 days prior to the examination have been used for many years in the preparation of patients for these procedures. Castor oil on the day prior to the examination and an enema on the morning of the test are widely used in the preparation for colonic radiology. The effectiveness of these standard preparatory procedures is directly related to the cooperation of the patient in taking the low residue diet for the required number of days and the medical or nursing staff administering an enema on the morning of the examination. Poor preparation is quite commonly a problem leading to poor results from the procedures. If a patient takes a chemically defined diet for several days prior to the examination good bowel preparation might be expected. The use of the elemental diet Vivonex® in the preparation of patients for colonic radiology has been successfully reported by Pincus[1] and Bunte,[2] although in neither case was a controlled study performed.

The preparation of the colon for colonoscopy has also proved to be a problem and several alternative regimes have been considered. A low residue diet, castor oil, and an enema on the morning of the procedure is widely used as a method of preparation[3] although whole gut irrigation is now used in some centers. The attraction of elemental diets is that they can be taken alone as a minimal residue dietary preparation which, over a few days, should lead to adequate preparation of the colon prior to the procedure. The use of a chemically defined diet for this purpose was reported by Dehyle and Demling.[4] A comparison of a standard low residue duet with the elemental diet Vivonex®, both administered for 5 days prior to colonoscopy, was reported by Teague and colleagues.[3] Both diets were found to be equally effective in producing a reasonably clean bowel for total colonoscopy. The satisfactory use of a peptide-based elemental diet for this purpose was also reported by Semler[5] in 1976.

A. Conclusions

Elemental diets, by virtue of their minimal residue nature, may be of value in the preparation of the colon for colonic radiology and colonoscopy, being given over a few days prior to the procedure being performed. Although it would appear that an elemental diet used in this way may be as good as a standard low residue diet, more specific preparation of the colon for colonoscopy with diet, castor oil, enema, or whole gut irrigation may prove to be more effective and practical in most cases, and controlled prospective studies are required. If a chemically defined diet is no more effective or practical than a standard low residue diet in colonic preparation, it may not find a regular place for this purpose as it is more expensive than a standard low residue diet. In general, effectiveness of colonic preparation for procedures such as colonoscopy and colonic radiology is directly related to the commitment of staff and patient to good preparative procedures, together with the availability of space for the preparation to be performed. These factors are more important than the specific mode of preparation used. Prospective controlled data is required to further study the place of elemental diets in colonic preparation.

III. ALLERGIES AND IMMUNOLOGICAL PROBLEMS

Early studies on elemental diets suggested that they might have hypoallergenic properties.[6] The effect of elemental diets on immunological mechanisms has been discussed in Chapter 8. All the work reported so far relates to animals and there is some evidence suggesting that the elemental diet, Vivonex®, when given to mice from shortly after birth, results in impaired humoral immunity, although cell-mediated immunity apparently remains unaltered. The results in animals may have little relevance to man as the animal models used in these studies bears more relationship to the development of immunological mechanisms in animals than to disease processes in man. No comparable information is available in the human subject, either in the normal state or in disease processes.

Elemental diets, because of their hypoallergenic effect, may have a part to play in the diagnosis and management of conditions associated with food allergy. They have also been considered as possible therapeutic agents in the management of diseases considered to have an immunological basis, such as coeliac disease and the nephrotic syndrome. The possible value of an elemental diet in the early management of patients with coeliac disease has been discussed in Chapter 12. Their potential value in the idiopathic nephrotic syndrome of childhood has been reported in a study investigating hypersensitivity to protein in patients with this condition.[7] This possible use is further discussed later in this chapter in the subsection on renal disease.

An early report of the successful therapeutic use of a chemically defined diet in an allergic condition was in its use in a patient with anergy, dysimmunoglobulinemia, and unexplained inflammation.[8]

There have been individual reports of success in using the elemental diet Vivonex® as a diagnostic and therapeutic agent in patients suffering from food allergy. In one patient the symptoms disappeared and the use of the chemically defined diet allowed testing for responsible allergens without affecting the patient's oral intake, thus maintaining adequate nutritional status.[9] Vivonex® has also been used to investigate food sensitivities of a group of patients with non-Meniere's, sensorineural hearing loss.[10] At about the same time, an evaluation of Vivonex® in nine institutionalized perennial asthmatic boys with food allergy revealed no clinical nor physiological improvement after 12 days on the diet.[11] The use of chemically defined diets to determine allergic sensitivity has been further discussed[12] and its value as a potential method for investigating food allergy and in the therapy of this condition reported by Galant and colleagues[13] in 1977. In this study Vivonex® was used in 21 patients suspected of food allergy. The clinical study was conducted over a 2- to 3-week period with full symptom and laboratory evaluation; no consistent significant improvement of allergic manifestations was seen while the patients received Vivonex®, although no marked side effects were noted either clinically or by laboratory measurements. The immunogenicity of the diet was studied using rabbits and

Vivonex® found to be not immunogenic either by a precipitin reaction or by passive cutaneous anaphalactic response. This study concluded that further similar investigations of young allergic children with clear-cut food sensitivity were indicated and may be of value.

A more recent study of Vivonex® as a diagnostic aid in food sensitivity and in determining which foods are involved has now been reported.[14] In this study Vivonex® was used to provide complete nutritional support for a 1-week period in 27 patients considered to have food allergy. Seventy percent of the allergic symptoms were relieved, thus supporting a diagnosis of predominant food allergy in these patients. In these subjects the diet was continued while selected foods were challenged orally. Safe diets were thus established within a 3-week period. Remission was achieved in 85% of the cases. While allergy testing was underway the patient could be fed satisfactorily and effectively by the elemental diet, and normal nutritional status maintained or improved during this period.

The use of a chemically defined diet in the management of a patient with the Cronkhite-Canada Syndrome has also been reported.[15]

A. Conclusions

Elemental diets are hypoallergenic and may have some value in determining the presence of food allergy, and by the use of individual selected food challenges while on an elemental diet, individual foods responsible for the allergic response may be identified. At the same time the elemental diets allow good nutritional status to be maintained by the normal oral route.

There is no convincing evidence of the value of elemental diets in the management of these conditions over a prolonged period, although short term remission of symptoms may occur.

Further prospective and controlled studies are required to investigate the place of elemental diets in the diagnosis and management of food allergy, and in other conditions which may be associated with allergic phenomena and alterations of immunological function.

IV. PHENYLKETONURIA AND MENTAL DEFICIENCY

Nutritional deficiency due to inadequate intake of a good nutritive diet is frequently a problem in the management of children with phenylketonuria or mental deficiency. Chemically defined diets may have a theoretical value in such patients in that if administered either orally or by means of an intragastric or intrajejunal tube, they may maintain the patients in an adequate nutritional state.

Long term treatment of phenylketonuric children with a phenylalanine-free chemically defined diet has been shown to be of considerable benefit.[16-18] These children gained weight and a reduction in the size and frequency of bowel motions was achieved, leading to more efficient and satisfactory institutional care. The incidence of abdominal discomfort and flatulence was also reduced. The use of phenylalanine-free chemically defined diets has recently been described in a review of the dietary management of phenylketonuria.[19] This is further discussed in Chapter 16. The preparations described are either based on hydrolyzed protein such as casein, from which phenylalanine has been removed, or of mixtures of pure amino acids. They are generally used as supplements to provide full protein requirements. All the preparations have added tyrosine as the body normally obtains much of its tyrosine from the breakdown of excess phenylalanine.

A similar beneficial effect of the use of the elemental diet Vivonex® in 11 patients with severe mental deficiency has also been reported.[20]

The benefit of elemental diets in such conditions is related to the improvement of calorie intake of the patients by their taking adequate amounts of the elemental diet compared to normal food. Adequate nutritional status can be maintained with the use of the liquid elemental diet, given via an intragastric or intrajejunal tube. It is probable that a similar beneficial effect would be obtained by the use of whole protein liquid support diets.

A. Conclusions

Elemental diets have been used successfully in the nutritional support of children with phenylketonuria and patients with mental deficiency. Whereas the provision of phenylalanine - free chemically defined diets may be of great value in patients with phenylketonuria, the problem in mentally deficient subjects is that of adequate intake of food rather than any specific value which an elemental diet may itself provide for the patient. Other forms of enteral nutritional support may be equally effective in this group of mentally deficient patients.

V. KWASHIORKOR

Malnutrition in childhood is a major problem in developing countries. The two principal syndromes of protein-calorie malnutrition which predominantly affect young children are kwashiorkor and marasmus. Chronic calorie deficiency leads to marasmus and results in the gradual wasting of muscle and subcutaneous fat. Classical kwashiorkor is the result of a protein-deficient diet which provides an adequate supply of calories and is characterized clinically by growth retardation, edema, skin and hair changes, anorexia, apathy, and irritability. These conditions are also often associated with other nutritional deficiencies and infections.[21] One additional problem in the management of kwashiorkor is the extensive damage to intestinal structure which may occur and which leads to malabsorption.[22] Mucosal atrophy of the small and large intestines may occur[23,24] and pancreatic atrophy may also be a feature.[25] Malabsorption of carbohydrate, fat, protein, and water may follow, together with impaired activities of intestinal enzymes and marked growth retardation.[26] Secondary parasitic infestation of the intestinal tract may occur in these patients. Standard oral dietary intake often causes diarrhea.

Twenty-one children with kwashiorkor have recently been treated with an elemental diet.[26,27] Thirteen of the 21 were given Vivonex® and eight received a standard diet with cow milk protein concentrate (Casilan). The children given Vivonex® were noted to have significantly less vomiting and reached minimum satisfactory weight faster than the group on a standard diet. Weight gain and diarrhea were similar in both groups. The rise of albumin and blood urea nitrogen were faster on the standard diet but a significant increase in hemoglobin was seen only in those given the elemental diet. It was considered that the lower total nitrogen content of the elemental diet might explain the observed slower rise of albumin and blood urea nitrogen, but the ready utilization of the elemental diet was indicated by the favorable weight changes. The high glucose concentration in the experimental diet was considered to cause some negative effects, and it is possible that other elemental diets with a formula containing lower concentrations of glucose may be more effective in this respect. The elemental diet was thus more effective in the treatment of children with Kwashiorkor than standard nutritional support, although no comparison was made with complete oral whole protein liquid diets. There appeared to be no increased risk of parasitic infestation in patients treated with the elemental diet as might be suggested by the immunological changes which have been reported in animal studies and which are described earlier in this chapter.

A. Conclusions

The elemental diet Vivonex® has been shown to be of value in the management of children with Kwashiorkor. Its use in this respect appears to be better than standard diets, but there are no controlled studies comparing a chemically defined diet with whole protein enteral nutritional support; such prospective studies are required. The expense of a chemically defined diet may be a disadvantage in underdeveloped countries and the problems of administration and motivation of patients receiving such a diet requires a commitment of medical and nursing staff which may not be feasible in areas where Kwashiorkor is common.

However, the nutritional value of elemental diets in this respect appears to be of value and their use can be recommended in this situation pending further data on the use of other forms of nutritional support.

VI. OBESITY

Total starvation has been advocated in the management of severe obesity when other methods fail.[28] However, there have been doubts regarding the long-term usefulness and safety of prolonged starvation.[29,30] Loss of lean body mass during starvation may be as great as the loss from the fat depots, and electrocardiographic changes suggestive of decreased heart size have been reported. Provision of a long-term low-calorie regime in the form of an elemental diet (based on Vivonex®) to correct the loss of lean body mass and avoid changes caused by negative nitrogen balance in total starvation has been reported.[31] In this study, five markedly obese subjects were treated for up to 1 year with the chemically defined diet Vivonex.® The optimal daily formulation containing 15 g amino acids and 30 to 45 g carbohydrate achieved positive nitrogen balance, only moderate ketosis, normal serum electrolytes and resulted in a mean weight loss of 1.8 kg/week. During treatment, patients developed postural hypotension and hypercholesterolemia. These findings reverted to normal on resuming a normal diet. This report suggests that an elemental diet may offer a more acceptable and safer form of weight reduction than complete starvation in patients with refractory obesity.

Vivonex® has also been used successfully for weight reduction prior to surgery so as to improve lung function and diminish operative risks.[32]

A. Conclusions

The management of severe and refractory obesity is unsatisfactory. Both total starvation and jejuno-ileal bypass surgery are potentially hazardous procedures and severe complications have followed both forms of treatment. The use of an elemental diet, provided committed administration is applied, may be helpful in the management of such patients, and should be considered as an alternative form of treatment. Prospective studies comparing chemically defined diets with other methods of managing such patients are required.

VII. HEPATIC INSUFFICIENCY AND FAILURE

Patients with hepatic insufficiency and hepatic failure, particularly those associated with alcohol, may also have nutritional deficiency. There are multiple causes for this in most patients, including poor oral nutritional intake and damaged small intestinal absorption mechanisms. The management of nutritional deficiency in hepatic disease is difficult because of the danger of overloading the liver with protein provided in any form of nutritional support which might be deemed necessary. The overriding issue in the management of such patients is prevention of protein overload of the liver but the problem of nutritional insufficiency is frequently not considered, especially in the initial phases of treatment. However, nutritional support is also important. Chemically defined diets as a nutritional source may have a theoretical place in the management of such patients in that ammonia-producing organisms in the colon may be reduced by their use.[33]

There have been few studies of the nutritional status of patients with hepatic insufficiency whether or not the cause is related to excessive alcohol ingestion, and thus little information is available as to the best way of improving nutritional deficiency which may be present in such patients. In one report, Muting treated four patients with hepatic cirrhosis and hyperammonemia exclusively with the chemically defined diet Vivonex®.[34] The nutritional status of the patients improved and a reduction of the blood ammonia level was achieved. This study was uncontrolled and more information is required on the effect of nutritional support of any kind, including elemental diets, in such patients.

A. Conclusions

Although there is no convincing evidence of any beneficial effect of chemically defined diets in patients with hepatic insufficiency, more information is required on the nutritional status of patients with hepatic disease, hepatic insufficiency, and encephalopathy, particularly those associated with excessive alcohol ingestion. When such data is available, and if nutritional deficiency defined by clinical and biochemical parameters shown to be a feature of such patients, then more information will require to be obtained on the value of particular nutritional support systems in the treatment of any deficiency which is present. At that stage there may be a case for controlled prospective studies on the value of elemental diets in such patients.

VIII. RENAL DISEASE

Elemental diets in which the protein is presented as amino acids have been suggested as being of possible value in the management of patients with chronic renal failure, acute renal failure, and the nephrotic syndrome.

Low protein diets have been an important feature of the management of chronic renal failure for many years. Controlled dietary treatment allows restriction of protein intake, definition of the type of protein ingested, maintenance of adequate energy intake from fat and carbohydrate sources and control of fluid and electrolyte intake.[35] Treatment with low protein diets leads to improvement of uremic symptoms and biochemical improvement. However, many of these patients may lose weight and become nutritionally deficient with the development of a negative nitrogen balance. This is generally related to a failure to ingest adequate amounts of the planned dietary regime. An oral elemental diet with nitrogen provided as amino acids has been shown to be successful in bringing patients into positive nitrogen balance.[36] In this study, an amino acid substituted diet was used in the form of tablets with a total nitrogen intake of 50 mg/kg body weight; a high energy intake of 55 kcal/kg body weight was achieved. Patients on long-term amino acid supplements or amino acid-substituted diets in chronic renal failure have also been reported to utilize the essential amino acids in protein synthesis, and exhibit no signs of protein depletion.[37] Complications such as peripheral neuropathy and a bleeding tendency are not seen on amino acid supplemented or substituted diets, but may occur in patients on long-term treatment with low-protein diets. These diets may thus be of some value in the management of chronic renal failure, when conservative management is indicated, and may be a useful dietary adjunct to hemodialysis.

The nutritional support of patients with acute renal failure has also been extensively studied, with particular reference to the value of intravenous nutrition. Many of these patients develop a catabolic state similar to patients with severe trauma or infection. Some of these patients may catabolize between 100 and 120 g of protein per day or more, equivalent to 16 to 19 g nitrogen.[38,39] They may also require frequent dialysis which further exacerbates their negative nitrogen balance. Intravenous nutrition providing essential and nonessential amino acids, and hypertonic glucose has been shown to be of value in the management of these patients.[40,41] Amino acid substituted diets of an elemental nature have also been shown to be of value in some of these individuals. Further work, however, is required to assess the value of this type of treatment in acute renal failure.

Elemental diets have also been used in six patients with the idiopathic nephrotic syndrome of childhood.[7] In these subjects, after initial treatment with prednisolone, elemental diet therapy (either Vivonex® or Flexical®) was given as sole diet. After proteinuria had decreased to a level less than 500 mg/24 hr on consecutive days, the patients were challenged with cow's milk, which resulted in the return of proteinuria and edema. Milk challenge was accompanied by acute alteration of plasma C3 complement component. Utilization of the hypoallergenic properties of elemental diets in this way in these patients suggest that in some individuals the nephrotic syndrome of childhood may be related to food hypersensitivity. As this study suggests that food allergens may be involved in the causation of symptoms in those patients, it is possible that longer-term treatment with an elemental diet may be of value, not only in the diagnosis, but also in the management, of some patients with the nephrotic syndrome. Further controlled work is required of the use of elemental diets in this group of patients.

A. Conclusions

Amino acid supplemented or substituted diets of elemental type may be of value in some individuals with chronic renal failure by providing a low protein diet while maintaining the patient in a good nutritional state. This treatment may be of some value when conservative management is indicated, or may be a useful adjunct to hemodialysis.

They may also be of help in acute renal failure of hypercatabolic type when nutritional support is required. Intravenous support may, however, be of more immediate value in that group of patients.

Elemental diets, by means of their hypoallergenic property, may be of value in the diagnosis and management of some patients with the nephrotic syndrome associated with hypersensitivity. More information is required on this possible use of elemental diets, especially under controlled conditions.

REFERENCES

1. **Pincus, I. J., Citron, B. P., and Haverback, B. J.,** Nutritional support of gastrointestinal problems with Vivonex 100 in a *Balanced Nutrition and Therapy*, Lang, K., Fekl, W., and Berg, G., Eds., Thieme, Stuttgart, 1971, 77.
2. **Bunte, H.,** Chemically defined diet during pre-operative preparation in *Balanced Nutrition and Therapy*, Lang, K., Fekl, W., and Berg, G., Eds., Thieme, Stuttgart, 1971, 124.
3. **Teague, R. H., Salmon, P. R., and Read, A. E.,** Fibreoptic examination of the colon. A review of 255 cases, *Gut*, 14, 139, 1973.

4. **Deyhle, P. and Demling, L.,** Colonoscopy — technique, results, indications, *Endoscopy,* 3, 143, 1971.
5. **Semler, P.,** Koloskopievorbereitung mit einer neuen vollbilanzierten, ballastfreien Peptiddiat, *Infusionstherapie,* 3, 216, 1976.
6. **Winitz, M. and Adams, R. F.,** Chemically defined diets. A new approach to metabolic nutrition in *Balanced Nutrition and Therapy,* Lang, K., Fekl, W., and Berg, G., Eds., Thieme, Stuttgart, 1971, 46.
7. **Sandberg, B. H., MacIntosh, R. M., Bernstein, C. W., Carr, R., and Strauss, J.,** Severe steroid-response of nephrosis associated with hypersensitivity, *Lancet,* 1, 388, 1977.
8. **Buckley, C. E.,** Anergy, dysimmunoglobulinaemia and unexplained inflammation. A new therapeutic approach with a chemically defined diet, *J. Allergy,* 44, 355, 1969.
9. **Berggren, E.,** Chemically defined diet (CDD) as a diagnostic and therapeutic aid in food allergy, *Infusionstherapie,* 2, 179, 1975.
10. **Hughes, E. C.,** Chemically defined diet in the diagnosis of food sensitivity. 1. With a panel of hearing impaired, *Trans. Am. Soc. Ophthalmol. Otolaryngol. Allergy,* 15, 60, 1975.
11. **Abrishami, M. A., Chai, H., Lynch, H. R., Miklich, D., and Denise, B.,** Evaluation of an elemental allergen free diet in chronic parennial asthmatic children, *J. Allerg. Clinical Immunol.,* 55, 85, 1975.
12. **Anon.,** Synthetic food diet shown effective as means to determine allergic sensitivities, *University of Southern California Health Science Record,* 1976, 8.
13. **Galant, S. P., Franz, M. L., Walker, P., Wells, I. D., and Lundak, R. L.,** A potential diagnostic method for food allergy: clinical application and immunogenicity evaluation of an elemental diet, *Am. J. Clin. Nutr.,* 30, 512, 1977.
14. **Hughes, E. C.,** Use of a chemically defined diet in the diagnosis of food sensitivities and the determination of offending foods, *Ann. Allergy,* 40, 393, 1978.
15. **Kindblom, L. G., Angervall, L., Santesson, B., and Selander, S.,** Cronkhite-Canada Syndrome. Case report, *Cancer,* 39, 2651, 1977.
16. **McKean, C. M.,** Growth of phenylketonuric children on a chemically defined diet, *Lancet,* 1, 148, 1970.
17. **McKean, C. M.,** The long-term effects of chemically defined diets on ambulatory phenylketonurics and bed-ridden severely retarded patients, in *Balanced Nutrition and Therapy,* Lang, K., Fekl, W., and Berg, G., Eds., Thieme, Stuttgart, 1971, 66.
18. **McKean, C. M.,** Effects of totally synthetic low phenylalanine diet on adolescent phenylketonuric patients, *Arch. Dis. Child.,* 46, 608, 1971.
19. **Coutts, J.,** The dietary management of phenylketonuria, *Proc. Nutr. Soc.,* 38, 315, 1979.
20. **Last, G.,** Experiences with Biosorbin MCT and Vivonex 100 in oligophenia. in *Balanced Nutrition and Therapy,* Lang, K., Fekl, W., and Berg, G., Eds., Thieme, Stuttgart, 1971, 126.
21. **Whitehead, R. G.** and **Alleyne, G. A. O.,** Pathophysiological factors of importance in protein-calorie malnutrition, *Br. Med. Bull.,* 28, 72, 1972.
22. **Herskovic, T.,** Protein malnutrition and the small intestine, *Am. J. Clin. Nutr.,* 22, 300, 1969.
23. **Stanfield, J. P., Hutt, M. S. R., and Tunnicliffe, R.,** Intestinal biopsy in Kwashiorkor, *Lancet,* 2, 519, 1965.
24. **Redmond, A. O. B., Kaschula, R. O. C., Freeseman, C., and Hansen, J. D. L.,** The colon in Kwashiorkor, *Arch. Dis. Child.,* 46, 252, 1968.
25. **Barbezat, G. O. and Hansen, J. D. L.,** The exocrine pancreas and protein-calorie malnutrition, *Paediatrics,* 42, 77, 1968.
26. **Habte, D., Persson, B., and Sterky, G.,** Chemically defined diets in the treatment of Kwashiorkor, *Acta Paediat. Scand.,* 64, 267, 1975.
27. **Persson, B., Demissie, H.,** and **Sterky, G.,** Chemically defined diet in the treatment of Kwashiorkor, *Infusionstherapie,* 3, 34, 1975.
28. **Bloom, W. L.,** Fasting as an introduction to the treatment of obesity, *Metabolism,* 8, 214, 1959.
29. **Spencer, I. O. B.,** Death during therapeutic starvation for obesity, *Lancet,* 1, 1288, 1968.
30. **Kahan, A.,** Death during therapeutic starvation, *Lancet,* 1, 1378, 1968.
31. **McLean Baird, I., Parsons, R. L., and Howard, A. N.,** Clinical and metabolism studies of chemically defined diets in the management of obesity, *Metabolism,* 23, 645, 1974.
32. **Bode, H. H., Botstein, P. M., Crawford, J. D., and Russell, P. S.,** Vergleich Mudizinischer und Chirurgischer Behandlung der Hypothalamischen Fettsucht im Kindesaltr, *Infusionstherapie,* 3, 7, 1975.
33. **Glotzer, D. J.,** Space diets, *Gastroenterology,* 61, 405, 1971.
34. **Muting, D.,** Influence of diets on liver insufficiency, in *Balanced Nutrition and Therapy,* Lang, K., Fekl, W., and Berg, G., Eds., Thieme, Stuttgart, 1971, 114.
35. **Lee, H. A.,** The nutritional management of renal diseases, in *Nutrition in the clinical Management of Disease,* Dickerson, J. W. T. and Lee, H. A., Eds., Edward Arnold, London, 1978, 210.
36. **Lee, H. A., Down, P. F., Fowell, E., and Hyne, B. E. H.,** Amino acid tablet substituted diets in the management of chronic renal failure, *Nutr. Metabol.,* 17, 154, 1974.
37. **Noree, L. O. and Bergström, J.,** Treatment of chronic uraemic patients with protein poor diet and oral supply of essential amino acids. II. Clinical results of long-term treatment, *Clin. Nephrol.,* 3, 195, 1975.

38. **Cameron, J. S., Ogg, C., and Trounce, J. R.,** Peritoneal dialysis in hypercatabolic acute renal failure, *Lancet,* 1, 1188, 1967.
39. **Silva, H., Pomeroy, J., Rae, A. I., Rosen, S. M., and Shaldon, S.,** Daily haemodialysis in 'hypercatabolic' acute renal failure, *Brit. Med. J.,* 2, 407, 1964.
40. **Blackburn, G. L., Etter, G., and MacKenzie, I.,** Criteria for choosing amino acid therapy in acute renal failure, *Am. J. Clin. Nutr.,* 31, 1841, 1978.
41. **Lee, H. A.,** The application of parenteral nutrition to renal failure patients. in *Current Concepts in Parenteral Nutrition,* Greep, J. M., Soeters, P. B., Wesdrop, R. I. C., Phaf, C. W. R., and Fischer, J. E., Eds., Martinus Nijhoff Medical Division, The Hague, Netherlands, 1977, 217.

Chapter 18

ADMINISTRATION AND HAZARDS OF ELEMENTAL DIETS

M. J. Hall and R. I. Russell

TABLE OF CONTENTS

I. INTRODUCTION

Elemental diets have been in widespread clinical use for over a decade. Their safety which was demonstrated by initial studies,[1,2,3] has been confirmed, subject to certain guidelines for their administration being followed and provided that careful supervision and monitoring are undertaken.[4,5]

II. ADMINISTRATION

There are two routes of administration available — by mouth or by fine bore enteral catheter — and the route selected will depend on the indications for the diet. When used as a supplement to normal food, the oral route is more suitable. However, when the elemental diet is the source of nutrition and prolonged feeding is anticipated, administration via a fine-bore tube is desirable.[6] Stephens and colleagues[7] found that patients experienced difficulty taking more than 2000 kcal/day orally for periods longer than 5 or 6 days and advocated the use of an infant feeding tube thereafter.

A. Oral Route

The greatest problem in oral administration is poor patient compliance due to the unpalatability of the diets. The unpleasant proteinaceous smell is due to organic amino acids and only limited success has been achieved in disguising the taste by commercial flavorings.[4,8] It is not uncommon for patients to decline further treatment because of palatability problems.[9]

1. Flavorings

Flavorings are made available by the manufacturers of commercial elemental diets but it should be noted that these increase osmolality and alter the pH of the solutions.[10] Some workers have experimented with their own flavorings, adding fruit juices, teas, soups, and spices, but the use of some of these detracts from the "elemental" nature of the diet.[11,12]

Behl et al.[13] undertook an extensive testing program of flavors designed to mask and improve the taste acceptability of Vivonex-HN. Using a tasting panel of volunteers who rated each solution on a scale of acceptability from 1 to 10, they found that in general those sweetened with sodium saccharin were more acceptable than unsweetened solutions. The top-rated solution was flavored with a mixture of sodium saccharin, rum, strawberry, and raspberry flavors and produced a mean score of 6.34 which in terms of descriptive phraseology lay between "like slightly" and "like moderately". This compared with a mean score of 1.75 obtained by unflavored Vivonex-HN and of 1.43 curiously obtained by Vivonex-HN flavored with "beef broth", one of Eaton Laboratories' own flavors. A comparison of the top-rated flavoring with and without Vivonex-HN produced no statistical difference suggesting that the flavor had an effective masking ability.

2. Preparation and Administration

Before administering the diet the reasons for giving this type of therapy should be fully explained to the patient; close cooperation between clinician, nurse, and a dietitian is the key to success.[5] Elemental diets are available in powder form and are reconstituted with water to the desired strength. For oral use, full strength is approximately 25% weight per volume giving 1 kcal/mℓ. They can be mixed by hand or by an electric blender up to 24 hr before administration and should be stored in a refrigerator until required. Because of high osmolality, a diet is administered initially in half-strength solution, and gradually increased in amount and concentration over 2 or 3 days.[14] A free intake of water is allowed but the diet is given according to a rigid schedule. The total prescribed daily intake should be divided into eight feedings and given to the patient individually at two hour intervals.[15,16] The use of small medicine cups is recommended at the start of therapy and this will allow a number of different flavors to be tried.[14] When full dosage is reached, larger polystyrene cartons with plastic lids have been used satisfactorily.[15] The diet should be sipped slowly and in small quantities over the 2-hr period.

There is greater acceptability of the liquid diet if it is served chilled, made up with iced water, and ice cubes added to each carton. Alternatively it can be given as a sorbet which is achieved by allowing a deep frozen carton of the diet to stand for 24 hr in the ward refrigerator.[15] Other modes of presentation which give some variety to the diet include soups, broths, puddings,[16] "ice-lollies" and jellies.[5]

B. Fine Bore Catheter Route

The use of a fine bore catheter for gastrointestinal (GI) feeding is not a new concept. Fallis and Barron[17] reported their experience with polyethylene tubes with an outside diameter of 1.9 mm and found that they were well tolerated for several months. They used a simple gravity drip apparatus although mechanical pumps were also available.[18] Jejunostomy feeding using fine bore tubing is also well-established.[19] More recently the development of silicone elastomer catheters has increased their comfort for prolonged feeding.[20,21,22]

As elemental diets are reconstituted into homogenous, nonviscous solutions they are ideal for administration via fine bore tubes.[8] The use of the latter is essential when prolonged high concentration therapy is contemplated.[14,23,24,25]

1. Surgically Placed Catheters

If postoperative elemental nutrition is indicated, an appropriate catheter can be sited at the time of operation through an esophagostomy, gastrostomy, or jejunostomy depending on the circumstances. An esophagostomy tube may be inserted into the pyriform sinus and is an alternative to, and simpler to perform than, a gastrostomy.[22] This latter approach is particularly useful when prolonged feeding is likely to be required, and the diet may be administered directly with a Y-tube open to air to act as a "pop-off" valve to avoid aspiration in the event of inadvertant rapid infusion.[26] The gastrostomy can be expected to close quickly and spontaneously on removal of the tube.[22]

The problem of leakage encountered with the use of a gastrostomy can be avoided by jejunostomy which also has the advantage that the diets bypass the stomach, pancreas, and biliary tract. The standard jejunostomy was the subject of modification by Liffman and Randall[27] who used a smaller diameter Witzel tunnel and also tunnelled the catheter through the subcutaneous tissues of the abdominal wall. Further modification was described by Delaney et al.[28] who used a needle to enter the jejunal wall 10 cm distal to the ligament of Treitz. The needle is inserted full length in the seromuscular layer of jejunum before entering the lumen along which the catheter is passed via the needle. This technique allows the catheter to be removed without risk of leakage of intestinal contents and has been used successfully in several centers for the administration of elemental diets.[4,8]

2. Nasally Passed Catheters

Although large bore tubes are easier to pass than fine tubes, the latter are more comfortable and any initial reluctance on the part of the patient to undergo the procedure is rapidly forgotten and tolerance for long periods is customary. Nasoesophageal tubes have been advocated as being less likely to cause reflux than when the tip is in the stomach,[22] but most workers have used the nasogastric or nasojejunal routes.[6,24]

The flexibility of modern catheters sometimes allows them to coil in the esophagus when being passed.[29] This can be avoided by prefreezing the tube or using a stylet.[22] Several catheters have a mercury olive at the distal end which allows a greater ease of placement.[24] Alternatively passage can also be effected by placing the fine bore tube alongside a standard nasogastric tube and cupping both distal ends with one half of a large gelatine capsule.[14] The larger tube acts as a splint for the feeding tube facilitating passage into the stomach. After 2 hr or so the capsule will have dissolved and the large tube can be withdrawn leaving the feeding catheter in position.

The tube should be marked at approximately 55 cm and passage to this mark will enable it to reach well into the body of the stomach. That the catheter has passed safely into the stomach can be confirmed at the bedside by injecting 50 mℓ of air through the tube and auscultating over the left upper quadrant of the abdomen.[8] It is wise to use a radiopaque catheter so that its position can be checked by lateral radiograph of the chest before infusion of the diet.[26] If nasojejunal placement is required a further length of the feeding tube is passed into the stomach and an appropriate interval allowed for the catheter to negotiate the pylorus and travel to the jejunum. A plain radiograph of the abdomen for confirmation of correct positioning should be obtained before commencement of the infusion.[24] Alternatively, the whole procedure can be performed using intermittent radiographic screening if the facilities are available. Recently direct endoscopic placement of the catheter in the duodenum has been advocated.[30]

Both intragastric and intrajejunal administration of elemental diet have been widely used with good results but each route has disadvantages. A nasogastric tube is quicker and easier to pass but the hypertonicity of the solution leads to gastric retention. Bury has suggested that the stomach should be aspirated twice daily and the infusion discontinued for a few hours if the gastric aspirate exceeds 300 mℓ.[25] On the other hand, because of side effects related to hyperosmolality initial jejunal infusion should be more dilute.[23,25] In general the intrajejunal route seems superior.

C. Preparation and Administration

Infusion of the diet can be controlled by a gravity drip method,[29,31] or by a pump.[24,25,32-34] The former is simple but is less reliable on a busy general ward especially during the night when supervision is minimal.[14] The use of a pump is the more usual technique and permits administration of the diet during sleep, although adding to the total expense involved. A method claiming to allow controlled infusion without the use of a pump has been described, but although inexpensive, it is cumbersome and complex.[35]

The control afforded by a reliable pump allows continuous infusion of the diet over 18 to 24 hr. daily and this is undoubtedly the technique of choice in both adults and children.[8,24,26,34] It results in better patient tolerance of the diet,[32] and is more efficient in the use of nursing time than a bolus method,[31] which has been shown to significantly delay gastric emptying with the risk of nausea, vomiting, and aspiration.[36]

The preparation of the diet for tube feeding is similar to that for oral administration except that flavorings are not required. Infusion should be commenced with small volumes of dilute solutions, 5 to 10% weight per volume for jejunal administration and 10 to 15% for intragastric catheters,[23] although patients fed by the latter route may tolerate 25% solution from the beginning.[25] Concentration should be increased by 5 to 10% every 1 or 2 days up to the recommended strength of approximately 25%, although up to 55% solutions have been tolerated without unfavorable effects.[32,33] It is mandatory that free water is allowed and that the patient can respond to thirst especially when these higher concentrations are given.[25] An infusion rate of 50 mℓ/hr is used initially,[14] and increased stepwise, once increments in concentration are tolerated, to the prescribed volume of between 2 and 5 ℓ daily depending on requirements.[6,23]

Continuous and assiduous supervision throughout the period of feeding will prevent complications. Methods of monitoring have been fully described in Chapter 4.

III. HAZARDS

It is important to be aware of the potential hazards of elemental diet therapy so that early recognition will enable appropriate measures to be taken. Many of the problems encountered are common to all forms of enteral nutrition.[37]

A. Gastrointestinal Side Effects

Nausea, vomiting, abdominal cramps, and distension occur frequently but are usually minor problems that can be alleviated by a reduction in the rate of infusion.[14,23,38] Delayed gastric emptying has been demonstrated and is due in part to hypertonicity although the L-amino acid content may be contributory.[36] However, a comparison of nonelemental diets of varied osmolalities has shown no differences in gastric emptying rates which, it is suggested, may be determined by caloric density.[39] Gastric retention was not observed in 30 patients fed elemental diets when rate of administration was less than 125 mℓ/hr,[40] and the problem can be avoided entirely by bypassing the stomach with intrajejunal feeding.

It is uncommon for diarrhea to be more than mildly troublesome if administration is controlled, and concentration and volume increased gradually.[40] Occasionally hyperosmotic diarrhea occurs rapidly and can lead to prerenal failure,[14] with fecal loss of fluid exceeding the total gut intake.[37] In the case of severe diarrhea, the diet should be discontinued for 24 to 48 hr, antidiarrheal agents prescribed and parenteral rehydration undertaken if necessary. The diet can normally be resumed thereafter without difficulty.[32]

B. Disturbances of Water Balance

Fluid retention sufficient to cause a dilutional fall in hematocrit has been reported,[23] but this phenomenon is more commonly seen in association with intravenous nutrition.[25,40] Indeed a significant increase in total body water has been demonstrated after intravenous nutrition but not after elemental diet therapy in a recent study of changes in body composition.[41]

Symptoms of dumping can occur especially in those with ablation of the normal pyloric mechanism.[42,43]

The nature of the diets introduces the danger of osmotic diuresis secondary to hyperglycemia and glycosuria.[44] Hypertonic dehydration has been reported in adults and infants, and unrestricted access to water is mandatory if this complication is to be avoided.[25,26,32] Hyperosmolar nonketotic coma may occur on elemental diet therapy, although often there are other precipitating factors.[45] Diabetic patients and those with pancreatic insufficiency are particularly at risk.[46]

C. Insulin Deficiency

Many of the patients in whom elemental diets are indicated are catabolic and can be expected to have a relative insulin lack.[47] Hyperglycemia, due to the high carbohydrate concentration of the diet, can be a particular problem in patients with diabetes mellitus, pancreatic insufficiency and those on steroids.[42,46] Regular monitoring of urine and plasma glucose is necessary and adjustment of insulin dosage may be required.[44]

D. Aspiration

The incidence of aspiration during nasogastric administration is of the order of 3%,[48] but only one fatality directly attributable to this complication has been reported.[29] Although gastroesophageal reflux is frequently a problem of large caliber tube administration,[24] fine-bore catheters do not interfere with antireflux mechanisms.[26,40] Elderly, obtunded, and unconscious patients are most at risk particularly when there is a pulmonary problem.[22] The hazard can be minimized by slow pump-controlled continuous feeding to prevent accumulation in the stomach, by raising the head of the bed, sitting the patient at an angle of 30 degrees or administering the diet intrajejunally.[8,14,21,40]

E. Nutritional Complications

Hypoprothrombinemia was a potential hazard of long-term therapy with the elemental diets originally available.[10] Many of them contained no vitamin K and, in others, interaction between menadione and cysteine ethyl ester (which was subsequently removed from the diets) resulted in vitamin K deficiency and hemorrhagic states in rats.[48,49] They may also have caused depression of bacterial synthesis of vitamin K due to alteration of bacterial flora in the GI tract.[42] GI hemorrhage has been reported in man but there was no evidence that the diets were causally related.[25] Commercially available elemental diets today contain adequate amounts of vitamin K and hypoprothombinemia does not appear to be a problem.[44]

Trace elements such as zinc, copper, and manganese are present in small quantities which, although adequate for nondeficient patients, may be inadequate for those patients with conditions which result in trace element deficiency and in which elemental diets may be particularly indicated.[44,50,51] Other essential trace elements, such as chromium and cobalt, are not present at all and this may be an important consideration if therapy for prolonged periods is planned.[10,14]

Elemental diets differ in their fat content and long-term administration of the low fat preparations may lead to the cutaneous changes of essential fatty acid deficiency,[52] although biochemical evidence may occur sooner.[53]

Metabolic studies in infants have demonstrated elevation of plasma amino acids and aminoaciduria during administration of a high nitrogen preparation.[54] Compensated metabolic acidosis and a normochromic normocytic anemia were also observed in some patients.

Both hypernatremia and hyponatremia have been observed,[26,32] but problems with electrolyte imbalance are more likely to occur because of the underlying condition. Excess losses from GI fistulas can be replaced easily but elemental diets may be unsuitable when sodium restriction is required in renal and/or hepatic disease.[10] Nutritional complications and deficiencies are more likely to be related to the underlying disease process than to the elemental diet therapy.

F. Effects on Specific Organs

Hepatic enzyme abnormalities have been reported with elevated aspartate and alanine aminotransferase and alkaline phosphatase levels, although they are often transient and only variably seen.[26,48,54] Studies of hepatic histology in rats fed elemental diets showed quite marked fatty infiltration in those fed standard Vivonex® compared to other preparations, although slight fatty change was also found with Flexical®.[55,62]

Necrotizing enterocolitis is an uncommon but serious complication in at-risk infants, and caution must be exerted on initiation of any type of hyperosmolar feeding including elemental diets in such patients.[34] The incidence of fecal impaction is unknown but the low residue nature of the diets and resulting infrequent bowel motions can be troublesome in some patients.[22] No information is available as to the effects on the myoelectric and mechanical activitiy of the small intestine in man although both are reduced in dogs fed an elemental diet,[56] and colonic mucosal atrophy in rats has been observed.[57]

Pancreatic acinar atrophy and fibrosis may occur in animals,[58,59] but autopsy studies in man have revealed no increase in pancreatic fibrosis in those fed elemental diets compared to a control group of patients with similar disease states. In both groups the changes were thought to be secondary to malnutrition.[48]

Transient skin rashes have occasionally been observed,[25] and if persistent, essential fatty acid or zinc deficiency should be excluded.[52]

G. Susceptibility to Drugs

Elemental diets appear to increase the GI toxicity of 5-Fluorouracil in rats,[60,61] and this important observation may be relevant to the use of cytotoxic agents in man and requires further study.

Colonic pseudo-obstruction was noted after an antidiarrheal agent containing diphenoxylate and atropine was prescribed for diarrhea resulting from elemental diet therapy.[37]

H. Conclusions

Flavorings, different modes of presentation, and encouragement to take small regular doses throughout the day are necessary for successful oral administration of elemental diets. For total nutritional support, continuous pump-controlled feeding via a fine bore catheter enables adequate quantities to be administered. The main hazards arise from the hyperosmolality and high carbohydrate content of the diets. Unrestricted access to water, regular monitoring of urine and plasma glucose, and careful supervision throughout the period of feeding allow elemental diets to be given for prolonged periods with a high degree of safety.

REFERENCES

1. **Winitz, M., Seedman, D. A., and Graff, J.,** Studies in metabolic nutrition employing chemically defined diets. I. Extended feeding of normal human adult males, *Am. J. Clin. Nutr.*, 23, 525, 1970.
2. **Winitz, M., Graff, J., Gallagher, N., Narkin, A., and Seedman, D.,** Evaluation of chemical diets as nutrition for man-in-space, *Nature*, 205, 741, 1965.
3. **Perrault, J., Devroede, G., and Bounous, G.,** Effects of an elemental diet in healthy volunteers, *Gastroenterology*, 64, 569, 1973.
4. **Andrassy, R. J. and Woolley, M. M.,** Progress in the use of elemental diets in infants and children, *Surg. Gynecol. Obstet.*, 147, 701, 1978.
5. **Russell, R. I. and Hall, M. J.,** The practical value of elemental diets, *Practitioner*, 222, 631, 1979.
6. **Voitk, A. J.,** The place of elemental diet in clinical nutrition, *Br. J. Clin. Pract.*, 29, 55, 1975.
7. **Stephens, R. V., Bury, K. D., and Randall, H. T.,** Clinical trials of an elemental, concentrated, liquid diet, *Rev. Surg.*, 29, 296, 1972.
8. **Page, C. P., Ryan, J. A., and Haff, R. C.,** Continual catheter administration of an elemental diet, *Surg. Gynecol. Obstet.*, 142, 184, 1976.
9. **Dickman, M. D., Chappelka, A. R., and Schaedler, R. W.,** Evaluation of gut microflora during administration of an elemental diet in a patient with an ileoproctostomy, *Am. J. Dig. Dis.*, 20, 377, 1975.
10. **Young, E., Heuler, N., Russell, P., and Weser, E.,** Comparative nutritional analysis of chemically defined diets, *Gastroenterology*, 69, 1338, 1975.
11. **Pichler, B.,** Geschmackliche Verbesserung der Bilanzierten Synthetischen Diat. (Flavour improvement of a balanced synthetic diet), *Infusionsther Klin Ernaehr*, 4, 52, 1977.
12. **Pichler, B.,** Geschmackliche Verbesserung der Vivasorb-Elementardiat. (Flavour improvement of the Vivasorb elemental diet), *Infusionsther Klin Ernaehr*, 4, 36, 1977.

13. **Behl, C. R., Agarwala, B. P., Giudici, R. A., and Galinsky, A. M.,** Improved taste acceptability for an oral hyperalimentation dosage form, *Am. J. Hosp. Pharm.*, 33, 1014, 1976.
14. **Freeman, J. B., Egan, M. C., and Millis, B. J.,** The elemental diet. *Surg. Gynecol. Obstet.*, 142, 925, 1976.
15. **Coubrough, H.,** A trial of elemental diets in a surgical ward, *J. Hum. Nutr.*, 31, 367, 1977.
16. **Miller, J. M. and Taboada, J. C.,** Clinical experience with an elemental diet, *Am. J. Clin. Nutr.*, 28, 46, 1975.
17. **Fallis, L. S. and Barron, J.,** Gastric and jejunal alimentation with fine polyethylene tubes, *Arch. Surg.*, 65, 373, 1952.
18. **Snyder, C. C.,** The continuous forced feeding pump; a new approach to nutritional therapy, *Plast. Reconstr. Surg.*, 8, 73, 1951.
19. **McDonald, H. A.,** Intrajejunal drip in gastric surgery, *Lancet*, 1, 1007, 1954.
20. **Keoshian, L. A. and Nelsen, T. S.,** A new design for a feeding tube, *Plast. Reconstr. Surg.*, 44, 508, 1969.
21. **Shils, M. E., Bloch, A. S., and Chernoff, R.,** Liquid formulas for oral and tube feeding, *Clin. Bull.*, 6, 151, 1976.
22. **Shils, M. E.,** Enteral nutrition by tube, *Cancer Res.*, 37, 2432, 1977.
23. **Voitk, A. J., Brown, R. A., McArdle, A. H., Hinchey, E. J., and Gurd, F. N.,** Clinical uses of an elemental diet: preliminary studies, *Can. Med. Assoc. J.*, 107, 123, 1972.
24. **Dobbie, R. P. and Hoffmeister, J. A.,** Continuous pump-tube enteric hyperalimentation, *Surg. Gynecol. Obstet.*, 143, 273, 1976.
25. **Bury, K. D., Stephens, R. V., and Randall, H. T.,** Use of a chemically defined liquid elemental diet for nutritional management of fistulas of the alimentary tract, *Am. J. Surg.*, 121, 174, 1971.
26. **Andrassy, R. J., Feldman, R. W., Ryan, J. A., Jr., and Ratner, I. A.,** Continual catheter administration of an elemental diet in infants and children, *Surgery*, 82, 205, 1977.
27. **Liffman, K. E. and Randall, H. T.,** A modified technique for creating a jejunostomy, *Surg. Gynecol. Obstet.*, 134, 663, 1972.
28. **Delaney, H. M., Carnevale, N. J., and Garvey, J. W.,** Jejunostomy by a needle catheter technique, *Surgery*, 73, 786, 1973.
29. **Voitk, A. J., Echave, V., Brown, R. A., and Gurd, F. N.,** Use of elemental diet during the adaptive stage of short gut syndrome, *Gastroenterology*, 65, 419, 1973.
30. **Allison, S. P., Walford, S. P., Todorovic, V., and Elliot, E. T.,** Practical aspects of nutritional support in *Developments in Clinical Nutrition*, Johnston, I. D. A. and Lee, H. A., Eds, MCS, London, 1979, 49.
31. **Woolfson, A. M., Pollard, B., Hardy, S. M., and Allison, S. P.,** Elemental diets, *Lancet*, 2, 1157, 1975.
32. **Stephens, R. V. and Randall, H. T.,** Use of a concentrated, balanced, liquid elemental diet for nutritional management of catabolic states, *Ann. Surg.*, 170, 642, 1969.
33. **Allardyce, D. B. and Groves, A. C.,** A comparison of nutritional gains resulting from intravenous and enteral feeding, *Surg. Gynecol. Obstet.*, 139, 179, 1974.
34. **Hartline, J. V.,** Continuous intragastric infusion of elemental diet. Experiences with 10 infants having small intestinal diseases, *Clin. Pediatr.*, 16, 1105, 1977.
35. **Gougeon, F. W.,** Enteral hyperalimentation: a new apparatus for administration, *Surgery*, 79, 697, 1976.
36. **Bury, K. D. and Jambunathan, G.,** Effects of elemental diets on gastric emptying and gastric secretion in man, *Am. J. Surg.*, 127, 59, 1974.
37. **McMichael, H. B.,** Complications of enteral nutrition, *Res. Clin. Forums*, 1, 107, 1979.
38. Elemental diets, *Drug Ther. Bull.*, 14, 23, 1976.
39. **Ruppin, H., Bar-Meir, S., Soergel, K. H., and Wood, C. M.,** Effects of liquid diets on proximal gastrointestinal function, *Gastroenterology*, 76, 1231, 1979.
40. **Rivard, J. and Lapointe, R.,** Clinical experience in using elemental diet in the management of various surgical nutritional problems, *Can. J. Surg.*, 18, 90, 1975.
41. **Yeung, C. K., Smith, R. C., and Hill, G. L.,** Effect of an elemental diet on body composition. A comparison with intravenous nutrition, *Gastroenterology*, 77, 652, 1979.
42. **Glotzer, D. J.,** Space diets, *Gastroenterology*, 61, 405, 1971.
43. **Morgan, A., Filler, R. M., and Moore, F. D.,** Surgical nutrition, *Med. Clin. North Am.*, 54, 1367, 1970.
44. **Russell, R. I.,** Progress report: Elemental diets, *Gut*, 16, 68, 1975.
45. **Brenner, W. I., Lansky, Z., Engelman, R. M., and Stahl, W. M.,** Hypersomolar coma in surgical patients: an iatrogenic disease of increasing incidence, *Ann. Surg.*, 178, 651, 1972.
46. **Pincus, I. J., Citron, B. P., and Haverback, B. J.,** Nutritional support of gastrointestinal problems with Vivonex-100 in *Balanced Nutrition and Therapy*, (Int. Symp. Nuremberg), Lang, K., Fekl, W., and Berg, G. Eds, Thieme, Stuttgart, 1971, 77.
47. **Allison, S. P., Hinton, P., and Chamberlain, K. J.,** Intravenous glucose-tolerance, insulin and free fatty acid levels in burned patients, *Lancet*, 2, 1113, 1968.
48. **Bury, K. D., Stephens, R. V., Cha, C., and Randall, H. T.,** Chemically defined diets, *Can. J. Surg.*, 17, 124, 1974.

49. **Campbell, A. H., Sewell, W. R., Chudkowski, M., Wilson, J. E., Lord, G. H., and Mohammed, K.,** The effects of feeding an elemental chemical diet to mature rats: toxicologic and pathologic studies, *Toxicol App. Pharmacol.*, 26, 63, 1973.
50. **Halsted, J. A. and Smith, J. C.,** Plasma zinc in health and disease, *Lancet*, 1, 322, 1970.
51. **Mills, P. R. and Fell, G. S.,** Zinc and inflammatory bowel disease, *Am. J. Clin. Nutr.*, 32, 2172, 1979.
52. **Berg, G., Wagner, H., and Weber, L.,** Bilanzierte ballastfreie Ernd'hrung bei Darmerkrankung (Balanced residue free diet in intestinal diseases), *Dtsch. Med. Wochenschr.*, 97, 826, 1972.
53. **Wene, J., Connor, W. E., and DenBesten, L.,** Essential fatty acid deficiency in healthy men fed fat-free diets intravenously and orally, *Clin. Res.*, 21, 890, 1973.
54. **Sherman, J. O., Hamly, C., and Khachadurian, A. K.,** Use of an oral elemental diet in infants with severe intractable diarrhea, *J. Pediatr.*, 86, 518, 1975.
55. **Young, E. A., Cioletti, L. A., Winborn, W. B., and Weser, E.,** The effect of defined formula diets on fat accumulation in the rat liver, *Gastroenterology*, 74, 1115, 1978.
56. **Moore, E. P., Copeland, E. M., Dudrick, S. J., and Weisbrodt, N. W.,** Effect of an elemental diet on the electrical activity of the small intestine in dogs, *J. Surg. Res.*, 20, 533, 1976.
57. **Janne, P., Carpentier, Y., and Williams, G.,** Colonic mucosal atrophy induced by a liquid elemental diet in rats, *Am. J. Dig. Dis.*, 22, 808, 1977.
58. **Geever, E. F., Seifter, E., and Levenson, S. M.,** Pancreatic pathology, chemically defined liquid diets and bacterial flora in the rat, *Br. J. Exp. Path.*, 51, 341, 1970.
59. **Levenson, S. M., Kan, D., Gruber, C., Crowley, L., Jaffe, E. R., Nakao, K., Geever, E. F., and Seifter, E.,** Hemolytic anaemia and pancreatic acinar atrophy and fibrosis conditioned by 'elemental' liquid diets and the ordinary intestinal microflora, *Ann. Surg.*, 1975, 469, 1971.
60. **Bounous, G., Pageau, R., and Regoli, D.,** Enhanced 5-FU mortality in rats eating defined formula diets, *Int. J. Clin. Pharmacol.*, 16, 265, 1978.
61. **Stanford, J. R., King, D., Carey, L., and Anderson, G.,** The adverse effects of elemental diets on tolerance for 5-FU toxicity in the rat, *J. Surg. Oncol.*, 9, 493, 1977.
62. **Nelson, L. M., Williamson, I., Russell, R. I.,** Elemental diet composition; effect on bile acid metabolism and hepatic lipids, *Gut*, 1981, in press.

SECTION IV

CONCLUSIONS

Chapter 19

SUMMARY OF CLINICAL INDICATIONS FOR THE USE OF ELEMENTAL DIETS

R. I. Russell

TABLE OF CONTENTS

I. INTRODUCTION

It is the purpose of this chapter to summarize the clinical indications for the use of elemental diets, which have been discussed in detail in Section III. A classification of the current clinical indications for the uses of elemental diets has thereby been devised.

II. SUMMARY OF CLINICAL USES OF ELEMENTAL DIETS

A. Surgical Conditions

Elemental diets appear to be effective in improving nutritional deficiency in association with head and neck surgery, trauma, and postoperative care. However, they are not any better in this respect than other forms of enteral nutritional support and data comparing the effectiveness of elemental diets with whole protein liquid diets and other dietary supplements reported in Chapter 11 indicates that whole protein liquid diets are at least as effective as elemental diets in improving the nutritional status of surgical patients.

Although elemental diets have been shown to be valuable in assisting the healing of gastrointestinal (GI) fistulas, it is probable that they are no more effective in this respect than other forms of low residue enteral nutrition such as whole protein liquid diets. A major factor in the healing of GI fistulas is improvement of the nutritional status of the patient in addition to the provision of low residue nutrition. Whole protein liquid diets are probably equally as effective as elemental diets in the healing of such fistulas although good comparative studies are still required.

Elemental diets appear to have some specific value in improving the nutritional status of surgical patients if given by jejunostomy. Jejunal feeding of ordinary nutritional preparations may result in inadequate mixing of the diet with pancreatic juice and bile so that adequate digestion does not occur; under these circumstances elemental diets may be of specific value as they require minimal digestion without pancreatic exocrine secretion or bile.

There appears to be no specific value of elemental diets in the preoperative nutritional management of patients, or in the preparation of the bowel prior to GI surgery. Elemental diets have no value over other forms of low residue and other nutritional support preparations for these purposes.

B. Maldigestion and Malabsorption States

1. Chronic Pancreatic Insufficiency and Other Pancreatic Diseases

Elemental diets have a distinct advantage over other forms of nutritional support in that they have minimal digestive requirements. They may thus be effective in improving nutritional deficiency associated with chronic pancreatic insufficiency and cystic fibrosis. They may also be helpful in improving nutritional insufficiency associated with pancreatic fistulas and pancreatic abscesses, and in assisting healing of pancreatic fistulas. They are of no value in the management of acute pancreatitis.

2. The Short Bowel Syndrome

Elemental diets are of value in the short bowel syndrome by providing nutritional support, while at the same time starting the process of intestinal adaptation by luminal nutrition. They are also of value in that they are assimilated rapidly in short lengths of intestine. Elemental diets may have an advantage over other forms of enteral nutrition in this respect.

3. Coeliac Disease and Other Chronic Malabsorption States

Although elemental diets are of value in providing adequate nutritional support if required in patients with coeliac disease and other chronic malabsorption states, they do not offer any specific value in the management of these conditions. There is no evidence that the hypoallergenic nature of elemental diets gives them any advantage over a gluten-free diet or other forms of enteral nutritional support.

4. Bile Acid Induced Diarrhea

The elemental diet Vivonex® has been shown to reduce fecal bile acid excretion and is helpful in the management of patients with bile acid-induced diarrhea. Although this observation may be of some value in the management of some of these patients, possibly in providing a break in the diarrhea while at the same time maintaining or improving the nutritional status of the patient, data are required on the effect of other low residue enteral nutritional preparations on bile acid metabolism. The principal value of this observation may be in focusing attention on the possible manipulation of bile acid metabolism by dietary means.

5. Other Diarrheal States

Elemental diets may be of some value in the management of those patients with irritable colon syndrome and postvagotomy diarrhea who have high fecal bile acid excretion, but it is unlikely that they will be of major value in the management of these conditions. There is no specific value of elemental diets in diverticular disease, in infective diarrhea or in prolonged infantile diarrhea, although they may be of value in providing nutritional support in some infants with intractable diarrhea.

C. Inflammatory Bowel Disease

Elemental diets may be helpful in the short- and long-term management of nutritional insufficiency associated with Crohn's disease, but are unlikely to be any better than other forms of enteral nutritional support or intravenous nutrition in this respect. By the provision of bowel rest with concomitant nutritional support, elemental diets are helpful in the management of local complications of Crohn's disease such as ano-rectal and perianal lesions, fissures, fistulas, subacute small intestinal obstruction, and in the healing of skin excoriations associated with an ileostomy. Elemental diets may not be more effective than whole protein liquid or complete oral diets in the management of these complications, although controlled prospective data is required. There is no convincing evidence of the value of elemental diets as "primary therapy" in Crohn's disease to date.

D. Cancer

Nutritional support is important in many patients with cancer, particularly those having treatment with chemotherapy or radiotherapy. Although elemental diets are effective in providing nutritional support in patients with cancer, they have not been shown to be any more effective than other forms of enteral nutrition.

E. Burns

The increased metabolic requirements associated with burn injuries can be supported adequately by the use of elemental diets, although it is likely that other forms of enteral nutritional support are as effective as elemental diets.

F. Pediatric Conditions

Elemental diets may be helpful in a range of pediatric conditions by providing adequate nutritional support. They may be effective in managing infants with the intractable diarrhea syndrome, the short bowel syndrome where the easy assimilation and intestinal adaptation are advantages in addition to nutritional support, and other conditions in infants and children which may be accompanied by nutritional insufficiency. They may not, however, be any better than other forms of enteral nutritional support in these conditions.

Elemental diets may have some value in the treatment of cystic fibrosis, although this requires to be more firmly established. Special diets of elemental type with special amino acid compositions may be helpful in infants with inborn errors of amino acid metabolism, such as phenylketonuria and maple-syrup disease. Improvement of children with glycogen storage disease has also been reported with Vivonex®.

The hypoallergenic nature of elemental diets may be of value in the diagnosis and management of children with food allergies and protein-sensitive enteropathies, although further work is required to confirm the value of these diets in this respect.

G. Preparation of the Colon for Diagnostic Procedures

By virtue of their minimal residue, elemental diets may be of value in the preparation of the colon for colonic radiology and colonoscopy, but they are not any better than other forms of low-residue diet preparations, and may be less effective than more active preparation regimes.

H. Allergies and Immunological Problems

Elemental diets, by virtue of their hypoallergenic nature, have been used in the diagnosis and management of food allergy, while maintaining the patients in good nutritional state. Although short-term remission of symptoms has been shown to occur in some patients there is no convincing evidence of the value of elemental diets over prolonged periods.

I. Hepatic Insufficiency and Failure

Although elemental diets may be helpful in improving the nutritional status of patients with hepatic disease, particularly those of alcoholic origin, there is no indication that they are superior to other forms of enteral nutrition in this respect.

J. Renal Disease

Amino acid-supplemented or substituted diets of elemental type may be of value in some patients with chronic renal failure by providing a low protein diet while maintaining the patient in a good nutritional state. It is unlikely that elemental diets will have a major part to play in correcting the nutritional insufficiency associated with other forms of renal disease such as acute renal failure. Other enteral nutritional support or intravenous nutrition is likely to be at least as good as elemental diets.

Because of their hypoallergenic nature, elemental diets have been considered to be of value in the diagnosis and management of some patients with the nephrotic syndrome. Further controlled data is required on this proposed use of elemental diets.

III. CLASSIFICATION OF INDICATIONS

A classification of the indications for elemental diets has been devised on the basis of their uses which have been described. These clinical uses can be classified into two groups:

1. Conditions in which elemental diets have been shown to be of clinical value.
2. Conditions in which elemental diets are of clinical value and have advantages over other forms of nutritional support.

The classification is summarized in Tables 1 and 2.

Table 1
CONDITIONS IN WHICH ELEMENTAL DIETS HAVE BEEN SHOWN TO BE OF VALUE, BUT ARE NOT NECESSARILY BETTER THAN OTHER FORMS OF ENTERAL NUTRITIONAL SUPPORT

Nutritional insufficiency
GI fistulas
Local complications of Crohn's disease
Colonic preparation
Bile acid-induced diarrhea
Chronic pancreatic insufficiency
Cystic fibrosis
Short bowel syndrome
Food allergy — diagnosis and management
? Nephrotic syndrome
Chronic renal failure
Inborn errors of metabolism

Table 2
CONDITIONS IN WHICH ELEMENTAL DIETS ARE OF VALUE AND HAVE ADVANTAGES OVER OTHER FORMS OF NUTRITIONAL SUPPORT

Chronic pancreatic insufficiency
Cystic fibrosis
Short bowel syndrome
Food allergy — diagnosis and management
? Nephrotic syndrome
Chronic renal failure
Inborn errors of metabolism

A. Conditions In Which Elemental Diets Have Been Shown to Be of Clinical Value But Are Not Necessarily Better Than Other Forms of Enteral Nutritional Support

1. Nutritional Insufficiency

Elemental diets are of value, if given in full doses, in improving the nutritional status of patients suffering from nutritional deficiency. The causes of severe nutritional insufficiency can be classified as follows:

- Trauma and surgery.
- GI and liver disease (severe diarrheal states, severe malabsorption and maldigestion states, prolonged vomiting, prolonged poor oral intake, GI surgery, pediatric conditions, severe liver disease and failure, particularly of alcoholic origin.)
- Severe renal disease and renal failure.
- Tumors.
- Burns.
- Sepsis.
- Kwashiorkor, mental deficiency.

Elemental diets are not particularly better in correcting nutritional insufficiency in these conditions than other forms of nutritional support such as complete oral liquid diets, provided both can be given in full dose schedules. The comparison of these and other forms of enteral nutrition is further discussed in Chapter 20, but complete oral liquid diets are probably easier to administer than elemental diets and are certainly less costly; they are as effective as elemental diets in providing nutritional support. In patients with GI failure or in patients with very severe nutritional insufficiency which is life-threatening, intravenous nutrition is indicated to improve nutritional status. In patients with moderate or even severe nutritional insufficiency in which GI function is normal, enteral nutrition may be successfully used in correcting nutritional insufficiency and should be considered as the first line of nutritional support therapy.

2. Clinical Uses

The following are specific clinical uses for elemental diets, based on their properties of low residue, minimal digestion requirements, and hypoallergenicity.

- GI fistulas.
- Management of local complications of Crohn's disease.
- Colonic preparation.
- Bile acid induced diarrhea.
- Chronic pancreatic insufficiency and cystic fibrosis.
- Short bowel syndrome.
- Diagnosis and management of food allergies, and possibly in nephrotic syndrome.
- Chronic renal failure — the use of special amino acid substituted diets.
- Inborn errors of metabolism — phenylketonuria, maple-syrup disease, glycogen storage disease.

B. Conditions In Which Elemental Diets Are of Clinical Value and Have Advantages Over Other Forms of Enteral Nutrition.

It has been shown that elemental diets, although effective in correcting nutritional deficiency, are not more effective in this than other forms of enteral nutritional support, such as complete oral liquid diets or nutritional supplements if administered in full doses; thus elemental diets cannot be regarded as being primarily indicated in the correction of nutritional insufficiency.

Complete oral liquid diets are also of low residue and elemental diets cannot thus be regarded as being the first choice treatment in conditions in which the low residue nature of the nutritional support regime is of importance, as in the management of GI fistulas, the local complications of Crohn's disease, or in colonic preparation. However the minimal digestion requirements and hypoallerginicity of elemental diets do allow them to offer advantages over preparations such as complete oral liquid diets. Specific uses of elemental diets are thus as follows:

- Chronic pancreatic insufficiency and cystic fibrosis.
- The short bowel syndrome.
- Bile acid induced diarrhea.
- Diagnosis and management of food allergy and protein-sensitive enteropathies, and possibly in the management of the nephrotic syndrome.
- Chronic renal failure, where amino acid substituted diets may be of value.
- Inborn errors of metabolism, where special diets of elemental type may be of value in phenylketonuria, maple syrup disease and glycogen storage disease.

The use of the low residue aspect of elemental diets in the management of intestinal fistulas, in the local complications of Crohn's disease, and in colonic preparation are likely to be equally effectively dealt with by means of complete oral liquid diets.

Chapter 20

ELEMENTAL DIETS IN RELATION TO OTHER NUTRITIONAL AIDS

R. I. Russell

TABLE OF CONTENTS

I. INTRODUCTION

The use of elemental diets must be considered in conjunction with other forms of nutritional support. Intravenous feeding was initially considered the best, and indeed the only, effective way of improving a patient's nutritional state when nutritional deficiency was first widely recognized. Although a number of supplemented oral preparations had been available for many years, the scientific use of enteral nutrition was not fully considered until the development of elemental diets. Then the choice lay between elemental diets and intravenous nutrition if full nutritional support was required. It is only in recent years that there have been further developments of other forms of enteral nutrition.

A summary of the clinical uses of, and indications for, elemental diets is given in Chapter 19. The purpose of this chapter is to compare the clinical uses of elemental diets with alternative forms of nutritional support — other forms of enteral nutrition and intravenous feeding. It has also been shown in preceding chapters that elemental diets have specialized uses other than improvement of the nutritional status of patients. Other forms of nutritional support must thus be considered in the light of these uses in addition to their basic purpose of improving the nutritional status of patients with nutritional insufficiency.

The selection of the most appropriate form of nutritional aid in any individual patient depends upon the severity of nutritional deficiency, the disease process present, the state of the GI tract, special indications for particular formulations, palatability, cost, and the back-up facilities which require to be available for adequate assessment and monitoring of nutritional status. It is thus relevant to compare the various forms of enteral nutrition with each other and with intravenous nutrition in relation to the effectiveness of nutritional support, specific clinical indications, ease of nutritional assessment, monitoring and administration, potential side-effects, and cost.

II. EFFECTIVENESS OF NUTRITIONAL SUPPORT

A. Intravenous Feeding and Enteral Nutrition

Intravenous nutrition, if correctly planned and executed, is effective in correcting severe nutritional insufficiency with associated protein-calorie malnutrition, whatever the underlying cause. However, a large number of patients who require some degree of nutritional support have normally functioning gastrointestinal (GI) tracts, and it is likely that some form of enteral nutrition will be adequate to correct the nutritional deficiency in most of these patients. Intravenous nutrition should be considered when the alimentary tract is nonfunctioning — alimentary failure — or if the patient has life-threatening nutritional insufficiency. It has been stated that the principal indication for intravenous feeding is GI failure and the only contraindication to enteral feeding is GI failure.[1] Life-threatening nutritional insufficiency is a positive indication for the prompt use of intravenous nutrition.[2] Under these circumstances intravenous feeding is more reliable and more rapidly effective than enteral nutrition in improving the patient's nutritional status. In such patients, once adequate nutritional status has been achieved by means of intravenous feeding, this can be phased out and replaced by a suitable form of enteral nutritional support which may then be able to maintain adequate nutritional status.

Intravenous feeding was the first effective way of correcting nutritional deficiency and much of the information on the assessment of nutritional support has been gained from studies on intravenous nutrition. The technique of intravenous feeding was successfully applied in animals by Dudrick and colleagues[3] in 1967 and the basic principles later defined.[4] There have been many reviews of the indications, techniques, regimes, and hazards of intravenous feeding.[2,5-9]

In view of the advances in recent years in the development of various enteral nutritional support preparations, ranging from dietary supplements to complete oral (whole protein) liquid diets and elemental diets, the place of intravenous feeding has been reassessed. Many enteral preparations are as good as intravenous nutrition in providing nutritional support in patients with normally functioning alimentary tracts who have nutritional deficiency. Enteral nutrition preparations are also easily available, are flexible in their use, are relatively cheap, simple, and effective.[10] Enteral nutrition is more physiological than intravenous nutrition and should be used whenever possible. Other advantages of enteral nutrition are ease of administration, fewer and less serious side-effects, better patient acceptability, cost-effectiveness, easier monitoring, and less personnel involvement.

It is as important to have a well-organized nutrition group for the provision of enteral nutrition as for intravenous nutrition. The combination of doctor, nurse, dietitian, pharmacist, and biochemist, each with experience and knowledge of the problems of enteral as well as intravenous nutrition, leads to greater success in the provision of any form of nutritional support. Full cooperation from the patient is essential in the successful provision of either enteral or intravenous nutrition and full explanation of the background and procedures requirements should be given to the patient. The patient should thus be regarded as an essential member of the team.

B. Elemental Diets and Other Forms of Enteral Nutrition

Enteral nutrition includes dietary supplements, blenderized whole food, complete oral (whole protein) liquid diets (which can be used either as supplements or for complete nutritional support), and elemental diets. A liquidized diet or blenderized whole food may be tolerated by the patient more readily than ordinary food and may be more effective than simple dietary supplements. Whole protein-diets such as Isocal®, Triosorbon-MCT, and Clinifeed® and Ensure® are provided ready for administration to the patient with only minimal preparation and are therefore more attractive than liquidized or blenderized foods which require to be specially prepared. Liquidized or blenderized foods are, however, cheaper than proprietary preparations.

The clinical uses of elemental diets have been considered in detail in Section II and summarized in Chapter 19. The question arises as to whether or not elemental diets have any advantages over dietary supplements, blenderized food or complete oral liquid diets in nutritional efficacy, or in improving nutritional deficiency. Dietary supplements are useful only as supplements to normal food in patients who have a minor degree of nutritional insufficiency. They will not be helpful in any patient with severe nutritional insufficiency. Complete oral liquid diets and blenderized food are probably as good as elemental diets in providing nutritional support in normal subjects and in patients with a minor or moderate degree of nutritional insufficiency. Complete oral liquid diets have minimal residue as have elemental diets, but they do have a major requirement for normal digestive processes which elemental diets do not have.

There is, however, little direct data in the literature to date comparing the nutritional efficacy of complete oral liquid diets and elemental diets in various disease processes, and good controlled studies of this kind are required. A few individual case reports have suggested adequate nutritional efficacy of complete oral liquid diets,[11,12] and long-term nutritional maintenance of a patient with severe Crohn's disease has been reported over many months by the use of an enteral nutrition regime using Isocal, after initial correction of severe nutritional deficiency with intravenous nutrition. In this patient, the enteral preparation was administered by means of a fine-bore nasogastric tube in the hospital and subsequently continued by the patient at home with regular visits to the hospital for clinical and biochemical monitoring.[13]

A few recent studies have compared elemental with other forms of enteral nutrition. In one report, an elemental and complete oral liquid diet were compared with a diet derived from low residue foods, the diets being given orally to normal volunteers for 7 days. The diet prepared from low residue food was the only one to maintain the subjects in a positive nitrogen balance during that period.[14] Although the results of this study are interesting, the information obtained was limited, as it was performed in normal subjects and the period of the study — 7 days — was too short to assess the effectiveness of the special nutritional preparations.

The comparison of whole protein liquid diets and elemental diets is discussed in Chapter 11. Patients in surgical practice generally have normally functioning GI tracts and are less likely to have very severe and long-lasting nutritional insufficiency. This study was performed in patients with head injuries.[15] Patients were either given an elemental diet (Vivonex® or Flexical®), a dietary supplement consisting of Albumaid and Caloreen, or the complete oral liquid diets Clinifeed 400 or Triosorbon MCT for a period of 12 days. The study was well-controlled, and nutritional assessment and monitoring performed at the beginning and throughout the study. The mean nitrogen balance remained negative in the groups given the elemental diets, but a positive nitrogen balance was achieved after about 7 or 8 days in patients given both Clinifeed 400 and Triosorbon MCT. The authors emphasized the difficulty in administering an enteral feed in catabolic patients in view of the fact that the feed has to be introduced at reduced strength and in many of these patients in which catabolism was severe, intravenous nutrition may be initially required. However, the study indicated that complete oral liquid diets did apparently offer some nutritional advantages over elemental diets in the patients studied. They also had the advantage of easier administration and better palatability.

In diseases in which the alimentary tract is functioning satisfactorily, it would appear that adequate dietary supplements or complete oral liquid diets may be at least as effective as elemental diets in improving the nutritional state of the patient, and may have an advantage in ease of administration and palatability. These diets may be of value in some patients in correcting short-term, minor nutritional deficiency as after trauma and in association with limited or minor surgery, but are less likely to be of value as complete nutritional support in severe nutritional deficiency or in nutritional insufficiency associated with severe, long-lasting disease.

Further prospective, controlled studies are required in various disease states to compare the nutritional efficacy of whole protein liquid diets and blenderized food with the various elemental diets.

III. SPECIFIC CLINICAL INDICATIONS

A. Elemental Diets and Other Forms of Enteral Nutrition

By definition, two essential features of elemental diets are their low or minimal residue and their minimal digestion requirements. These two aspects have led to the use of elemental diets in conditions in which low residue may be of value (as in the management of GI fistulas) and in those conditions in which minimal digestion requirements may be deemed an advantage (as in maldigestion secondary to chronic pancreatic insufficiency). These uses have been considered in detail in earlier chapters, and summarized in Chapter 19.

The provision of a low residue nutritional source can be effectively achieved by means of intravenous nutrition, but other forms of enteral nutrition other than elemental diets should also be considered in this respect. Complete oral liquid diets also have minimal residue and may therefore be as valuable as elemental diets in diseases in which minimal residue may be of value.

One of the earliest reported indications for the use of elemental diets was in the healing of fistulas by the provision of bowel rest with adequate nutritional support.[16] Other reports of the successful use of elemental diets in GI fistulas followed.[17,18] Voitk and colleagues[17] gave an elemental diet through a nasogastric or enterostomy tube in 29 patients and reported that two esophageal and three gastroduodenal fistulas healed spontaneously; seven of eight colonic, and five of six pancreatico-biliary fistulas also healed satisfactorily. It was also noted that small bowel fistulas did less well, fewer than 50% of these closing, and that the elemental diet altered the fistula fluid so that it became inoffensive and that skin excoriations tended to heal. Allardyce and colleagues[19] evaluated elemental or intravenous feeding in the treatment of fistulas and concluded that an elemental diet given via a jejunal stoma was the most effective means of providing long-term nutritional support while allowing healing of the fistula. The relationship of complete oral liquid diets and elemental diets in the healing of fistulas is reflected in the question asked in Chapter 11, "Does the food need to be truly elemental in terms of nonresidue, low fat, amino acids, and glucose?" Few adequate investigations into the use of other nutritional support regimes in the treatment of fistulas have been published to date, although Smith and Lee[20] reported healing of fistulas using a feed based on partially hydrolyzed milk protein with glucose and alcohol, and Celestin[11] reported results in the healing of fistulas which were as good with complete oral liquid diets as with elemental diets. Improvement of nutritional status of the patient may be as important as, if not more important, than low residue in the healing of GI fistulas. Further studies are required. It may well be that complete oral liquid diets are as good as elemental diets and have an advantage in being more palatable and less costly.

There would also appear to be no specific value of elemental diets in the pre- and postoperative care of patients, low residue diets of any type being effective in preoperative preparation, and nutritional support being given in simpler ways by complete oral liquid diets in the postoperative group. A similar conclusion must be drawn in bowel preparation for colonic surgery, in which any form of low residue diet which maintains adequate nutrition is likely to be as effective as elemental diets, and may have advantages in relation to cost, ease of administration, and palatability.

In the management of local complications of Crohn's disease, other forms of low residue enteral nutrition may be as effective as elemental diets. Thus, complete oral liquid diets may be of value in the management of complications such as anorectal lesions, fistulas, and fissures, by means of their low residue properties, although controlled studies are required. The use of bowel rest as "primary therapy" for Crohn's disease is a more complex problem, and is discussed in Chapter 13. The provision of bowel rest in Crohn's disease has been considered by a number of authors to be of value as "primary therapy" in inducing a remission of the disease.[21-23] Intravenous nutrition has also been considered to be of some value as "primary therapy" in Crohn's disease, although good controlled studies have not been performed either for intravenous nutrition or for elemental diets. There are no data on the value of complete oral liquid diets as "primary therapy" in Crohn's disease, and it is possible that these preparations may be of some value in this respect because of their minimal residue, resting the bowel and inducing a remission of the disease. However, bowel rest may be better achieved by means of intravenous nutrition and elemental diets than by complete oral liquid diets. Some recent papers have suggested that there may be a specific effect of elemental diets in inducing remission of Crohn's disease, although this requires to be confirmed. If confirmation is obtained, it may be due to a combination of bowel rest, nutritional support and the hypoallergenic nature of the elemental diets. If this latter aspect is confirmed as being an important factor, it is likely that elemental diets will be preferable to complete oral liquid diets in Crohn's disease.

The hypoallergenic nature of elemental diets may be helpful in the diagnosis and management of food allergy, or of the nephrotic syndrome. Complete oral liquid diets and other forms of enteral nutrition are unlikely to be hypoallergenic because of their "whole" protein source and are, therefore, unlikely to be of value in these diseases.

In conditions in which the minimal digestion characteristic of elemental diets has been utilized therapeutically, as in maldigestion states, whole protein liquid diets and other forms of enteral nutrition are unlikely to be as helpful as elemental diets. Complete oral liquid diets require to undergo considerable digestion before absorption occurs, whereas elemental diets are presented to the alimentary tract in a form in which easy assimilation can take place. It is thus likely that elemental diets, rather than other forms of enteral nutrition, will be of value in the management of chronic pancreatic insufficiency, cystic fibrosis, and pancreatic abscess, and may also help to heal pancreatic fistulas. In the presence of severe nutritional insufficiency, intravenous nutrition will be helpful in these conditions.

In the short bowel syndrome, which may lead to severe nutritional insufficiency and malabsorption, nutritional support may be required initially by means of intravenous feeding, but enteral nutrition should be started as early as possible so that adaptive changes in the remaining gut can be stimulated by the presence of luminal nutrition while at the same time continuing nutritional support. Complete oral liquid diets may be as effective as elemental diets in providing luminal nutrition sufficient to speed intestinal adaptation and at the same time maintain nutritional support during the period of adaptation. Elemental diets, however, may be more effectively absorbed from small areas of remaining intestine than complete oral liquid diets by virtue of their more basic formulations and minimal digestion requirements.

The elemental diet Vivonex® has been shown to be successful in the reduction of fecal bile acid excretion in patients suffering from severe bile-acid induced diarrhea. Although the mechanism of alteration of bile acid metabolism and fecal excretion of bile acids by this elemental diet require to be further studied, it is possible that other elemental diets and other minimal residue preparations such as complete oral liquid diets which are fiber-free, may be of value in this group, although this has yet to be demonstrated.

IV. EASE OF NUTRITIONAL ASSESSMENT, MONITORING, AND ADMINISTRATION

A. Assessment and Monitoring of Nutritional Status

Whatever nutritional support system is used, whether it be intravenous feeding, elemental diets, or other form of enteral nutrition, it is important that a full nutritional assessment based on clinical, anthropometric, biochemical, and immunological factors should be performed before the nutritional support regime is started. On the basis of this initial assessment, together with knowledge of the underlying disease process and the state of the GI tract, the nutritional support system most suited to that individual patient should be selected. The regime should be planned on the basis of the requirements of the patient, depending upon the deficiencies which are present and the underlying disease process leading to nutritional deficiency. Throughout the course of nutritional support, regular monitoring of clinical, biochemical, anthropometric, and immunological features should be performed, following the protocol described in Chapter 4. By so doing, the ideal duration of nutritional support can be worked out for each individual patient, and the nutritional regime phased out when adequate clinical improvement has occurred and nutritional parameters have reached normality. Base-line nutritional assessment and regular monitoring is thus important in any nutritional support program. Ideally, there should be no essential differences in the requirements for nutritional assessment and monitoring between intravenous nutrition and any form of enteral feeding, including elemental diets, although it is probable that less extensive monitoring may be adequate for enteral nutrition regimes.

The selection of an appropriate nutritional support regime in any individual patient depends not only upon the severity of nutritional insufficiency, the underlying disease process and the state of the GI tract, but also on the ability of the hospital to provide adequate back-up facilities to ensure that treatment is successfully performed. This includes good laboratory facilities to allow of adequate baseline assessment and continuous monitoring during the course of treatment and a well-organized and experienced team of medical, nursing, biochemical, pharmacy, and dietetic personnel who are experienced in planning regimes and looking after these patients. It is probable that enteral nutrition, if applicable in any individual patient, may be preferable to intravenous nutrition for reasons of lack of experience or the absence of adequate nutritional personnel who are experienced and well-organized in the planning and running of nutritional support regimes. There is no essential difference between the use of dietary supplements, complete oral liquid diets, and elemental diets in this respect. The existence of such experience in a hospital will clearly be of value in the management of all patients, whether it be on any form of enteral nutritional support or intravenous feeding.

B. Ease of Administration

Another important aspect is ease of administration. The methods of administration of elemental diet regimes have been discussed in Chapter 18. The use of fine-bore nasogastric or nasojejunal tubes may be superior to the oral use of elemental diets. Palatability has always been a problem in the clinical use of chemically defined diets, principally because of the presence of amino acids in these preparations. The use of various flavoring products and the provision of elemental diets as jellies or as iced preparations does not significantly improve their palatability. However, the introduction of fine-bore tubes has made the use of elemental diets more satisfactory and successful. One undoubted advantage of blenderized food and complete oral liquid diets is that they are more palatable than elemental diets when given orally and there is thus greater patient acceptance of this type of regime. This aspect may be of paramount importance in selecting an enteral nutrition regime for any individual patient. In general, however, controlled fine-bore tube administration of elemental diets, complete oral liquid diets and other tube feeds have advantages over oral administration. There is no essential advantage of one form of enteral nutrition over any other as regards administration when fine-bore tubes are used.

V. HAZARDS

The potential side-effects of intravenous nutrition are more severe than those likely to be encountered with any form of enteral nutrition. A wide range of side-effects associated with intravenous nutrition have been reported.[24-27]

1. Complications of central venous catheterization — pneumothorax, hemothorax, superior vena cava syndrome, subcutaneous emphysema, hepatic vein thrombosis, catheter embolism, superior vena cava thrombosis, and injuries to arteries, nerves or lymphatics.
2. Septic complications — septicemia and local infections.
3. Metabolic problems — hyperosmolar syndrome, hyperglycemia, hypoglycemia, hyperammonemia, hyperchloraemic acidosis.
4. Electrolyte abnormalities, mineral, trace element, and vitamin deficiencies.

5. Essential fatty acid deficiency (if a fat emulsion is not used in the regime).
6. Hepatic complications — a cholestatic syndrome, enzyme abnormalities, and fatty change in the liver.

These complications can be prevented or minimized by good technique, a well-planned approach, experienced operators, and good monitoring facilities. Good clinical experience in the insertion of central venous lines and in the assessment and monitoring of patients lessen the incidence of side effects.

The risk of serious complications is greater than with enteral nutrition, and the seriousness of such complications when they do occur is a further reason for the use of enteral nutrition whenever possible.

A number of complications may also be associated with the use of enteral feeding. The side-effects which may occur in association with the use of elemental diets have been described in Chapter 18. Problems such as nausea, vomiting, abdominal discomfort, diarrhea, and gastric retention may be a problem, but can generally be prevented by carefully planned administration of elemental diets, starting off with lower concentrations and working up to full doses after some days. Disturbances of water balance such as dumping, hypertonic dehydration, and hyperosmolar, nonketotic coma are rare if elemental diets are used with care. Rarer complications include essential fatty acid deficiency, skin rashes and complications of nasogastric or nasoduodenal tubes such as nasopharyngeal ulceration, gastric erosions, and aspirations. These latter complications can be largely avoided by the use of a thin, fine-bore nasogastric tube. Trace element and mineral deficiency may be more common during prolonged elemental diet treatment as most elemental diet preparations are basically low in these substances. It should also be remembered that elemental diet regimes are given to patients who generally have some degree of nutritional insufficiency, in which trace element and mineral deficiency may itself be a feature. These may be worsened during prolonged elemental diet therapy and supplements may be required to avoid deficiencies.

Other forms of enteral nutrition such as complete oral liquid diets, dietary supplements, and other tube feeds may also be associated with side-effects. The most common of these is diarrhea and this is usually associated with the use of full-strength preparations too early in a planned regime. As with elemental diets, a planned gradual introduction of the nutritional support preparations should be made to avoid diarrhea. However, these preparations are often iso-osmolar, in contradistinction to elemental diets, and are, therefore, theoretically less liable to cause diarrhea. Nausea, vomiting, abdominal distension, and alterations of gastric emptying may also occur with the use of these preparations, and trace element and mineral deficiency may also develop. Complete oral liquid diets have, like elemental diets, low levels of trace elements and minerals, and deficiencies can occur if these preparations are used as the sole source of nutrition over a long period of time. This is more common if the underlying disease process, as in chronic GI disease, is associated with trace metal and element deficiencies. Used properly and backed up by experience and good monitoring, complete oral liquid diets and elemental diets can be used without the development of any major side effect which may necessitate stopping treatment.

VI. COST

The cost-effectiveness of any nutritional support regime is clearly important to establish. The relative costs of blenderized food preparations, various dietary supplements, complete oral liquid diets, elemental diets, and intravenous nutrition are assessed in Table 1. Intravenous nutrition regimes are very expensive and the cost of elemental diets

Table 1
COST OF NUTRITIONAL SUPPORT PREPARATIONS
(April 1981)

	Product	Approximate daily cost (full recommended regime)
Dietary supplements	Blenderized food	£ 2.00—£ 3.00
	or tube foods	£ 2.00
	Caloreen	£ 2.00
	Casilan	£ 2.00
	Complan	£15.00
	Aminutrin	
	Calonutrin	
Complete oral liquid diets	Isocal	£ 5.75
	Clinifeed 400	£ 6.15
	Clinifeed 500	£ 7.80
	Triosorbon MCT	£ 6.00
	Ensure	£ 6.50
Elemental diets	Vivonex	£11.00
	Vivonex HN	£16.60
	Flexical	£14.00
Intravenous nutrition (standard regime)	Synthamin (or vamin) glucose, intralipid	£50—£75

is considerably more than complete oral liquid diets, blenderized foods, or dietary supplements. The costs listed in the table refer to the cost of the preparations themselves on a daily basis, but the total expense of regimes must also include the cost of nutritional monitoring and staff associated with the planning and execution of nutritional regimes. This is likely to be more extensive for intravenous nutrition rather than for any form of enteral feeding. However, to provide ideal nutritional support, similar assessment and monitoring facilities should also be available when elemental diets and complete oral liquid diets are used.

Cost-effectiveness, however, also relates to the correct and appropriate management for individual patients. Cost should be considered only when there is a choice of regime which is likely to lead to equally good results in the management of the patient. When enteral nutrition is indicated, the use of complete oral liquid diets or blenderized foods may have better cost-effectiveness than elemental diets.

REFERENCES

1. **Lee, H. A.,** Why enteral nutrition?, in *Developments in Clinical Nutrition,* Johnston, I. D. A. and Lee, H. A., Eds., MCS Consultants, London, 1979, 17.
2. **Johnston, I. D. A.,** Metabolic foundations of intravenous nutrition, in *Advances in Parenteral Nutrition,* Johnston, I. D. A., Ed., MTP Press, Lancaster, 1976, 3.
3. **Dudrick, S. J., Wilmore, D. W. and Vars, H. N.,** Long term parenteral nutrition with growth in puppies in positive nitrogen balance, *Surg. Forum,* 18, 356, 1967.

4. **Dudrick, S. J. and Ruberg, R. L.,** Principles and practice of parenteral nutrition, *Gastroenterology,* 61, 901, 1971.
5. **Dudrick, S. J., MacFadyen, B. V., Van Buren, C. T., Rouberg, R. L., and Maynard, A. T.,** Parenteral hyperalimentation — metabolic problems and solutions, *Ann. Surg.,* 176, 259, 1972.
6. **Wretlind, A.,** Intravenous nutrition, in *Scientific Foundations of Surgery,* 2nd ed., Wells, C., Kyle, J., and Dunphy, E., Heinemann, London, 1974, 626.
7. **Shenkin, A. and Wretlind, A.,** Parenteral nutrition, *World Rev. Nutr. Diet.,* 28, 1, 1978.
8. **Fischer, J. E., Yoshimura, N., Aguirre, A., James, H., Cumings, M. G., Abel, R. M. and Deindoerfer, F.,** Plasma amino acids in patients with hepatic encephalopathy. Effects of amino acid infusion, *Am. J. Surg.,* 127, 40, 1974.
9. **Greep, J. M., Soeters, P. B., Wesdorp, R. I. C., Phaf, C. W. R., and Fischer, J. E.,** *Current Concepts in Parenteral Nutrition,* Martinus Nijhoff, The Hague, 1977.
10. **Heymsfield, J. B., Bethel, R. A., Ansley, J. D., Nixon, D. W., and Rudman, D.,** Enteral hyperalimentation: an alternative to central venous hyperalimentation, *Ann. Int. Med.,* 90, 63, 1979.
11. **Celestin, L. R.,** Residue — sense and nonsense, *Res. Clin. Forum.,* 1, 91, 1979.
12. **Allison, S. P., Walford, S., Todorovic, V., and Elliott, E. T.,** Practical aspects of nutritional support, *Res. Clin. Forum.,* 1, 49, 1979.
13. **Main, A. N. H., Morgan, R. J., Russell, R. I., Hall, M. J., Shenkin, A., and Fell, G. S.,** Home enteral tube feeding with a liquid diet in the long-term management of inflammatory bowel disease and intestinal failure, *Scot. Med. J.,* 25, 312, 1980.
14. **Bondy, R. A., Beyar, P. L., and Rhodes, J. B.,** Comparison of two commercial low residue diets and a low residue diet of common foods, *J. Parenteral Enteral Nutr.,* 3, 226, 1979.
15. **Jones, D. C., Rich, A. J., Wright, P. D., and Johnston, I. D. A.,** A comparison of proprietary elemental and whole protein diets, *Br. Med. J.,* 280, 1493, 1980.
16. **Bury, K. D., Stephens, R. V., and Randall, H. T.,** Use of a chemically-defined, liquid, elemental diet for nutritional management of fistulas of the alimentary tract, *Am. J. Surg.,* 121, 174, 1971.
17. **Voitk, A. J., Echave, V., Brown, R. A., McArdle, A. H., and Gurd, F. N.,** Elemental diet in the treatment of fistulas of the alimentary tract, *Surg. Gynaecol. Obstet.,* 137, 68, 1973.
18. **Rocchio, M. A., Cha, C. M., Haas, K. F., and Randall, H. T.,** Use of chemically-defined diets in the management of patients with high output gastrocutaneous fistulas, *Am J. Surg.,* 127, 148, 1974.
19. **Allardyce, D. B. and Groves, A. C.,** A comparison of nutritional gains resulting from intravenous and enteral feeding, *Surg. Gynaecol. Obstet.,* 139, 179, 1974.
20. **Smith, D. W. and Lee, R. M.,** Nutritional management and duodenal fistulas, *Surg. Gynaecol. Obstet.,* 103, 666, 1956.
21. **Voitk, A. J., Echave, V., Feller, J. H., Rowan, R. A., and Gurd, F. N.,** Experience with elemental diets in the treatment of inflammatory bowel disease, *Arch. Surg.,* 107, 329, 1973.
22. **Rocchio, M. A., MoCha, C., Haas, K. F., and Randall, H. T.,** Use of chemically defined diets in the management of patients with acute inflammatory bowel disease, *Am. J. Surg.,* 127, 469, 1974.
23. **Bounous, G., Devroede, G., Haddad, H., Beaudray, R., Perey, B. J., and Lejeune, L. P.,** Use of an elemental diet for intestinal disorders and for the critically ill, *Dis. Colon Rectum,* 17, 157, 1974.
24. **Fischer, J. E.,** Complications of parenteral nutrition, in *Current Concepts in Parenteral Nutrition,* Greep, J. M., Soeters, P. B., Wesdorp, R. I. C., Phaf, C. W. R., and Fischer, J. E., Eds, Martinus Nijhoff, The Hague, 1977, 171.
25. **Law, D. H.,** Current Concepts in Nutrition — Total Parenteral Nutrition, *N. Engl. J. Med.,* 297, 1104, 1977.
26. **Ota, D. M., Imbembo, A. L., and Zuidema, G. D.,** Total parenteral nutrition, *Surgery,* 83, 503, 1978.
27. **Russell, R. I.,** Intravenous nutrition and elemental diets, in *Scientific Foundations of Gastroenterology,* Sircus, W. and Smith, A. N., Eds., Heineman, London, 1980, 130.

INDEX

INDEX

C

D

E

F

G

H

N

O

P

R

S

T

U

V

W

Z